Cytokine Cell Biology

A Practical Approach

Edited by

Fran Balkwill

ICRF Translational Oncology Laboratory,
St Bartholomews and the Royal London
Hospital School of Medicine and Dentistry,
Biological Sciences Building,
Charterhouse Square,
London EC1M 6BQ, U.K.

OXFORD
UNIVERSITY PRESS

OXFORD

UNIVERSITY PRESS

Great Clarendon Street, Oxford OX2 6DP

Oxford University Press is a department of the University of Oxford.
It furthers the University's objective of excellence in research,
scholarship, and education by publishing worldwide in

Oxford New York

Athens Auckland Bangkok Bogotá Buenos Aires Calcutta Cape Town
Chennai Dar es Salaam Delhi Florence Hong Kong Istanbul Karachi
Kuala Lumpur Madrid Melbourne Mexico City Mumbai Nairobi Paris
São Paulo Singapore Taipei Tokyo Toronto Warsaw

with associated companies in Berlin Ibadan

Oxford is a registered trade mark of Oxford University Press in the UK
and in certain other countries

Published in the United States by Oxford University Press Inc., New York

A catalogue record for this title is available from the British Library

Library of Congress Cataloguing in Publication Data
Cytokine cell biology : a practical approach / edited by Fran Balkwill.
(The practical approach series)
Includes bibliographical references and index.
1. Cytokines.   2. Cytokines–Research–Methodology   I. Balkwill, Frances R.   II. Series.
QR185.8.C95 C956 2000   616.07'9–dc21   00-057472
1 3 5 7 9 10 8 6 4 2

ISBN 0 19 963860 8 (Hbk)
ISBN 0 19 963859 4 (Pbk)

Typeset in Swift by Footnote Graphics, Warminster, Wilts
Printed in Great Britain on acid-free paper
by The Bath Press,

Preface

During the past 10 years the study of cytokines has become central to biomedical research. Cytokines form a chemical signalling language in multicellular organisms that regulates development, tissue repair, haemopoiesis, inflammation, and the immune response. Potent cytokine polypeptides have pleiotropic activities and functional redundancy. They act in a complex network where one cytokine can influence the production of, and response to, many other cytokines. This bewildering array of effector molecules and associated cell-surface receptors has been simplified by the assignment of cytokines and their receptors into structural superfamilies; elucidation of convergent intracellular signalling pathways; and molecular genetics, especially targeted gene disruption to the 'knock-out' production of individual cytokines in mice.

It is also now clear that the pathophysiology of infectious, autoimmune, and malignant disease can be partially explained by the induction of cytokines, and that the subsequent cellular response and functional polymorphisms of cytokine genes contribute to the genetic programming of responses to pathogenic stimuli.

Cloning of cytokine and cytokine receptor genes has allowed the production of milligram quantities of purified protein for use in pre-clinical and clinical studies of acute and chronic infection, inflammatory disease, autoimmune disease, and cancer. Manipulation of the cytokine network with these recombinant proteins or other cytokine regulators provides a range of novel approaches to treating acute and chronic disease.

Cytokine Molecular Biology and *Cytokine Cell Biology* are the third editions of this popular book. The importance of the field is reflected in the expansion of the book into two volumes. Both volumes contain up-to-date methods for the study of cytokines, their receptors, and cytokine-driven processes; the first focusing mainly on molecular biology, the second on cell-biology techniques.

The third editions of *Cytokine Molecular Biology* and *Cytokine Cell Biology* contains important new chapters, and revised and additional techniques have been added to the original chapters. Apart from the wide range of methods covered in the second edition, these two books also describe proteomics; conditional deletion of cytokine genes; measurement of intracellular signalling via the Jak/STAT and

MAPK pathways; purification of cytokine proteins; analysis of cytokine gene polymorphisms; intracellular fluorescent staining for cytokine protein; and biological assays for the newer cytokines.

With 192 protocols and 21 chapters in the two volumes, *Cytokine Molecular Biology* and *Cytokine Cell Biology* are not only essential for cytokine research, but are comprehensive guides to a wide range of techniques employed in biomedical research.

London   F.R.B.
September 2000

Contents

CONTENTS

CONTENTS

10 **Flow cytometric detection of intracellular cytokines**   171

*Alasdair M. J. Pennycook, Pietro Pala, Steve Matthews, Tracy Hussell, and
Peter J. M. Openshaw*

11 **Development of antibodies to cytokines**   181

S. Poole

Protocol list

XV

Abbreviations

%CV	percentage variation of the mean
%II	percentage of the integrated intensity of the individual protein spot of the sum of the integrated intensities of all spots on the 2D gel
[^{3}H]TdR	tritiated thymidine
2-ME	2-mercaptoethanol
2D	two-dimensional
2DGE	2-dimensional gel electrophoresis
4-MUH	4-methylumbelliferyl heptanoate
A-SMase	acidic, endosomal sphingomyelinase
AET	aminoethylisothiouronium bromide (?hydrombromide?)
AML	acute myeloid leukaemia
AP	alkaline phosphatase
APAAP	anti-alkaline phosphatase
APC	antigen-presenting cell
APS	ammonium persulfate
ATCC	American Tissue (or Type) Culture Collection
BCDF	B-cell differentiation factor
BCG	bacille Calmette–Guérin
BCGF	B-cell growth factor
BCIP	5 Bromo-4-chloro-Indoxyl phosphate
BDT	bis-diazotolidine
BFU-E	burst-forming units—erythroid colonies
BHK	baby hamster kidney
BLAST	basic local-alignment search tool
bo	bovine
Boc	t-butyloxycarbonyl
bp	base pair
BrdU	bromodeoxyuridine
BSA	bovine serum albumin
BSS	balanced salt solution
BTG	bovine thyroglobulin
c.p.m.	counts per minute
CAPK	ceramide-activated protein kinase

ABBREVIATIONS

CAPP	protein phosphatase 2A
CD40L	CD40 ligand
CFC	colony-forming cells
CFU-E	colony-forming units—erythroid progenitors
CHAPS	(3-[(3 cholamidopropyl)dimethylammonio]-1-propane-sulfonate)
CHEF	contour-clamped horizontal electrical field
CHO	chinese hamster ovary (cells)
CID	collision-induced dissociation
cM	centimorgan
CM	conditioned medium
CMC	cell-mediated cytotoxicity
CMV	cytomegalovirus
ConA	concanavalin A
CPER	cytopathic effect reduction
CPG	controlled-pore glass
CPP32	(caspase 3)-like apoptotic protease
$CrC1_3 \cdot 6H_2O$	chromium chloride hexahydrate
Cre	*causes recombination*
CSF	colony-stimulating factor
CTL	cytotoxic T lymphocytes
CTSD	cathepsin D
CV	coefficient of variation
d.p.m.	disintegrations per minute
DAB	diaminobenzidine tetrahydrochloride
DAG	diacylglycerol
DEAE	diethylaminoethyl
DEPC	diethyl pyrocarobonate
dFCS	dialysed fetal calf serum
DIC	differential interference contrast optics
DIG	digoxigenin
DME	Dulbecco's Modified Eagle's Medium
DMEM	Dulbecco's Modified Essential Medium
DMSO	dimethylsulfoxide
DSS	disuccinimidyl suberate
DTT	dithiothreitol
E^-	non rosette-forming lymphocyte
E^+	E rosette-forming T cell
EBV	Epstein–Barr virus
EC	endothelial cells
ECGS	endothelial cell-growth supplement
EDA	eosinophil differentiation assay
EDMF	endothelial factor able to induce EC migration
EDTA	ethylenediaminetetraacetic acid
EGF	epidermal growth factor
EIA	enzyme immunoassays
ELAM-1	endothelial leucocyte adhesion molecule-1

ELISA	enzyme-linked immunoabsorbent assay
ELISpot	enzyme-linked immunospot assay
EMCV	encephalomycarditis virus
EMEM	Eagle's Minimum Essential Medium
EMSA	electrophoretic mobility-shift assay
Eo-CFC	eosinophil colony-forming cell
EP	eosinophil peroxidase
Epo	erythropoietin
EqS	equine serum
ERK 1,2	extracellular signal-regulated kinases
ES	embryonic stem cells
ESR	erythrocyte sedimentation rate
EST	expressed sequence tag
FACS	fluorescence-activated cell sorter
FALS	forward-angle light scatter
FBS	fetal bovine serum
FCA	Freund's 'complete' adjuvant
FCS	fetal calf serum
FDA	fluoroscein diacetate
FDG	fluorescein digalactosidase
FGF	fibroblast growth factor
FHS	Fischer's medium plus horse serum
FIA	Freund's 'incomplete' adjuvant
FITC	fluorescein isothiocyanate
Fmax	fluorescence at very high calcium
Fmin	fluorescence at very low calcium
fMLP	formylmethionyl-leucylphenylalanine
Fmoc	9-fluorenylmethoxycarbonyl
FRET	Förster resonance energy transfer
FSH	follicle-stimulating hormone
G-CFC	granulocyte colony-forming cells
G-CSF	granulocyte colony-stimulating factor
GAM	goat anti-mouse
GAPDH	glyceraldehyde phosphate dehydrogenase
GCP	granulocyte chemotactic protein
GFP	green fluorescent protein
GM-CFC	granulocyte and macrophage colony-forming cells
GM-CSF	granulocyte and macrophage colony-stimulating factor
Gp	G protein
GST	glutathione S-transferase
GuSCN	guanidinium thiocyanate
HBBS	Hanks' buffered salt solution
huCG	human chorionic gonadotropin
Hepes	4-(2-hydroxyethyl)-1-piperazine-ethanesulfonic acid
HFF	human foreskin fibroblast
HMP	4-hydroxymethyl-phenoxymethyl-copolystyrene

HPLC	high-performance (or pressure) liquid chromatography
HPTLC	high-performance thin-layer chromatography
HR	homologous recombination
HRP	horseradish peroxidase
HRR	haplotype relative-risk analysis
HS	horse serum
HSA	human serum albumin
hu	human
huIFN	human IFN
huTNF	human TNF
huVEC	human umbilical venous endothelial cells
ICAM-1	intercellular adhesion molecule-1
ICCS	intracellular cytokine staining
IDDM	insulin-dependent diabetes mellitus
IEF	isoelectric focusing
IFN	interferon
IGIF	interferon-γ inducing factor
II	integrated intensity
IKKs	IkB kinases
IL	interleukin
IL-1ra	IL-1 receptor antagonist (product of *IL1RN*)
IL1RN	IL-1 receptor antagonist gene
IMDM	Iscove's Modified Dulbecco's Medium
iNOS	inducible nitric oxide synthase
IP	intraperitoneal
IP$_3$	inositol 1,4,5-trisphosphate
IPG	immobilized pH gradient
IPG	immobilized pH gradient
IRMA	immunoradiometric assay
ISH	*in situ* hybridization
IV	intravenous
Jak	Janus activated kinase
JNK	c-Jun N-terminal kinase
K_d	dissociation constant
KLH	keyhole limpet haemocyanin
KSR	kinase suppressor of Ras
LAB	labelled avidin–biotin
LAK	lymphokine-activated killer cell
LAL	Limulus amoebocyte lysate assay
LBD	ligand binding domain
LCR	locus control region
LDH	lactate dehydrogenase
LFA-1	lymphocyte function associated antigen 1
LGL	large granular lymphocyte
LIF	leukaemia inhibitory factor
*lox*P	*lo*cus of *x*-ing over *P*1

LPBA   liquid-phase binding assays
LPS   bacterial lipopolysaccharide
LR   ligand/receptor
LSIMS   liquid secondary ion mass spectometry
LT   lymphotoxin
LTB4   leukotriene B4
LU   lytic units
M-CFC   macrophage colony-forming cell
M-CSF   macrophage colony-stimulating factor
mAb   monoclonal antibodies
MAC   monoclonal anti-cytokine
MACS   magnetic cell sorter
MAPK   p38 mitogen-activated protein kinase
MAPKAPK   MAPK-activated protein kinase
MAR   mouse anti-rabbit
MBP   myelin basic protein
MBS   maleimidobenzoic acid N-hydroxysuccinimide
MCCG   Monte Carlo composite genotype test
MCP   monocyte chemotactic protein
Meg-CFC   megakaryocyte colony-forming cell
MEM   Minimal Essential Medium
MF   mating factor
MFI   median fluorescence intensity
MFR   mannosyl fucosyl receptor
MHC   major histocompatibility complex
MKK   MAPK kinase
MKKK   MAPK kinase kinase
MLP   major late promoter
MMLV   Molony murine leukaemia virus
MMR   macrophage mannosyl receptor
MNC   mononuclear cells
$MNPV$ nuclear polyhedrosis virus containing many nucleocapsids
Mø   macrophage
MOPS   3-N-morpholinopropanesulfonic acid
M_r relative molecular weight
MS   mass spectroscopy
MTBE   methyl t-butyl ether
MTT   (3-[4,5-dimethylthiazol-2-ys]-2,5-diphenyl tetrazolium salt
mu   murine
muTNF   murine TNF
MW   molecular weight
MWCO   molecular weight cut-off
N-SMase   neutral plasma membrane-bound sphingomyelinase
NAC   N-acetyl cysteine
NADG N acetyl-D-glucosamine
NBB   Naphthol Blue Black

NBS	*N*-bromosuccinimide
NBT	nitrobluetetrazolium
NCI	National Cancer Institute
NCS	newborn calf serum
NEPHGE	non-equilibrium pH gradient gel
NFκB	nuclear factor-κB
NGF	nerve growth factor
NGS	normal goat serum
NHS	normal human AB serum
NIBSC	National Institute for Biological Standards and Controls
NK	natural killer (cell)
NMMA	N^g-monomethylarginine
NMP	*N*-methylpyrrolidone
NMS	normal mouse serum
NPP	*p*-nitrophenylphosphate
NSD	neutral sphingomyelinase (activation) domain
NTA	nitrilotriacetic acid
OD	optical density
OLB	oligo-labelling buffer
OMP	orotidine monophosphate
OPD	orthophenylenediamine
ori	origin of replication
OVA	ovalbumin
PA	phosphatidic acid
PA-Ptase	phosphatidic acid-phosphatase
PAF	platelet activating factor
PAGE	polyacrylamide gel electrophoresis
PBA	phosphate-buffered saline + 0.1% bovine serum albumin
PBL	peripheral blood lymphocytes
PBMC	peripheral blood mononuclear cells
PBS	phosphate-buffered saline
PC	phosphatidylcholine
PC-PLC	phosphatidylcholine-specific phospholipase C
PC-PLD	phosphatidylcholine-specific phospholipase D
PCA	procoagulant activity
Pchol	phosphorylcholine
PCR	polymerase chain reaction
PdB	phorbol dibutyrate
PDGF	platelet-derived growth factor
PDQUEST	Protein Databases Quantitative Electrophoresis Standardized Test
PE	phycoerythrin
PEG	polyethylene glycol
PEth	phosphatidylethanol
PFA	paraformaldehyde
PFU	plaque-forming units

PG1$_2$	prostacyclin
PHA	phytohaemagglutinin
pI	isoelectric point
PI	phosphoinositol
PIP$_2$	phosphatidyl inositol bisphosphate
PK	proteinase K
PKA, -B, -C	protein kinases A, B, and C
PL	phospholipase
PLAP	placental alkaline phosphatase
PLC, -D	phospholipase C, -D
PMA	phorbol myristate acetate
PMC	2,2,5,7,8-pentamethylchroman-6-sulfonyl
PMEF	primary mouse embryo fibroblasts
PMN	polymorphonuclear cells
PMS	pregnant mare serum
PMSF	phenylmethylsulfonyl fluoride
PmT	polyoma middle T
pNPP	p-nitrophenylphosphate
PPD	purified protein derivative
PrA	protein A
PrA-sRBC	PrA-conjugated sRBC
PRP	platelet-rich plasma
PTH	phenylthiohydantoin
PVDF	polyvinylidene difluoride
PVP	polyvinyl pyrrolidone
R	recombinant
ra	rat
RA	rheumatoid arthritis
RAC	rabbit anti-cytokine
RACE	rapid amplification of cDNA ends
RALS	right-angle light scatter
RAM	rabbit anti-mouse IgG
RANTES	regulated upon activation, normal T-cell expressed and secreted chemokine
RBC	red blood cells
RFLP	restriction fragment length polymorphism
RHPA	reverse haemolytic plaque assay
RIA	radioimmunoassay
RP-HPLC	reversed phase-HPLC
RPA	RNase protection assay
RR	NIBSC reference reagent
RT-PCR	reverse transcriptase polymerase chain reaction
SAC	staphylococcus aureus-Cowan
SAPK	stress-activated protein kinase
SC	subcutaneous

SCF	stem-cell factor
SD	standard deviation
SDS	sodium dodecyl sulfate
SDS-PAGE	sodium dodecyl sulfate-polyacrylamide gel electrophoresis
SEB	staphylococcal enterotoxin B
Sf	*Spodoptera frugiperda*
SF	synovial fluid
SFV	Semlike Forest virus
SG	specific gravity
SL	specific lysis
SLE	systemic lupus erythematosus
SM	sphingomyelin
SMase	sphingomyelinase
SPBA	solid-phase binding assays
sRBC	sheep red blood cells
SSC	saline–sodium citrate (buffer)
SSCP	single-stranded conformation polymorphism
STAT	signal transducer and activator of transcription
Sv	simianvirus
TBP	tributylphosphine
TBP	tributylphosphine
T_c	cytotoxic T cell
TCA	trichloroacetic acid
TCR	T-cell receptor complex
TDT	transmission disequilibrium test
TEMED	N,N,N',N'-tetramethylenediamine
TESPA	3-aminopropyltriethoxysilane
TFA	trifluoroacetic acid
TG	triglyceride
TGF-α, -β	transforming growth factor-α, -β
T_H	T-helper cell
T_{HP}	T-helper precursor cells
TIL	tumour-infiltrating lymphocytes
TLC	thin-layer chromatograhy
TMC	tonsillar mononuclear cells
TNF	tumour necrosis factor
TP	thyroid peroxidase
Tpo	thrombopoietin
TR	TNF receptor
TRAF	TNF receptor-associated factor
TRF	T-cell replacing factor
TT	tetanus toxoid (vaccine)
TUNEL	terminal transferase dUTP nick end labelling
UNG	uracil-DNA N-glycosylation
VCAM	vascular cell-adhesion molecule

VEGF	vascular endothelial growth factor
VNTR	variable number of tandem repeats
VSV	vesicular stomatitis virus
WGA-FITC	wheat-germ agglutinin–fluorescein isothiocyanate
YAC	yeast artificial chromosome

Chapter 1

Measurement of proliferative, cytostatic, and cytolytic activity of cytokines

Frances Burke and Frances R. Balkwill

Biological Therapy Laboratory, Imperial Cancer Research Fund, Lincoln's Inn Fields, London WC2A 3PX

1 Introduction

Most cytokines have proliferative, cytostatic and/or cytolytic activity depending on the context in which they are acting. IFN-α, -β, and -γ, TNF-α and -β, IL-1, and IL-4, have all been shown to have proliferative, cytostatic, and cytolytic activity depending on the conditions (1). Synergistic interactions between cytokines can often produce powerful antiproliferative and cytotoxic effects (2), as can a combination of cytokines and inhibitors of transcription. For some cytokines, such as IFN-γ, the cytokine has to be continually present in the tissue culture medium for two or more days to have an irreversible effect on cell growth (3). Other cytokines such as Fas ligand and TRAIL can induce apoptosis within hours. Some of the methods used to assess the above parameters will be described in this chapter. Other assays for measuring the action of cytokines on cell growth are described in Chapter 13, this volume.

2 Effects of cytokines on cell growth *in vitro*

The protocols described in this chapter all require basic tissue culture experience and sterile technique. It is strongly recommended that all cell lines are grown under pyrogen-free conditions when studying the effects of cytokines. For this, sterile disposable plastic pipettes, dishes, flasks, and tubes should be used and glassware and Pasteur pipettes triple-baked. Batches of fetal calf serum with a minimal endotoxin content should be chosen.

Reagents for general tissue culture:

(a) Trypsin 0.25% in Tris–saline pH 7.7 (filter-sterilized and stored at $-20\,°C$), for 1 litre:

- Trypsin   2.5 g
- NaCl   8.0 g

- KCl (19% solution (w/v) in distilled water)   2.0 ml
- Na_2HPO_4 0.1 g
- Dextrose   1.0 g
- Trizma base   3.0 g
- Phenol red (1% solution (w/v) in distilled water)   1.5 ml
- Penicillin 1×10^5 units
- Streptomycin   0.1 g

Adjust the pH to 7.7 with 1 M HCl

(b) Versene in PBS pH 7.2 (autoclave and store at 4 °C); for 1 litre:

- EDTA (disodium salt)   0.2 g
- NaCl   8.0 g
- KCl   0.2 g
- Na_2HPO_4 1.15 g
- KH_2PO_4 0.2 g
- Phenol red (1% solution (w/v) in distilled water)   1.5 ml

Use at 1:4 trypsin:versene

(c) Relevant defined medium (e.g. RPMI-1640 or DMEM)

(d) Fetal calf serum

Equipment for general tissue culture

- 37 °C humidified incubator in an atmosphere of 5% CO_2
- waterbath
- inverted microscope

NB: Specialized reagents and equipment in addition to those outlined above will be listed within each protocol.

2.1 Direct cell counting

Direct cell counting is valuable for assessing cell viability and doubling time. In our laboratory we use this routinely in preference to any other assay. However, to assess whether a cytokine induces proliferation or is cytostatic or cytotoxic at specific stages during the cell cycle, more extensive analysis is required.

Two methods will be described for direct cell counting. The simplest method is to count a suspension of cells on a haemocytometer. Although this can be very time consuming, especially when comparing the effects of different concentrations and/or combinations of cytokines, we find it extremely accurate. An alternative method involves the use of a Coulter counter. The disadvantage of this method is that it does not distinguish viable cells from dead cells. This is not so important for cells growing in monolayers since dead cells become detached and float off, thus being removed by the washing procedure prior to trypsinization.

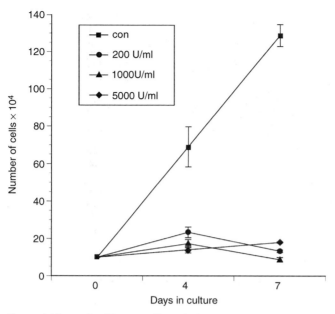

Figure 1 The antiproliferative effect of IFN-γ on human ovarian cancer cells measured by direct cell counting.

2.1.1 Direct cell counting using an improved Neubauer haemocytometer

This procedure is described in *Protocol 1*. In our laboratory the cells are routinely grown in six-well plates. Each cell line or timepoint is set up in triplicate and cells are allowed to seed overnight prior to the addition of cytokine. It is important that untreated control cells are not confluent and contact-inhibited at the end-point of the experiment, otherwise this may skew the results. A typical experiment examining the antiproliferative effect of a range of doses of IFN-γ in an ovarian cancer cell line is shown in *Figure 1*.

Protocol 1

Direct cell counting using an improved Neubauer haemocytometer

Equipment

- Improved Neubauer haemocytometer with coverslip
- Needles and syringes
- Phase-contrast microscope

Method

1 Trypsinize the cells if adherent, spin down, and resuspend in an appropriate volume for counting. For cells growing in suspension, pellet by spinning at approximately 210 g for 5 min and resuspend as appropriate.

3

Protocol 1 continued

2   Obtain a single-cell suspension by dispersing the cells with a 19-gauge needle. This will ensure accuracy when counting.

3   Wash the haemocytometer in detergent and water followed by an alcohol rinse.

4   Moisten the edge and position the coverslip until stable Newton's rings are obtained. Using a Pasteur pipette add one drop of cell suspension under the coverslip to fill the haemocytometer (do not allow fluid to enter the channels).

5   The central 25 squares of the grid have an area of 1 mm^2. Count all the cells in this area under phase contrast, count cells that fall on top and left middle lines, but not those that fall on the right and bottom middle lines. Viable cells will appear bright and refractive, whilst dead cells will appear dull. Count approximately 100 cells to ensure accuracy. Dilute and recount if necessary.

6   Calculate the cell count/ml using the following equation:

Cell count/ml = number in the central 1 mm^2 area $\times 10^4 \times$ dilution factor.

7   Use the mean of the triplicates to draw graphs.

2.1.2 Direct cell counting using a Coulter counter

This method makes use of an electronic means of cell counting. An electric current is passed through a 100 μm aperture in a probe, which is subsequently placed into a single-cell suspension using isoton as a buffering solution. The cells are drawn through the probe by a mercury manometer-controlled pump, this alters the resistance to the current flow and produces a series of pulses which are counted and displayed on a digital readout. The change in resistance produced is thus proportional to the volume of the cell passing through the probe. Using the manufacturer's instructions a threshold is set so that background counts from cell debris are excluded.

In our laboratory 6-well plates (3.5 $\times$ 1.0 cm) are used, each containing 10^5 cells per plate. All parameters are assayed in triplicate and counts are made at various time points to obtain a cell growth curve.

Protocol 2

Direct cell counting using a Coulter counter

Equipment and reagents

- Accuvettes (Coulter Electronics Ltd)
- Coulter counter (source as above)
- Isoton IC Saline

Method

1   Trypsinize the cells if they are adherent. Use a 0.5 ml solution to disperse the cells and stop the action of trypsin/versene (see Section 2(b)) with 1.5 ml of isoton/2% fetal calf serum. If cells grow in suspension, spin down, and resuspend in 2 ml of isoton/2% fetal calf serum.

2 Obtain a single-cell suspension by dispersing the cells with a 19-gauge needle and wash the dish with up to 8 ml of isoton. Transfer the final volume, which will be 10 ml, into an Accuvette.

3 Allow the Coulter counter to warm up and prepare it for use following the manufacturer's instructions.

4 Count the contents of each Accuvette and multiply by 20.[a]

5 Calculate the mean of triplicate samples and plot growth curves.

[a] This can accurately measure up to 10 000 cells. The accuracy will decrease if the total number of cells exceeds this as a result of the coincident passage of cells through the probe aperture. In this case a conversion chart provided by the manufacturer must be referred to.

3 Determination of the effects on growth of cytokines using indirect methods

Two protocols will be outlined. One method uses a fluorogenic assay, whilst the other is a kit adaptation of the conventional MTT assay as also described in Chapter 13 of this volume.

3.1 The alkaline phosphatase assay

Protocol 3 is based on a fluorogenic enzyme assay which measures alkaline phosphatase activity, a membrane-bound enzyme present in most human cell types. This enzyme is found in three main forms: in the placenta; in the intestine and liver; and in the bone or kidney. The assay conditions allow the non-fluorogenic substrate 4-methylumbelliferyl phosphate to react with all forms of the enzyme to produce free phosphate and the fluorogenic compound 4-methyl umbelliferylerone. The fluorescence is then measured on a multiscan plate reader where the total enzyme activity given is directly proportional to the cell number. The activity of alkaline phosphatase increases proportionately with cell number and is not affected by time in culture.

This assay has been reported to accurately assess as few as 10^4 cells. The cells are plated in 96-well plates in the range of 10^4 to 10^5 cells/per well. Cells are grown as monolayers and analysed at defined time points.

Protocol 3

Alkaline phosphatase assay

Equipment and reagents

- Dynatech Fluor Tm reader (Dynatech products)
- Phosphate-buffered saline (PBS)
- Assay solution: 0.2 M boric acid, 1 mM $MgCl_2$, 1.2 mM 4-methyl umbelliferyl phosphate

Method

1 Wash the cells twice in PBS to remove any dead cells.

2 Add 200 μl of freshly prepared assay solution to each well.

3 Incubate at 37 °C for 3 h.

4 Measure the relative fluorescence using a Dynatech Fluor Tm reader (Dynatech products) according to the manufacturer's instructions.

3.2 The MTT-type assay

The conventional MTT assay is described in Chapter 13. We have used a Promega kit^{96TM} which is a modified version of the conventional MTT assay. The data from the Promega, cell titre, non-radioactive, cell proliferation/cytotoxicity assay is analysed at 570 nm on a standard plate reader.

4 Measurement of cell lysis using crystal violet

The cytotoxic effect of cytokines can be simply measured using a microtitre plate and staining the viable cells with crystal violet. This procedure can be used in various biological assays that look for cellular cytokine secretion or for the presence of cytokines in serum. The WEHI 164 cell-line assay described below can be used for measuring TNF-α. The WEHI assay using cell lysis and crystal violet is outlined in *Protocol 4*.

Protocol 4

WEHI assay for TNF-α production

Equipment and reagents

- Dynatech Fluor Tm reader (Dynatech products)
- Methanol
- 1% aqueous crystal violet
- 96-well Costar plates
- TNF-α (R and D systems)

Method

1 To a 96-well Costar plate add 5×10^4 cells/100 μl RPMI and 10% FCS/well. Leave for 2–3 h in a 37 °C incubator.

2 Dilute the TNF-α stock solution in RPMI only (no FCS) using ten-fold dilutions so that the final concentrations range from 100 ng/ml to 1 pg/ml, or lower if required.

3 Add 100 μl of the above to the plate in duplicate.[a]

4 Add 100 μl RPMI to four control wells.

5 Add the test samples at a 1:5 dilution to duplicate wells.

Protocol 4 continued

6 Transfer the plate to the 37 °C incubator and leave for 18–24 h.

7 Flick out the medium and fix the cells by filling the wells with methanol for 30 sec.

8 Remove the methanol, add 100 µl of 1% aqueous crystal violet to each well, and leave for 5–20 min.

9 Flick out the stain and wash the wells with distilled water. Invert the plate over a paper towel for a few minutes to allow to dry.

10 Measure the optical density at 620 nm on a multiscan plate reader, following the manufacturer's instructions.

[a] Remember the final concentration will be half that put in

5 Cell-cycle studies

As described in Section 2, cell counting provides simple growth curves which can be used to assess cell viability and doubling time. However, the effect of a cytokine on specific stages during the cell cycle must be studied by more complex techniques.

De novo synthesis of DNA can be quantified by measuring the incorporation of tritiated thymidine (present in the culture medium) during S phase. Incorporated label is subsequently detected by autoradiography or liquid scintillation counting. Incubating cells with the cytokine for a range of times followed by pulsing with tritiated thymidine provides information on the effect of the cytokine from the early phases of the cell cycle through to S phase. It is not, however, an indication of quiescence. Another way to examine increases or decreases in DNA synthesis in a cell population is to use cytofluorimetry, staining the nuclei with dyes such as propidium iodide. These protocols are outlined below. Quiescent cells can be obtained from fibroblasts and primary cultures. Fibroblasts, for example Swiss 3T3 cells, are plated and incubated for a further 4–7 days before use in the assay described in *Protocol 5*. At this time the cells are arrested in G_1 as judged by cytofluorometric analysis and by the fact that less than 1% of the cells are autoradiographically labelled after a 40-h exposure to [³H]thymidine (see *Protocol 5*).

5.1 Measurement of [³H]thymidine incorporation into acid-insoluble material

This section refers particularly to the effects of murine cytokines or cross-species reactive cytokines on murine fibroblast cell lines. Other medium and conditions will be required for different cell lines. The incorporation of [³H]thymidine into acid-insoluble material has been widely used as a convenient method for assessing the stimulatory and inhibitory effects of various agents on the growth of

7

many different cells. However, this technique not only assesses effects on DNA synthesis, but can also reflect alterations in the transport of thymidine across the plasma membrane, and in the phosphorylation of this nucleotide by thymidine kinase which occurs before it can be incorporated into DNA. In some systems, agents previously thought to have antiproliferative activity have subsequently been shown merely to inhibit thymidine transport. An easy way to circumvent any effects on thymidine transport is to vary the concentration of thymidine used in the experiment (e.g. from 1 μM to 10 μM). If the apparent inhibition of DNA synthesis is entirely due to a decrease in thymidine transport, then the effect should be overcome by increasing the concentration of this nucleoside, because at high concentrations the nucleotide permeates the cell membrane by simple diffusion rather than by carrier-mediated transport. Thus, this technique provides a convenient measurement of changes in DNA synthesis, provided that appropriate controls are included. The assay described in *Protocol 5* is carried out on Swiss 3T3 cells in the absence of serum in DMEM medium supplemented with Waymouth's medium, which contains additional amino acids and vitamins present in serum but that are lacking in DMEM (4). The protocol should be adapted for other cells as appropriate.

Protocol 5

Measurement of [^{3}H]thymidine incorporation into acid-insoluble material

Equipment and reagents

- Scintillation counter and Picoflor
- Waymouth's medium (MB 752/1 powdered formula plus 1.6 mM FeSO$_4$)
- [^{3}H]thymidine (Stock 37 MBq/ml 1 mCi/ml)
- 5% trichloroacetic acid (TCA)

- Phosphate-buffered saline: 0.15 M NaCl in 0.1 M potassium phosphate buffer, pH 7.4
- 0.1 M NaOH, 2% Na$_2$CO$_3$, 1% sodium dodecyl sulfate (SDS)

Method

1   Wash confluent and quiescent cultures of Swiss 3T3 cells twice with DMEM medium at 37 °C to remove residual serum.

2   Incubate the cultures in 2 ml of DMEM/Waymouth's medium (1:1) containing [^{3}H]thymidine (1 μCi/ml; 1 μM) for 40 h at 37 °C.[a]

3   Wash the cultures twice with ice-cold phosphate-buffered saline and remove acid-soluble radioactivity by a 2-min treatment with 5% TCA at 4 °C.

4   Wash the cultures twice with ethanol and solubilize the cells by a 30-min incubation in 1 ml of 0.1 M NaOH containing 2% Na$_2$CO$_3$ and 1% SDS.

5   Determine the radioactivity incorporated into the acid-insoluble material by liquid scintillation counting in Picoflor.

6 To determine the rate of DNA synthesis pulse-label the cultures with [^{3}H]thymidine (e.g. for 5–15 min), but bear in mind that this measurement is meaningful only if the specific radioactivity of the precursor pool is taken into consideration.

[a] After 40 h, [^{3}H]thymidine incorporation reaches saturation and thus ensures that the maximum response of the cell population is being determined rather than variations in the rate of DNA synthesis.

5.2 Autoradiography of labelled nuclei

To substantiate further that neither the transport nor the phosphorylation of thymidine is affected by a cytokine, the proportion of cells actually synthesizing DNA can be measured by autoradiographic techniques. This method is much less sensitive to changes in the specific radioactivity of the precursor pool. Furthermore, it is possible to stimulate DNA synthesis in quiescent mouse fibroblasts by the addition of growth factors without completion of the cell cycle, i.e. arrest occurs after completion of S phase when highly radioactive [^{3}H]thymidine is present (1 μM, 1 μCi/ml). Mitotic cells do not accumulate under these conditions because of radiation damage due to the incorporation of [^{3}H]thymidine into DNA. The cells progress to G$_2$, remain arrested there due to radiation effects, and very few cells detach. Thus, with the highly radioactive [^{3}H]thymidine generally used in these protocols (1 μM, 1 μCi/ml) most cells never reach mitosis and they remain firmly attached to the dish after one round of DNA replication. To determine the duration of G1 and the rate at which the cell population starts DNA synthesis (rate of entry into S phase) the percentage of labelled nuclei should be determined after various times of growth-factor stimulation in the continuous presence of the labelled precursor. *Protocol 6* describes the autoradiography of labelled nuclei quiescent cultures of Swiss 3T3 cells. The protocol should be adapted for other cell lines.

Protocol 6

Autoradiography of labelled nuclei

Equipment and reagents

- Waymouth's medium (MB 752/1 powdered formula plus 1.6 mM FeSO$_4$)
- [^{3}H]thymidine (Stock 37 MBq/ml 1 mCi/ml)
- Chrome alum solution: heat 5 g of gelatine in 40 ml distilled water to dissolve; dissolve 0.5 g chrome alum separately in 400 ml of water. Mix the solutions when cool, and make up to 1 litre.
- Isotonic saline
- 5% TCA
- Ethanol
- Kodak AR10 stripping film
- Kodak D19 developer
- Hypam fixer (Ilford)
- Giemsa stain

Protocol 6 continued

Method

1 Wash confluent and quiescent cultures of Swiss 3T3 cells and incubate as described in *Protocol 5*, except that [³H]thymidine is added to a concentration of 1 μM and 5 μCi/ml.

2 After a 40-h incubation, wash the cultures twice with isotonic saline, extract with 5% TCA twice for 5 min each time, wash three times with ethanol, and dry. Coat the dishes with chrome alum solution and leave to dry.

3 Lay Kodak AR10 stripping film on the dishes and store them in the dark for 1–3 weeks.

4 Develop the film under a red safe light with Kodak D19 developer (4 min) and fix for 5 min with Hypam fixer diluted 1:4 with distilled water.

5 Stain the cells with Giemsa stain.

Following this protocol, the nuclei engaged in DNA synthesis become intensively labelled. Labelled and unlabelled cells in several microscopic fields are counted and the results expressed as follows:

% labelled nuclei = no. of labelled cells × 100/total no. of cells.

5.3 Cytofluorimetry

To confirm that the [³H]thymidine incorporation method is an accurate reflection of the state of DNA synthesis an independent technique such as cytofluorimetry can be used. This interrupts the progression of the cells through the cell cycle in mitosis. In this manner, the proportion of cells that move from G_1 to M after treatment can be precisely assessed. Although colchicine does stimulate the incorporation of [³H]thymidine into DNA in 3T3 cells, it has been shown that its mitogenic activity is lost if it is added to the cells once S phase has been initiated, i.e. 20 h after stimulation with other factors. By adding colchicine, which blocks the cells in mitosis but does not potentiate DNA synthesis if added 20 h after the factors, the effect of growth factors and cytokines on the movement of the cells through the cycle from G_1 through S phase and into G_2 can be readily assessed.

Protocol 7

Cytofluorimetry

Equipment and reagents

- Fluorescence-activated cell sorter (Becton Dickinson, FACS-1)

- 1 mM colchicine

- Lysis buffer: 0.5% Triton X-100, 4 mM $MgCl_2$, 0.6 M sucrose, 10 mM Tris–HCl pH 7.5

- Nuclei buffer: 0.25 M sucrose, 5 mM $MgCl_2$, 20 mM Tris–HCl pH 7.4

- RNase A

- 0.05 mg/ml propidium iodide in 0.1% trisodium citrate

Protocol 7 continued

Method

1   Treat cultures of quiescent cells with various agents as indicated and incubate for 20 h at 37 °C.

2   To ensure that cells which were stimulated to synthesize DNA are arrested in G_2, add the microtubule disrupting agent colchicine at 1 μM, and incubate for a further 20 h (total incubation time = 40 h). Note that colchicine has no mitogenic effect when added so late after the commencement of the experiment.

3   Trypsinize the cells from the monolayer, wash, pass through a 19-gauge needle to ensure a single-cell suspension, and incubate in lysis buffer for 3 min at room temperature.

4   Incubate the nuclei at 37 °C for 30 min in nuclei buffer containing 0.5 mg/ml ribonuclease A.

5   Stain with propidium iodide for 20 min.

6   Spin down the stained nuclei at 840 g at 4 °C for 5 min, resuspend in cold PBS, and immediately measure the DNA content on a fluorescence-activated cell sorter at 488 nm excitation.

5.4 Measurement of bromodeoxyuridine incorporation to assess cell-cycle changes *in vivo*

A useful method to assess cell proliferation *in vivo* in experimental animals involves labelling cells with bromodeoxyuridine, BrdU, a thymidine analogue which is incorporated into DNA during the S-phase of the cell cycle. Subsequently, immunohistochemistry can be performed on excised tissue. Both growth inhibitory and

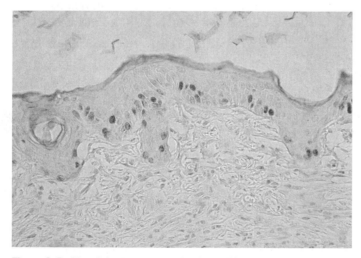

Figure 2 BrdU staining to measure *in vivo* proliferation in a section of mouse skin. Cells synthesizing DNA are darkly stained. Magnification × 20.

stimulatory cytokines can be investigated. We have used this method to look at the effects of IFN-γ on the growth of solid tumours (6) in nude mice and to investigate the effects of tumour promoters on the skin of TNF-$\alpha^{-/-}$ mice (7). The method we used to study proliferation in TNF$^{-/-}$ mice is outlined in *Protocol 8*, and a typical section is shown in *Figure 2*. The DNA needs to be denatured so the BrdU can be exposed to the specific antibody. This denaturation is usually with acid, but it can result in poor tissue morphology. The incubation period for the denaturation procedure is critical.

Protocol 8

In vivo labelling of tumours/tissues with BrdU and subsequent immunohistochemistry

Caution: DAB may cause severe eye and skin irritation. Wear gloves and make up in a fume hood. DAB is light-sensitive.

Equipment and reagents

- Bromodeoxyuridine made up in saline immediately before use (1 M stock)
- General immunohistochemistry reagents (reagents for immunohistochemistry are widely available, e.g. our reagents were obtained from DAKO or Sigma)
- Anti-rat BrdU (Seralab)
- Goat anti-rat horseradish peroxidase (HRP)
- ABC/HRP (Dako)
- Formol saline
- Diaminobenzidine tetrahydrochloride (DAB)
- Poly-L-lysine coated slides (see Chapter 3 Vol. 1 *Protocol 9*)
- Xylene
- 0.1% hydrogen peroxide in methanol
- 1 M HCl
- PBS pH 7.6
- Mayer's haematoxylin
- DPX mountant

Method

1. Inject 50 mg/kg of BrdU in 0.1 ml intraperitoneally into mice. Leave for 45–60 min.
2. Kill the mice by cervical dislocation and remove tumours into formol saline.
3. Cut sections on to poly-L-lysine coated slides. Then treat slides as follows.
4. Xylene for 10 min.
5. 95% alcohol for 2 min.
6. 50% alcohol for 2 min.
7. Tap water for 2 min. Block endogenous peroxidase with 0.1% hydrogen peroxide in methanol at room temperature.
8. Wash in tap water and transfer to freshly prepared trypsin pre-heated to 37 °C (pH 7.8).
9. Denature the DNA by immersing the slides in 1 M HCl for 10 min at 60 °C.
10. Wash in tap water for 5 min.

Protocol 8 continued

11 Flood the slides with PBS pH 7.6 for 5 min. Tip off and wipe around the sections.

12 Incubate with anti-BrdU diluted 1:1000 for 35 min.

13 Wash three times in PBS.

14 Add goat anti-rat HRP-conjugate diluted 1:200 for 35 min.

15 Wash three times in PBS. Add ABC/HRP complex prepared according to manufacturer's instruction, wash in PBS.

16 Add DAB solution made up as per manufacturer's instructions. Leave on for approximately 5–10 min. Rinse in PBS, followed by tap water for 10 min.

17 Counterstain in Mayer's haematoxylin, followed by tap water for 3–4 min. Note that the staining time is dependent on the age and frequency of use of the reagent, but is in the range of 10 sec to 2 min.

18 Fix in 1% HCl/alcohol in and out, then in running tap water for 5 min.

19 Dehydrate through 50% (2 min), 95% (2 min), and absolute alcohol (in and out).

20 Leave in xylene for 2 min.

21 DPX mount.

5.5 Mitotic index

This technique looks at the rate of entry into mitosis and thus completes the picture of the cell cycle and the effects that cytokines may have. The main disadvantage of this procedure is that mitoses occur rapidly, usually only lasting 45 min, and therefore frequent time points have to be studied. The procedure involves the gentle lysis of cells. Any resulting 'mitotic spreads' are fixed and stained and examined under a low-power microscope. The procedure is outlined in *Protocol 9*.

Protocol 9
Determination of the mitotic index

Equipment and reagents

- 0.684% trisodium citrate in distilled water
- Carnoy's fixative: one part glacial acetic acid plus three parts absolute alcohol
- 30 mm tissue culture dishes
- Orcein acetate (filtered)
- Absolute alcohol

Method

1 Aspirate the medium.

2 Add 1.9 ml of trisodium citrate to the Petri dishes followed by 0.4 ml of distilled water dropwise. Mix the contents by very gently swirling the dish and leave at room temperature for 10 min.

13

3   Add 2.3 ml of Carnoy's fixative, pour off and repeat, leave at room temperature for 10 min.

4   Pour off the fixative and air-dry.

5   When dry, stain with filtered orcein acetate for 10 min.

6   Wash off the stain with absolute alcohol and air-dry.

7   Observe under low-power magnification. Mitotic nuclei should be visible.

8   Count 1000 cell nuclei (200 per field of view) per dish and calculate the percentage of mitoses.

6 DNA fragmentation

Duke *et al.* (1983) have shown that during target-cell lysis by sensitized T-cells, fragmentation of target-cell DNA may occur within 10 min of exposure (5). This fragmentation occurs in a specific manner resulting in the formation of 200 base pairs or multiples of 200 base pairs, indicating that the DNA is being cleaved at susceptible points between condensed regions of chromatin. The DNA fragmentation observed in the Duke system has been shown to act via the activation of an endonuclease and has since been observed in lytic events mediated by cytokines such as TNF-α (2). Analysis of DNA fragmentation may provide useful information on mechanisms of cytokine-mediated killing.

The assay described in *Protocol 10* is a modification of that described by Duke *et al.* (5)

Protocol 10

DNA fragmentation

Equipment and reagents

- 24-well plates
- [^{3}H]thymidine 37 MBq/ml 1 mCi/ml
- Cytokines of interest
- 25 mM sodium acetate buffer pH 6.6
- 19-gauge needle and syringe
- Scintillation counter and scintillant

Method

1   Seed the target cells at a density of 1×10^5 cells in 2 ml of medium in 24-well plates.

2   Leave to attach for 6 h.

3   Incubate for 18 h with 5 μCi/ml [^{3}H]thymidine.

4   Wash the cells three times with culture medium.

5   Incubate for 30 min on ice in culture medium.

Protocol 10 continued

6 Remove unincorporated [³H]thymidine by further washing.

7 Culture at a range of time points with the cytokine of interest.

8 At each time point remove and retain the culture medium.

9 Treat the cultures for 1 h with 25 mM sodium acetate buffer, pH 6.6

10 Using a 19-gauge needle, syringe the contents of the dishes to detach the cells and centrifuge for 15 min at 27 000 g at RT. This will separate the intact chromatin (which will form a pellet) from the fragmented DNA.

11 Count the radioactivities of the target-cell DNA present in the culture medium, in the 27 000-g supernatant, and in the 27 000-g pellet, using a beta scintillation counter.

12 Calculate the specific fragmentation using the formula below:

$$\% \text{ DNA fragments} = \frac{\text{c.p.m. DNA fragments}^{a} - \text{c.p.m. spontaneous DNA fragments}^{a}}{\text{total c.p.m.}^{c} - \text{c.p.m. spontaneous DNA fragments}^{b}};$$

where:

[a] = c.p.m. in the culture medium + c.p.m. in the 27 000-g supernatant of cytokine treated cells retained in step 8;

[b] = c.p.m. in the culture medium + c.p.m. in the 27 000-g supernatant of parallel control cells;

[c] = c.p.m. in the DNA fragments + c.p.m. in the 27 000-g pellet of the cytokine treated cells.

Specific labelling of DNA fragmentation can also be investigated *in vivo* using immunohistochemical methods. *Protocol 11* is based on the terminal transferase dUTP nick end-labelling (TUNEL) assay published by Gavrieli *et al.* (9), and allows the effects of cytokines such as IFN-γ to be investigated in this way. Sections are prepared for staining as described in *Protocol 8* up to step 9. This method is now available in kit form from Promega.

Protocol 11

Specific labelling of DNA fragmentation *in vivo*

Equipment and reagents

- Slide box

- 20 µg/ml proteinase K

- Terminal transferase (Boehringer Mannheim (now Roche))

- Biotin-16-dUTP (Boehringer Mannheim (now Roche))

- Bovine serum albumin (BSA)

- TDT buffer (Boehringer Mannheim (now Roche))

- TB buffer: 300 mM sodium chloride, 300 mM sodium citrate

- General immunohistochemistry reagents (see *Protocol 8*)

Protocol 11 continued

Method

1 Follow *Protocol 8* to step 9.

2 Incubate tissue sections with 20 µg/ml proteinase K for 15 min at RT.

3 Wash four times in distilled water.

4 Inactivate endogenous peroxidase activity by incubating with 0.1% hydrogen peroxide for 15 min at RT.

5 Rinse the sections in distilled water and immerse in TDT buffer.

6 Add TDT and biotinylated dUTP diluted in TDT buffer to sections and incubate for 60 min at RT (Need 50 µl/slide of 45 µl TDT buffer, 5 µl Biotin-16-dUTP 1 µl enzyme TDT).

7 Terminate the reaction by immersing the slides in TB buffer for 15 min at room temperature. Rinse the sections with distilled water.

8 Add a 2% solution of BSA for 10 min at room temperature.

9 Rinse in distilled water.

10 Immerse the sections in PBS for 5 min at room temperature.

11 Follow *Protocol 8*, steps 18–21.

References

1. Burke, F., Naylor, M. S., Davies, B., *et al.* (1993). *Immunol. Today*, **14**, 165.
2. Dealtry, G. B., Naylor, M. S., Fiers, W., *et al.* (1987). *Eur. J. Immunol.*, **17**, 689.
3. Burke, F., Smith, P. D., Crompton, M. R., *et al.* (1999). *Br. J. Cancer*, **80**, 1236.
4. Mierzejewski, K. and Rozengurt, E. (1977). *Exp Cell, Res.*, **106**, 394.
5. Duke, R. C., Chervenak, R., and Cohen, J. J. (1983). *Proc. Natl Acad. Sci. USA*, **80**, 6361.
6. Burke, F., East, N., Upton, C., *et al.* (1997). *Eur. J. Cancer*, **33**, 1114.
7. Moore, R. J., Owens, D. M., Stamp, G., *et al.* (1999). *Nature Medicine*, **5**, 828.
8. Gavrieli, Y., Sherman, Y., and Ben Sasson, S. A. (1992). *J. Cell Biol.*, **119**, 493.

Chapter 2
Human B-cell responses to cytokines

Robin E. Callard and Karolena T. Kotowicz
Institute of Child Health, 30 Guilford St, London WC1N 1EH

1 Introduction

B-lymphocyte responses are determined by complex interactions between antigen, cell-surface ligands, and soluble growth and differentiation factors (cytokines) binding to specific receptors on the cell surface. To date, at least 17 out of more than 40 recombinant cytokines are known to stimulate B-cell activation, proliferation, and/or differentiation (*Table 1*). Many of these cytokines are derived from T cells and are involved in T-cell/B-cell collaboration, but some are made by B cells, monocytes, and a variety of non-lymphoid cells such as endothelial cells and fibroblasts. Two important properties of cytokines need to be taken into account when considering their action on B cells:

(a) Cytokines usually lack specificity for cells of any one lineage and none are specific for B cells.

(b) Any one cytokine may have more than one biological effect on B cells, depending on the stage of B-cell differentiation and state of activation.

IL-4 for example can activate resting B cells, promote cell division by activated B cells and T cells, and stimulate the production of IgE and IgG4 in humans (IgE and IgG1 in mice) by inducing heavy-chain switching (1). Similarly, IL-2 is a growth and differentiation factor for human B cells and T cells (2, 3), whereas TGF-β inhibits B-cell proliferation and IgG secretion (4), but enhances IgA secretion, probably by inducing alpha heavy-chain switching (5, 6). This diversity of function is further complicated by the fact that two or more cytokines often act in concert, and the possibility that different B-cell subpopulations may not all respond in the same way. Another property of cytokines that may have far-reaching implications is that several come in pairs with very similar but non-identical properties. These include IL-1α and -β; IL-2 and IL-15; IL-4 and IL-13; and TNF-α and -β. The similar, and in some cases indistinguishable, activity of these pairs of cytokines raises interesting and important questions about the nature of the receptors involved and may be related to where the cytokines are made. For example, only T cells make IL-2, whereas most cell types except T cells make

Table 1 Responses of human B cells to cytokines

Type of response Cytokine	Activation	Proliferation	Differentiation	TRF	Isotype regulation
IL-1	(+)[a]	(+)	(+)	no	no
IL-2	+	+	+	+	no
IL-3	?	+ (pre B)	+	no	no
IL-4	+	+	+	no	+ (IgE/IgG4)
IL-5[b]	no	no	no	no	?
IL-6	+	+	+	no	no[c]
IL-7	?	+ (pre B)	?	no	?
IL-10	(+)[d]	+	+	no	+ (IgG3/IgA)
IL-13	+	+	+	no	+ (IgE/IgG4)
IL-14	?	+	−	?	?
IL-15	?	+	+	+	?
IFN-α	?	+	±	no	?
IFN-β	+	+	+	no	?
IFN-γ	±	+	+	no	− (IgE)
NGF	?	+	+	?	+ (IgG4)
TGF-β	?	−	−	no	+ (IgA)
TNF-α	?	+	±	no	?
TN F-β	?	+	+	no	?

[a] Positive response +; negative response −; no response no; unknown or not reported ? The (+) for IL-1 indicates some controversy. TRF = T-cell replacing factor.

[b] IL-5 has no effect on human B cells but it does on murine B cells.

[c] IL-6 may be required for IgE and IgA responses.

[d] IL-10 increases MHC class II on resting murine B cells, but not on human B cells.

IL-15. Unfortunately, it is beyond the scope of this introduction to discuss the nature of the cytokine receptors and the reader is referred to references 7 and 8 for further information.

In this chapter, assays for measuring human B-cell activation, proliferation, and differentiation in response to cytokines are described. In appropriate combinations, these assays can be used to distinguish between different B-cell growth and differentiation factors, and help to determine their action on different populations of normal and malignant B cells.

2 Reagents used for *in vitro* experiments with human B cells

2.1 Culture media

For most B-cell assays, RPMI-1640 (Gibco) supplemented with 25 mM Hepes, 2 mM glutamine, and 5% fetal calf serum (FCS) can be used. In some cases, however, particularly CD40-induced Ig secretion, Iscove's modified Dulbecco's medium (IMDM) (Gibco) can give better responses than RPMI-1640. Gentamicin at 50 μg/ml should be used to inhibit the bacterial growth that can occur with B cells prepared from tonsils. Gentamicin from some sources has been found toxic to B cells. In our hands, the most reliable form is the cidomycin sterile solution from Roussel Laboratories. For specific antibody responses, RPMI-1640 with 10% horse serum (EqS) should be used. The horse serum must be aliquoted and kept frozen. The RPMI-1640 medium should be purchased as either liquid medium with Hepes included, or made up from powdered medium with Hepes included. In both these formulations, the NaCl concentration is reduced to compensate for the increased osmolarity arising from the addition of Hepes buffer. This can be crucial for specific antibody responses, which may be absent or significantly reduced if ordinary RPMI-1640 with added Hepes is used.

2.2 Holding medium

For preparing cells, and holding on the bench before culture, use RPMI-1640 (GIBCO 31800) supplemented with 25 mM Hepes and 5% fetal calf serum (FCS). Some workers use a balanced salt solution (BSS), but we find that human B cells do not do so well in BSS compared to medium. Gentamicin at 50 μg/ml is routinely used with tonsil-cell preparations since these frequently harbour some bacteria. This medium contains no bicarbonate and is used exclusively for preparing, washing, and holding cells before culture.

2.3 Lymphocyte separation medium

Ficoll–Hypaque or Ficoll–sodium metrozoate at 1.077 kg/l, such as Lymphoprep (Nycomed) or Ficoll-Paque (Pharmacia), are used to prepare mononuclear cells from blood or tonsils. Percoll (Pharmacia) is used to separate E-rosetting (E^+) cells from non-E-rosetting (E^-) cells and for separating low- and high-density B cells on discontinuous density gradients.

Protocol 1

Preparation of Percoll for E-rosette separation and discontinuous density gradients

NB: Percoll solutions for discontinuous density-gradient centrifugation are commonly made to a predetermined percentage by mixing with buffered saline or medium. However, the density of stock Percoll varies slightly, as do the various diluting solutions, and a given percentage of Percoll does not always result in the same density. For this reason, Percoll solutions should be prepared from solutions of known densities (specific gravities). Specific gravities are determined easily and accurately by weighing in specific gravity bottles.

2.12 Recombinant cytokines

Purified recombinant human cytokines are available from a variety of different sources, such as R&D Systems advertised in most of the major immunology journals.

3 Preparation of human B cells

The way in which B cells are prepared from human lymphoid tissues can be critical for assaying B-cell growth and differentiation factors. It is important to appreciate that completely pure preparations of B cells can never be obtained from normal tissues, even by cell sorting. The degree of contamination with other cell types may interfere with the assays, and should always be determined. T-cell depletion of tonsillar mononuclear cells by rosetting will routinely give preparations of greater than 95% B cells, which can be used in assays for proliferation and antibody production without further purification. Similar preparations from venous blood usually yield much lower proportions of B cells (10–20%), but these can be used in certain circumstances, for example to test for T-cell helper activity in specific antibody responses. If required, further purification can be achieved by depleting adherent cells. Negative selection of other unwanted cells with monoclonal antibodies and depletion by magnetic beads or complement lysis can also be used to improve B-cell purity. Subpopulations of B cells can be obtained by fractionation on density gradients or by sorting after staining with selected monoclonal antibodies. In addition to purified normal B cells, selected B cell- lines can also be used as indicators for human B-cell growth and differentiation factors (BCGF and BCDF).

Protocol 2

Preparation of mononuclear cells from tonsils (TMC) and venous blood (PBMC)

Equipment and reagents

- Medium (see Section 2.2)
- Lymphocyte separation medium (Section 2.3)
- Syringe fitted with a 21-gauge needle
- Preservative-free heparin
- Ficoll–sodium metrozoate: (Section 2.3)
- Benchtop centrifuge
- Sterile plastic Universal tubes, pipettes, pipette tips, Petri dishes
- Microscope and haemocytometer
- Trypan Blue solution
- Sterile scalpel
- 70% alcohol

A. Preparation of tonsillar mononuclear cells (TMC)

Tonsils can be readily obtained with ethical approval from most hospitals. They should be collected in a sterile container and used the same day.

Protocol 2 continued

1 Surface-sterilize the excised tonsil with 70% alcohol for 5 sec, and then rinse in RPMI-1640 holding medium.

2 Put the tonsil into a Petri dish with 20 ml of RPMI-1640 holding medium containing 50 μg/ml of gentamicin, then tease out the mononuclear cells by scraping from the connective tissue with a sterile scalpel.

3 Pipette the cell suspension into a plastic Universal tube and allow any clumps of tissue to settle for 1 min.

4 Remove the suspended cells and layer on to 8 ml of the lymphocyte separation medium (1.077 kg/litre) (Section 2.3) in a plastic Universal tube. Centrifuge at 1000 g for 15 min at room temperature.

5 Collect the mononuclear cells from the interface, taking a portion of the Ficoll–Hypaque layer below, and wash by centrifugation at 200 g for 10 min.

6 Wash the cells a second time (200 g) and resuspend in 10 ml of RPMI-1640 holding medium containing 5% FCS and gentamicin.

7 Remove a small aliquot and count on a haemocytometer. Viability determined by Trypan Blue exclusion should always be in excess of 90%.

B. Preparation of peripheral blood mononuclear cells (PBMC)

1 Take blood from volunteer donors into a syringe wetted with preservative-free heparin.

2 Dilute blood with an equal volume of RPMI-1640 holding medium containing 10 IU/ml of preservative-free heparin but without FCS, and layer on to lymphocyte separation medium (Section 2.3) (2 vol. of diluted blood to 1 vol. of separation medium) and centrifuge at 1000 g for 15 min at room temp. Make sure the centrifuge brake is off to prevent disturbance of the interface.

3 Collect the mononuclear cells from the interface, taking a portion of the Ficoll–Hypaque layer below, and wash at 200 g for 15 min with at least an equal volume of holding medium containing 10 IU/ml of preservative-free heparin, but without FCS. (The slow wash in the presence of heparin will leave most of the platelets in the supernatant and prevent clumping of the mononuclear cell pellet.)

4 Wash the cells a second time at 200 g in RPMI-1640 holding medium with 5% FCS, and resuspend to 5×10^6 cells/ml.

5 Remove a small aliquot and count on a haemocytometer. Viability determined by Trypan Blue exclusion should be in excess of 95%.

3.1 Mononuclear cell preparation

The first step in the preparation of human B cells is to obtain mononuclear cells free of red blood cells, platelets, and polymorphonuclear cells (PMN). These are prepared from peripheral blood or tonsils as described in *Protocol 2*. Splenic B cells can also be obtained in a similar manner.

3.2 Depletion of T cells by E-rosetting

Human T cells and some natural killer (NK) cells express cell-surface CD2 antigen which binds to specific receptors on sheep erythrocytes (E) resulting in the formation of E rosettes. Separation of E-rosette-forming cells (E$^+$) from non-rosette-forming (E$^-$) cells by density-gradient centrifugation is the simplest and most effective method of depleting T cells from mononuclear cell preparations.

Protocol 3

Depletion of T cells by E-rosetting with AET-treated sheep red blood cells (sRBC)

Equipment and reagents

- Gey's Haemolytic Balanced Salt Solution:
  Solution A: 35.0 g NH$_4$Cl, 1.85 g KCl, 1.5 g Na$_2$HPO$_4$·12H$_2$O, 0.119 g KH$_2$PO$_4$, 5.0 g glucose, 0.005 g Phenol Red, 25.0 g gelatine (Difco), made up to 1 litre in double-distilled water
  Solution B: 4.2 g MgCl$_2$·6H$_2$O, 1.4 g MgSO$_4$·7H$_2$O, 3.4 g CaCl$_2$, made up to 1 litre in double-distilled water
  Solution C: 22.5 g NaHCO$_3$, made up to 1 litre in double-distilled water.
  Sterilize all three solutions by autoclaving and store at 4 °C. As required, make up Gey's solution fresh by mixing 7 vol. of sterile double-distilled water with 2 vol. of Solution A (warmed at 37 °C for 5 min

before use to melt the gelatine), 0.5 vol. of Solution B, and 0.5 vol. of Solution C.
- 40.2 mg/ml AET (S-2 aminoethyliso-thiouronium bromide hydrobromide) in water, pH 9.0 adjusted with 1 M NaOH and filter-sterilized.
- Sheep's blood in Alsever's solution (Section 2.4)
- Sterile 0.14 M NaCl
- Holding medium (Section 2.2) with and without FCS
- Percoll (Section 2.3 and *Protocol 1*)
- Sterile pipettes, pipette tips, plastic Universal tubes
- Refrigerated benchtop centrifuge

A. Preparation of AET-treated sRBC

E rosettes are best formed using sheep red cells treated with S-2-aminoethylisothiouronium bromide hydrobromide (AET) to stabilize rosettes as described by Kaplan and Clark (9).

1 Wash sheep's blood (stored in Alsever's solution for up to 3 weeks) three times in sterile 0.14 M NaCl by centrifuging at 200 g for 7 minutes at room temperature. Remove all the supernatant and any buffy coat on each wash.

2 After the last wash, remove all residual supernatant and incubate 1 vol. of the packed sRBC pellet with 4 vol. of freshly prepared AET solution at 37 °C for 15 min.

3 Wash five times in sterile 0.14 M saline by centrifuging at 200 g for 7 minutes at room temperature and resuspend in RPMI-1640 holding medium (without FCS) to give 10% AET-sRBC. These may be stored at 4 °C for up to 3 weeks.

B. E-Rosette formation and separation

1 Mix 10 ml of mononuclear cells at 5 × 10^6/ml with 2.5 ml of 10% AET-SRBC and 1 ml of FCS in a plastic Universal tube. Centrifuge at 200 g for 15–20 min at 4 °C with the

Protocol 3 continued

brake off. Ensure that a good cell pellet is obtained with no SRBC in the supernatant. If necessary, centrifuge for a longer time but not at higher speed.

2   Incubate for 60 min on ice.

3   Resuspend the rosettes by gently rotating the centrifuge tube. Do not resuspend by pipetting as this will disrupt some rosettes.

4   Layer on to 7–8 ml of Percoll (SG 1.080) (Section 2.3) in a plastic Universal tube and centrifuge at 1000 g for 20 min at room temp. with the brake off.

5   Remove the E⁻ fraction from the interface along with about 75% of the Percoll. Be careful not to disturb the red cell pellet.

6   Dilute with at least an equal volume of holding medium and wash twice by centrifuging at 200 g for 7 minutes at room temperature.

7   To recover the E⁺ cells, remove all the Percoll from above the SRBC and resuspend the pellet with 5 ml of Gey's haemolytic balanced salt solution for 1–2 min. Immediately after red cell lysis, dilute with holding medium, and wash twice by centrifuging at 200 g for 7 minutes at room temperature)

8   Resuspend the E⁺ and E⁻ fractions in 2–5 ml of holding medium, and count the cells. It is most important to check each preparation for purity by determining the percentages of B cells, T cells, and monocytes (Section 3.7). Discard preparations with unacceptable numbers of contaminating T cells (more than 2%).

More effective T-cell depletion can be obtained if Percoll rather than Ficoll–Hypaque is used to separate E-rosette forming (E⁺) cells from non-rosette forming (E⁻) cells (10). The E⁻ fraction of TMC obtained by this method should contain less than 1% of CD3⁺ (T) cells. Two cycles of E-rosetting may be required to reduce the proportion of T cells to this level when PBMC are used. T-cell contamination must be reduced to this level in the E⁻ preparations used in most B-cell assays to avoid indirect action through residual T cells. Poor T-cell depletion may be obtained with some batches of SRBC even after AET treatment. In this case it is best to discard the offending batch of SRBC and start afresh. Analyses of typical E⁻ cell preparations from TMC and PBMC cells are given in *Table 2*.

3.3 Depletion of monocytes by adherence

Blood E⁻ cells contain 60–80% monocytes compared with only 1–2% in tonsillar E⁻ cell preparations. These can be depleted by adherence on tissue-culture grade, plastic Petri dishes. If recovery of the monocytes is required, plates coated by microexudate (extracellular matrix) from the BHK cell-line should be used. Contamination by monocytes in the non-adherent fraction is usually reduced to between 2 and 10% using this method. Better depletion may be obtained by passing cells through columns of Sephadex G-10, or by cell sorting, or cytotoxicity using antimonocyte monoclonal antibodies, but this is not usually necessary. In some assays, for example the antigen-specific antibody response to influenza virus (Section 6), small percentages of monocytes (about 0.5%) are essential, presumably for antigen presentation.

Table 2 Phenotype of fractionated E⁻ lymphocytes

Cell type	% Fluorescence-positive cells				
	CD20	CD3	CD14	CD57	CD16
Blood E⁻					
2 × rosetted	21	< 2	75	< 1	6
Light fraction	13	< 2	78	< 1	10
Heavy fraction	92	< 2	1	< 1	3
Tonsil E⁻					
1 × rosetted	95	< 1	2	2	1
Light fraction	98	< 1	1	nd	nd
Heavy fraction	98	< 1	< 1	nd	nd

Antibodies used were: B1 (CD20); UCHT1 (CD3); UCHM1 (CD14); HNK-1 (CD57); Leu 11 (CD16). nd × not done.

Protocol 4

Depletion of adherent cells on microexudate plates

Equipment and reagents

- Holding medium and culture medium (Sections 2.1 and 2.2)
- Holding medium containing 3 mM EDTA
- PBS containing 10 mM EDTA
- BHK cell line
- Sterile plastic 90-mm Petri dishes, pipettes, pipette tips
- Bactericidal UV light source

A. Preparation of BHK microexudate coated Petri dishes

1 Prepare microexudate dishes by growing baby hamster kidney (BHK) cells to confluence on 90-mm tissue-culture grade, plastic Petri dishes.

2 Remove the BHK cell monolayer with 10 mM EDTA in PBS.

3 Wash dishes vigorously several times with PBS, and sterilize with a bactericidal UV light source for 5 min. If desired, seal the treated dishes with tape and store at 4 °C.

B. Depletion of adherent cells

1 Incubate 2×10^7 E⁻ cells in 10 ml of holding medium containing 10% FCS on the microexudate dishes for 45 min at 37 °C.

2 Resuspend the non-adherent cells by gently rocking the dishes, and remove by pipette. Repeat this procedure at least twice with 10 ml of warm medium carefully added to the dish.

3 To remove the adherent cells, incubate for 15 min with medium containing 3 mM EDTA at 37 °C, and pipette vigorously.

3.4 Preparation of heavy and light B cells

In many B-cell activation and proliferation experiments, E⁻ cells are fractionated on discontinuous Percoll gradients to give light (<1.074 kg/litre) and heavy (>1.074 kg/litre) populations. The small heavy B cells are generally considered to be resting (G_0) cells, but there is some evidence to suggest that some of these cells are already activated (11). Because of this, some investigators prefer even higher density B cells to exclude activated cells in G_0 (12).

Protocol 5

Density-gradient fractionation of human B lymphocytes

Equipment and reagents

- Holding medium (Section 2.2)
- Percoll (Section 2.3)
- Trypan Blue solution
- Refrigerated benchtop centrifuge
- Sterile pipettes, pipette tips, Universal tubes
- Microscope and haemocytometer
- Conical centrifuge tubes

Method

1 Layer up to 3×10^7 cells in 2–3 ml of holding medium on to 3 ml of Percoll (SG 1.074) in a 10 ml conical centrifuge tube, and centrifuge at 1000 g for 20 min at room temperature. If using blood E⁻ cells, first deplete monocytes.

2 Remove the low-density B cells from the interface.

3 Discard most of the Percoll supernatant leaving about 0.2 ml. Take care not to remove all the supernatant or disturb the pellet as the cells in the pellet tend to be very loose.

4 Resuspend the high-density B cells in the remaining Percoll.

5 Wash each fraction twice by centrifuging at 200 g for 7 minutes at room temperature, and resuspend the cells in 1–2 ml of holding medium containing 5% FCS.

6 Count viable cells using Trypan Blue exclusion method, viability should be >95%.

3.5 Separation of B-cell subpopulations with monoclonal antibodies

Various methods have been described for preparing B-cell subpopulations defined by monoclonal antibodies. These include complement-mediated cytotoxicity, panning on antibody-coated plastic plates, rosetting with antibody-coated ox red blood cells, magnetic beads, and fluorescence-activated cell sorting (FACS). A major disadvantage with most of these methods is the difficulty in recovering labelled cells (positive selection) in sufficient numbers and condition suitable for cell culture. The magnetic separation technique (MACS) uses very small (100 nm) paramagnetic beads, which make positive selection as easy as negative selection. Moreover, the beads are biodegradable so they do not interfere with the cells in culture, and their small size does not noticeably change the light-scattering properties of the cells on FACS analysis. The method for MACS separation of B-cell subpopulations is as follows.

Protocol 6

MACS separation of B-cell subpopulations identified by monoclonal antibodies

The MACS magnetic cell sorter obtained from Miltenyi Biotec comes with magnet, columns, and biotinylated paramagnetic beads. Cell labelling is achieved with a sandwich of biotinylated monoclonal antibody followed by fluoresceinated streptavidin and then biotinylated beads. The streptavidin is FITC- (or PE-) conjugated to allow labelling to be checked by FACS analysis.

Equipment and reagents

- Holding medium (Section 2.2)
- PBS containing 0.01% sodium azide and 5 mM EDTA at pH 7.4 (PBS–EDTA)
- PBS containing 1% BSA and 5 mM EDTA at pH 7.4 (PBS–BSA)
- 70% and 95% ethanol
- Double-distilled or Milli-Q (Millipore) water
- Biotinylated monoclonal antibodies, FITC– or PE–streptavidin

- Mild detergent
- 10 ml syringe, 25-gauge short needles, and 21-gauge needles
- Three-way stopcock to fit the column and syringe
- MACS apparatus with biotinylated paramagnetic beads and columns of appropriate size
- Sterile pipettes and Universal tubes

A. Column preparation

1   Attach a three-way stopcock to the MACS column. Fill the column with 70% ethanol slowly from the bottom using a syringe fitted to the stopcock, tapping frequently to dislodge bubbles. Replace the ethanol by running in PBS–BSA from the top. Leave at 4 °C until required. (This filling method avoids bubbles in the column.)

2   Connect a 25-gauge short needle vertically and a 10 ml syringe of PBS–BSA to the three-way stopcock attached to the column. Use the PBS–BSA to flush through the needle if it becomes blocked.

3   Cool the column by passing through 3 column vol. of ice-cold PBS–BSA before use.

4   To regenerate the column after use, rinse by suction with 500 ml of mild detergent followed by 1 litre of double-distilled water then 500 ml of 95% ethanol. Dry the column completely. (The columns can be sterilized by autoclaving at 120 °C, but this does shorten the column life. Columns can normally be used about 10 times.)

B. Cell staining and separation

1   Wash the cells in ice-cold PBS–EDTA and centrifuge at 200 g for 5 minutes at 4 °C. Keep an aliquot for FACS analysis.

Protocol 6 continued

2   Add 100 μl of biotinylated monoclonal antibody to the washed pellet of 10^6 cells, mix, and incubate for 10 min at 4 °C.

3   Wash the cells in PBS–EDTA, centrifuge at 200 g for 5 minutes at 4 °C then add 10 μl of FITC–streptavidin and incubate for 10 min at 4 °C. Treat the aliquot put aside in step 1 as a negative control in the same way.

4   Wash the cells once in PBS–EDTA centrifuge at 200 g for 5 minutes at 4 °C and resuspend in 200 μl of PBS–EDTA (if using more than 4×10^7 cells, add an extra 50 μl per 10^7 cells). Add 1 μl of concentrated biotinylated MACS beads to each 100 μl of cell suspension, mix, and incubate for 5 min at 4 °C.

5   Add 400 μl of PBS–BSA to each 100 μl of cell suspension and apply immediately to the MACS column fitted with a short 25-gauge needle. Note that the column flow rate is determined by the needle gauge. Keep an aliquot of unseparated cells at this stage for FACS analysis.

6   As soon as the cells have been applied to the column, place the column in the magnet. Open the stopcock and add 5 column vol. of PBS–BSA to the top of the column. Allow the unbound cells to pass through the column and collect into a container on ice. Do not let the column run dry.

7   Replace the 25-gauge needle with a 21-gauge needle (to increase the flow rate) and run through 5–10 column vol. of PBS–BSA. Discard this wash.

8   To remove bound cells, remove the column from the magnet, attach a 10 ml syringe to each end of the column (one filled with PBS–BSA) and vigorously squirt PBS–BSA back and forth through the column to dislodge the bound cells. Wash this bound fraction into a container on ice.

NB: The use of sodium azide as described and keeping the cells at 4 °C is important to prevent capping and shedding of the antibody. The azide is removed by washing the cells and does not affect subsequent viability or function.

Separation purity should always be checked by FACS analysis of cells incubated with FITC–streptavidin only (background), stained unseparated cells, stained unbound cells, and stained bound cells. Better purity of unbound cells can sometimes be obtained by passing through the column twice.

3.6 Immunofluorescence analysis of B-cell preparations

It is essential to monitor all human B-cell preparations used to investigate responses to cytokines for purity, since unacceptable contamination can sometimes occur and interfere with the assay. This is best done by indirect immunofluorescence using well-defined monoclonal antibodies to B cells, T cells, monocytes, and NK cells. For small numbers of cells, staining is carried out in round-bottomed microtitre wells, or round-bottomed flexible PVC microtitration plates which can be cut to the required number of wells and supported on a rigid microtitre tray. Larger numbers of cells can be stained in 12×75 mm Falcon tubes.

Protocol 7

Immunofluorescent staining of B-cell preparations

Equipment and reagents

- Holding medium (Section 2.2) containing 2% FCS and 0.01% NaN_3
- Monoclonal antibodies (second-layer antibody if required)
- Plastic round-bottomed microtitre trays, Falcon tubes (cat. no. 2052), pipettes, and pipette tips
- Refrigerated benchtop centrifuge fitted with a microtitre plate holder
- Whirlimixer
- Flow cytometer such as the FACScan
- Paper tissue

A. Monoclonal antibody staining of cells in microtitre wells

1 Dispense between 1 and 3×10^5 cells per well of a non-sterile, round-bottomed microtitre tray. Include wells for each monoclonal antibody as well as negative and positive controls.

2 Centrifuge the cells into a pellet at 200 g for 2 min using a microtitre plate attachment available for most centrifuges.

3 Remove supernatants by inverting the plate with a *single* flicking motion over a sink. Do not repeat this action as the cells will become resuspended and lost. Carefully wipe any droplets of medium from the surface of the plate using a paper tissue, then resuspend the cells by holding the plate firmly on to a vortex Whirlimixer.

4 Add 50 μl of monoclonal antibody diluted in holding medium containing 2% FCS and 0.01% NaN_3. When checking for B-cell purity, include CD19 antibody for B cells, CD3 antibody for T cells, and a monocyte-specific antibody such as UCHM1 (CD14). For the negative control, use medium alone or a monoclonal antibody known not to react with human leucocytes. For the positive control, use an anti-common leucocyte (CD45). Mix each well individually when adding the antibody. Do not use the Whirlimixer as antibody will spill over the sides into adjacent wells.

5 Incubate on ice for 30 min.

6 Wash the cells three times by adding 200 μl of medium to each well, centrifuging at 200 g for 2 min, and removing the supernatant by inverting the plate with a *single* flicking motion over a sink. Resuspend the cells by holding the plate firmly on a vortex Whirlimixer. After each wash, carefully remove any droplets remaining on the surface of the plate with a paper tissue. Take extra care at this stage to prevent any spill-over of antibody from one well to the next.

7 If directly conjugated antibodies are used, go to step 10. Otherwise, to the resuspended cells add 50 μl of pre-titrated FITC-conjugated F(ab')$_2$ goat anti-mouse Ig adsorbed against human serum proteins (Section 2.10) in medium containing 2% FCS, 0.01% NaN_3, and 2% normal goat serum (NGS) to inhibit Fc receptor binding.

8 Incubate on ice for 30 min.

9 Wash three times as in step 6.

10 Resuspend the cells and make up to 0.5 ml in Falcon tubes with holding medium containing 2% FCS and 0.01% NaN$_3$. The stained cells can be kept on ice for 2–3 h before analysis on a flow cytometer such as the FACScan. If it is necessary to delay the FACS analysis, fix the cells as described in *Protocol 8*; they can then be kept for several days without loss of fluorescence.

B. Monoclonal antibody labelling of larger numbers of cells

For larger numbers of cells, staining can be done in Falcon tubes.

1 Incubate 0.5×10^6 cells with 100 µl of pre-titrated monoclonal antibody in Falcon tubes for 30 min on ice.

2 Wash twice in cold medium containing 2% FCS and 0.01% NaN$_3$.

3 For directly conjugated antibodies go to step 4. Otherwise incubate the cells with 100 µl of pre-titrated FITC-conjugated goat anti-mouse Ig for a further 30 min on ice.

4 Wash twice, then resuspend the cells in 0.5 ml of holding medium and analyse samples by flow cytometry.

NB: In some cases, phenotypic analysis of B cells, which have been cultured in the presence of another monoclonal antibody, is required. To avoid detection of this antibody one can use either directly conjugated monoclonal antibodies for staining, or a second layer specific for the IgG subclass of the staining (e.g. IgG2a) but not the other (e.g. IgG1) monoclonal antibody.

Protocol 8
Fixing FITC-labelled cells

Equipment and reagents

- Paraformaldehyde
- 1 M sodium hydroxide solution
- PBS
- Holding medium (Section 2.2)
- 80 °C waterbath

- Plastic pipettes, pipette tips, Falcon tubes (cat. no. 2052)
- Benchtop centrifuge
- FACScan

Method

1 Make up 0.1 g of paraformaldehyde with 2 drops of 1 M NaOH and 0.2 ml of H$_2$O.

2 Heat to 80 °C in a waterbath. Do not boil.

3 Cool, and add 9.8 ml of PBS.

4 Wash labelled cells in PBS centrifuge at 200 g for 5 minutes at 4 °C and then resuspend pellet in 200 µl of fixative at 4 °C for 20 min, then wash twice in holding medium as before.

5 Resuspend the cells to 0.5 ml in holding medium containing 5% FCS before reading on the FACScan.

3.7 Human B cell-lines for assaying B-cell growth and differentiation factors

In some circumstances, continuous B cell-lines may offer certain advantages over purified B cells for measuring growth and differentiation in response to cytokines:

(a) Continuous B cell-lines are free of the non-B-cell contamination, which can cause problems even with FACS-selected preparations.

(b) B cell-lines are more homogeneous than normal B-cell preparations, which generally consist of ill-defined B-cell subpopulations, and/or B cells at different stages of activation.

These advantages are offset to some extent by the abnormal physiological status of B cell-lines and the uncertain relevance of their responses to normal B-cell growth and differentiation. For this reason, B cell-lines are best used in conjunction with other assays.

By the judicious selection of indicator B cell-lines, it is possible to distinguish between different factors. For example, the mouse B9 hybridoma cell-line proliferates in response to very low concentrations of IL-6, (13), see Vol. 2, Chapter 13. In addition, responses to particular cytokines can be confirmed by using specific blocking antibodies. Of the numerous B cell-lines that respond to cytokines, we have selected four based on their responses in different assays. One of the best characterized of these is CESS, a lymphoblastoid line used for detecting B-cell differentiation factors such as IL-6 (14). In addition, we have identified three other lines (HFB1, L4, and BALM 4) which proliferate and/or differentiate (secrete immunoglobulin) in response to different cytokines. There are many other lines, however, that can be used according to the investigator's needs and preferences. Of particular importance are those representing different stages of B-cell maturation.

3.7.1 Maintenance of B cell-lines used in assays for B-cell growth and differentiation

The B cell-lines used in proliferation and differentiation assays described in Sections 5 and 6 were grown in medium RPMI-1640 supplemented with 25 mM Hepes, 2 mM glutamine, and 10% FCS in 25 cm² or 75 cm² flasks at 37 °C in an atmosphere of 5% CO_2 in air. Other lines may require different media and culture conditions. Small numbers of cells can be grown in 24-well Costar plates. Antibiotics are not normally necessary, but gentamicin at 50 µg/ml can be used without interfering with the assays. The lines should be split regularly to keep the cells in log-phase growth.

One important problem, which must be closely monitored, is that of mycoplasma contamination which can interfere with responses to B-cell growth factors. Interpretation of [³H]TdR-incorporation results may be impossible if the responding cell-lines are contaminated. Under these circumstances, cell proliferation can be determined with the MTT test (15). The Epstein–Barr virus (EBV) transformed line, CESS, is often contaminated with mycoplasma, but this does not seem to inhibit its ability to respond to IL-6. Mycoplasma-free lines should be checked routinely for infection. If possible, contaminated and mycoplasma-free lines should be dealt with completely separately to reduce the possibility of cross-contamination. If separate facilities are not available, mycoplasma-free cultures should be handled only after fumigation of the laminar flow cabinet with formaldehyde, preferably overnight. This is most easily done by leaving an open dish of formaldehyde in the closed cabinet with the fan off. It is also important to use separate stocks of medium and other reagents, and to keep the incubator clean and free of mycoplasma infected cultures. There are fewer problems with contamination, especially fungi and mycoplasmas, if the incubators are kept dry.

4 B-cell activation

Activation of B cells by ligand binding to receptors on the cell membrane, such as anti-Ig or IL-4, involves a series of biochemical events—beginning with receptor-mediated signal transduction and stimulation of second-messenger cascades, followed by activation and/or synthesis of transcription factors responsible for gene regulation, and leading to synthesis of RNA and the expression of activation antigens. The cell then leaves G_0 and enters G_1, but in the absence of a second signal does not normally synthesize DNA or divide. The early signalling events of B-cell activation, such as protein tyrosine phosphorylation and hydrolysis of phosphatidylinositol bisphosphate (PIP_2) in response to anti-Ig (16), and the elevation in cAMP that follows stimulation with IL-4 (17) occur within minutes and are dealt with in Chapter 6 (this volume). Later events, such as c-myc expression, synthesis of RNA, size increase, and expression of cell-surface activation antigens involve more complex cell functions and occur within hours or days.

4.1 Measurement of RNA synthesis

Activation of B cells to leave G_0 and enter G_1 is accompanied by RNA synthesis. Most of this is ribosomal RNA not mRNA and is part of the cells preparation for protein synthesis. *De novo* RNA synthesis can be easily measured by the incorporation of [^{3}H]uridine.

Protocol 9

Measurement of RNA synthesis

Equipment and reagents

- Culture medium (Section 2.1)
- [^{3}H]uridine (specific activity 25–30 Ci/mmol)
- Sterile, flat-bottomed microtitre trays for tissue culture
- CO_2 incubator
- Sterile pipettes, pipette tips, Universal tubes
- Cell harvester with glass-fibre filters
- Liquid scintillation counter, scintillant, and capped counting tubes

Protocol 9 continued

Method

1 Prepare small resting B cells (*Protocol 5*) and culture at 10^6 cells/ml in 200 μl of culture medium in flat-bottomed microtitre wells with and without the cytokine to be investigated. Also include control cultures in medium alone and with a non specific B-cell activator such as PMA (10 ng/ml).

2 Incubate for 18 h at 37 °C in an atmosphere of 5% CO_2, then add 1 μCi of [^{3}H]uridine to each well and incubate for a further 6 h at 37 °C.

3 Harvest the labelled cells on to glass-fibre discs with an automated cell harvester, and count the amount of incorporated [^{3}H]uridine in a liquid scintillation counter. Correct the results for quenching and efficiency and express as disintegrations per minute (d.p.m.).

4.2 Measurement of B-cell activation by expression of surface activation antigens such as CD23 and surface IgM

Activation of B cells with cytokines such as IL-4 or IL-13 results in increased expression of activation antigens including CD23, surface IgM, CD40, and, in some cases, MHC class II antigens. These can easily be measured by monoclonal antibody labelling and flow cytometry. The most commonly used B cells for activation experiments are small, heavy, tonsillar E$^-$ cells isolated on discontinuous Percoll gradients (*Protocol 5*), but unfractionated tonsillar B cells are usually satisfactory. Other sources of B cells such as spleen can be used, but peripheral blood B cells are not very satisfactory because of the relatively small numbers of B cells obtained, and the difficulties in removing the high proportion of monocytes, NK, and null cells (*Table 2*). The technique for activating B cells and measuring the expression of activation antigens is described in *Protocol 10*.

Protocol 10

Expression of human B-cell activation antigens

Equipment and reagents

- Culture medium (Section 2.1)
- Lymphocyte separation medium (e.g. Ficoll–Hypaque) at 1.077 kg/litre (Section 2.3)
- PMA
- Monoclonal antibodies to activation antigens (e.g. CD23, CD40, CD86, and IgM)
- Sterile 24-well Costar plates, 12 × 75 mm Falcon tubes, Universal tubes, pipettes and pipette tips, Pasteur pipettes
- 5% CO_2 incubator
- Benchtop centrifuge
- Flow cytometer (FACScan)

Method

1 Prepare T-cell depleted E$^-$ cells as described in Section 3, and resuspend to 1×10^6 cells/ml with culture medium containing 5% FCS, 25 mM Hepes, and 50 μg/ml of gentamicin.

2   If small numbers of activated cells are required, use 2 ml cultures at 10^6 cells/ml in 24-well Costar plates. For activation with cytokines such as IL-4, add 50 μl of an appropriate dilution in culture medium. A final concentration of IL-4 of 100 units/ ml is optimal. Use PMA at a final concentration of 0.5–10 ng/ml for positive control cultures. Note that, normally, 10 ng/ml of PMA will both activate and induce cell division, whereas 0.5 ng/ml will activate without significant DNA synthesis. To prevent the cultures from drying out, put sterile water into the outer wells, and place the Costar plate inside an unsealed plastic box. For larger numbers of cells, set up the cultures at 10^6 cells/ml in tissue-culture flasks.

3   Incubate at 37 °C for 72 h in a dry incubator with an atmosphere of 5% CO_2 in air.

4   At the completion of the culture period, resuspend the cells and centrifuge at 1000 g for 20 min at room temperature over Ficoll–Hypaque (1.077 kg/litre) to remove dead cells and debris. For small numbers of cells, this can be done in 12 × 75 mm Falcon tubes containing 1.5 ml of Ficoll–Hypaque, otherwise use plastic Universal containers with at least 7 ml of Ficoll–Hypaque.

5   Carefully remove the cells from the interface with a Pasteur pipette, then wash twice by centrifuging at 200 g for 7 minutes at room temperature and resuspend to 2×10^6 cells/ml in holding medium.

6   To assess the expression of activation antigens, stain the cells with the appropriate monoclonal antibody as in *Protocol 7*, and analyse on a flow cytometer.

Note: Appropriate negative controls for B cells activated with cytokine or PMA are B cells cultured under the same conditions but without the activation signal. About 20% more cells are required in control cultures as they do not survive as well as activated cells. Freshly prepared E⁻ cells are not suitable controls.

An example of B-cell activation with IL-4 is given in *Figure 1*. After stimulation with IL-4 for 72 h the cells were stained for surface CD23 and IgM expression. The FACScan histograms clearly show an increase in expression of CD23 and surface IgM by B cells activated with IL-4. Much lower concentrations of IL-4 are required for optimal surface IgM expression compared with CD23 expression (18).

The enhanced expression of surface activation antigens detected by FACS analysis can be expressed in three different ways:

(a) The fluorescent channel subdividing the histogram into two equal proportions (median) can be compared. This is usually known as the median fluorescence intensity (MFI).

(b) The fluorescent channel showing the peak fluorescence (mode) can be compared.

(c) The proportion of activated cells labelled can be given by setting the marker at the base of the peak obtained with control cells.

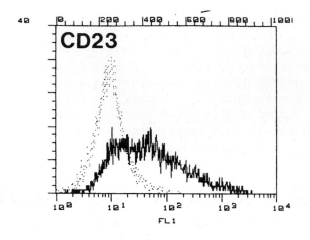

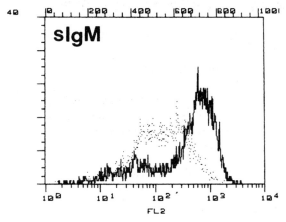

Figure 1 FACS histogram of small, heavy, tonsillar B cells cultured with medium alone or IL-4 for 3 days and then stained for CD23 and sIgM expression.

Of these, MFI is the preferred measurement. Changes in cell size on activation can be determined by comparing forward-angle scatter histograms in the same way.

5 Assays for B-cell proliferation in response to cytokines

Cytokines which promote the growth of B cells can be assayed in different ways. The two most common methods are co-stimulation of normal (tonsillar) B lymphocytes, and enhancement of cell division in indicator B cell-lines.

5.1 Cytokine stimulation of B-cell proliferation

This assay depends upon the co-stimulation of small, heavy (resting) B cells with cytokine and a second activation signal such as anti-IgM, anti-CD40, or PMA.

Under the right conditions, co-stimulation with both signals will result in B-cell proliferation, whereas each signal alone will have little or no effect. Several different methods for activating resting B cells to respond to growth-promoting cytokines have been described. Most of these use either soluble or particular preparations of anti-immunoglobulin, *Staphylococcus aureus* Cowan 1 preparations (SAC), anti-CD40 monoclonal antibodies, or phorbol esters (PMA). We have found the most reliable to be anti-IgM coupled to polyacrylamide beads and anti-CD40 monoclonal antibodies. These are used in the co-stimulation assay for B-cell growth factors as follows (see also Vol. 2, Chapter 13).

Protocol 11

Proliferation of resting B cells in response to co-stimulation with cytokine and anti-IgM or anti-CD40

Equipment and reagents

- Culture medium (Section 2.1)
- Anti-IgM beads or CD40 monoclonal antibody (Sections 2.6 and 2.12)
- [^{3}H]TdR (Section 2.9)
- Sterile, 96-well flat-bottomed microtitre plates for tissue culture
- Hamilton Stepper syringe
- CO_2 incubator
- Cell harvester with glass-fibre filters
- Liquid scintillation counter, scintillant, and capped counting tubes
- Saline

Method

This method describes the co-stimulation of tonsillar B cells

1   Prepare small resting tonsillar E$^-$ cells as described in Section 3.2, and resuspend to 10^6 cells/ml in culture medium supplemented with 5% FCS and 50 µg/ml of gentamicin.

2   Dispense 100 µl (10^5) of the cell suspension into sterile, flat-bottomed microtitre wells. To triplicate wells, add 50 µl of each cytokine to be tested plus 50 µl of anti-IgM beads (10 µg/ml final concentration) or CD40 monoclonal antibody (1 µg/ml). For each experiment, include control cultures with medium alone, and anti-IgM beads (or anti-CD40 monoclonal antibody) alone. If using a dry incubator, fill the outer wells with sterile water and place the plate in an unsealed plastic box to minimize evaporation.

3   Incubate for 72 h at 37 °C in an atmosphere of 5% CO_2 in air.

4   Add 1 µCi of [^{3}H]TdR in 10 µl of saline to each culture well using a 0.5 ml Hamilton Stepper syringe, and incubate at 37 °C for 6–8 h.

5   Harvest the labelled cells on to glass-fibre discs with an automated cell harvester, and count the incorporated [^{3}H]TdR in a liquid scintillation counter. Correct the results for quenching and efficiency and express as disintegrations per minute (d.p.m.).

Table 3 Co-stimulation of B cells with anti-IgM and IL-4

Anti-IgM beads	IL-4	Response ([^{3}H]TdR d.p.m.)
–	–	1286 ± 187[a]
×	–	2612 ± 297
–	×	1879 ± 241
×	×	87 345 ± 1223

[a]± 1 standard error of the mean [SEM]

A typical result from an IL-4 co-stimulation experiment is given in *Table 3*. In this case, tonsillar B cells were stimulated with anti-IgM beads and IL-4 (100 units/ml). A 10-fold stimulation index with counts up to 30 000 is typical for this sort of experiment.

It is important to note that the choice of activation signal in these experiments is not just a matter of convenience. Different B-cell activators may have quite different effects and prime B cells to respond in different ways to the various B-cell growth-promoting cytokines. For example, PMA, but not anti-IgM, is a powerful inducer of the CD23 antigen. Similarly, CD40 is a good co-stimulator for IL-4 and IL-13, whereas anti-IgM is good for IL-4 but not for IL-13. It may be important therefore to try different activation signals when screening for unknown B-cell growth factors.

5.2 Cytokine stimulation of proliferation by B cell-lines

When grown at low cell densities, some B cell-lines depend upon the addition of exogenous growth factors for continual proliferation. Using selected B cell-lines such as HFB1, L4, and BALM 4, this property can be exploited to assay for growth-promoting cytokines (see also Vol. 2, Chapter 13).

Protocol 12

Cytokine stimulation of growth by B cell-lines

Equipment and reagents

- Culture medium (Section 2.1)
- [^{3}H]TdR (Section 2.9)
- Sterile, 96-well flat-bottomed microtitre plates for tissue culture
- Hamilton Stepper syringe
- 5% CO_2 incubator
- Cell harvester with glass-fibre filters
- Liquid scintillation counter, scintillant, and capped counting tubes

Method

This method describes the measurement of proliferation by B cell lines

1   Harvest cells from a vigorous log-phase growth culture of the cell line. Subculture the cells 24–48 h beforehand. Do not use cultures that contain many dead cells, or are growing slowly, they will not perform well in this assay. Wash the cells once and resuspend to 10^6 cells/ml in culture medium.

Protocol 12 continued

2   Add 100 μl of cells to give final cell concentrations ranging from 10^3 to 10^5 cells/ml in six replicate microtitre wells. Add 100 μl of cytokine to six replicate cultures at each cell concentration. Add medium only to one set of six wells as a negative control.

3   If using a dry incubator, fill the outer wells with sterile water, and put the plate in an unsealed plastic box to minimize evaporation. Incubate for 48 or 72 h at 37 °C in an atmosphere of 5% CO_2 in air.

4   Add 1 μCi/well of [^{3}H]TdR in 10 μl of saline using a 0.5 ml Hamilton Stepper syringe and incubate for a further 6–8 h.

5   Harvest the cells on to glass-fibre discs with an automatic cell harvester, and count the incorporated [^{3}H]TdR in a liquid scintillation counter.

NB: In these experiments, the starting cell concentration is critical. If the cell concentration is too high, cells proliferate well without any exogenous factor. On the other hand, if the concentration is too low, the cells will die even in the presence of added cytokine. We routinely use at least three cell concentrations of each cell-line. With the normal day-to-day variation, any of the three concentrations may give an optimal response.

6 Assays for cytokines that stimulate human B-cell differentiation (Ig secretion)

Cytokines that stimulate antibody secretion by human B cells (B-cell differentiation factors) can be measured in co-stimulation assays with SAC or anti-Ig-activated B cells (19) and on indicator B cell-lines (14). CD40 activated cells can also be used. Other assays have also been developed for cytokines which stimulate the production of immunoglobulin isotypes and those which can replace T cells in specific antibody responses called T-cell replacing factors (TRF). It is worth bearing in mind that B-cell differentiation could, in principle, also refer to other B-cell responses such as memory cell production or antigen presentation. Assays to measure the cytokine control of these other functions have not yet been developed.

6.1 Co-stimulation assays for cytokines that stimulate immunoglobulin secretion (B-cell differentiation factors)

These are set up in exactly the same way as described for proliferation (Section 5.1) except that SAC, CD40 monoclonal antibodies, or CD40 ligand (CD40L) are more commonly used than anti-Ig to activate the B cells, and the cultures normally run for 5–7 days rather than 3–4 days. At the end of the culture period, supernatants are removed and assayed for Ig as described in Section 8. A typical result using SAC-activated B cells and IL-6 or IL-2 as B-cell differentiation factors is given in *Table 4*.

Table 4 SAC co-stimulation assay for B-cell differentiation factors

SAC	IL-2 (ng/ml)	IL-6	Response Proliferation ([^{3}H]TdR d.p.m.)	IgG
–	–	–	800 ± 280^a	18 ± 6
$\times$	–	–	2000 ± 780	52 ± 11
$\times$	–	$\times$	1850 ± 540	1876 ± 230
$\times$	$\times$	–	66400 ± 6260	2360 ± 420

$^a\pm$ 1 SEM

Note that IL-2 stimulates both [^{3}H]TdR uptake (proliferation) and Ig secretion, whereas IL-6 stimulates only Ig secretion. IL-6 is therefore a true B-cell differentiation factor, whereas in this experiment the increased Ig secretion obtained with IL-2 may have been due to an increase in the number of B cells and not differentiation. This distinction should be taken into account when assaying for B-cell differentiation factors.

6.2 Assays for B-cell differentiation factors using B cell-lines

Immunoglobulin secretion by B cell-lines such as L4, BALM 4, and CESS may be increased in the presence of B-cell differentiation factors (21). With CESS it was originally reported that the minor population of surface IgG positive cells were more responsive to BCDF than unseparated CESS cells (14), but we have not found it necessary to isolate this subpopulation. The assay is carried out in exactly the same way as described for those cytokines that stimulate proliferation (*Protocol 12*), except that the cultures are extended to 5–7 days. Supernatants are then harvested and assayed for immunoglobulin content as described in Section 7. CESS, L4, and BALM 4 are all suitable cell lines for measuring immunoglobulin secretion in response to cytokines, but other cell lines can also be used. Lower concentrations of immunoglobulins are secreted by L4 and BALM 4, and it may be necessary to culture for a longer period (6–7 days) and at a higher cell concentration.

6.3 Assays for cytokine regulation of Ig isotype responses

A number of different assays have been used to investigate cytokine regulation of Ig class and IgG subclass responses in humans. Co-culture of B cells and T cells with IL-4 has been used to show that IgE production depends on IL-4, activated T cells, and other cytokines (IL-6) (22–24). CD40 antibody or ligand (CD40L) binding to CD40 on B cells has been shown to be an essential signal for heavy-chain switching by human B cells (25, 26). Co-stimulation of B cells with anti-CD40 antibody (or CD40L) and cytokine has since emerged as a suitable assay for Ig class and IgG subclass regulation. IgE and IgG subclass secretion can also be obtained by polyclonal activation of B cells with EBV at days 10–12 and IL-4 in the absence of CD40 activation, but this is probably not switching (27). EBV used in this way is a polyclonal activator and transformation has not occurred at this time point. Other polyclonal B-cell activators such as PMA have also been used to investigate the cytokine regulation of Ig isotype production (28, 29). The effect of cytokines on isotype and IgG subclass production can be determined by specific ELISA described in Section 7.

Protocol 13

Assays for cytokine regulation of immunoglobulin isotype production

Equipment and reagents

- EBV-containing supernatant from the marmoset B95–8 cell-line: Grow the B95–8 line in RPMI culture medium until the cultures are bright yellow, then centrifuge to remove the cells and filter the supernatant through a 0.45 micron filter. The EBV-containing supernatant can be aliquoted and stored at $-70\,°C$ until required.

- IMDM culture medium (Section 2.1)
- CD40 antibody or CD40L
- 5% CO_2 incubator
- Sterile, flat-bottomed 96- and 48-well microtitre plates, pipettes, pipette tips

A. Co-stimulation with CD40 antibody and cytokine

1   Prepare T-cell depleted E– cells from PBMC as described in *Protocol 3* and make up to 10^6 cells/ml in IMDM culture medium (Section 2.1) with 5% FCS.

2   Dispense 100 μl (10^5 cells) into each well of a 96-well flat-bottomed microtitre plate.

3   Add 50 μl of purified anti-CD40 antibody to give a final concentration of 1 μg/ml and 50 μl of cytokine to be tested. Include control cultures with CD40 antibody alone. If available, CD40L can be used instead of CD40 antibody.

4   Culture at $37\,°C$ in 5% CO_2 for 8–9 days then collect the supernatant for Ig class and IgG subclass assay as described in Section 7.

B. Ig isotype responses by B cells stimulated with EBV and cytokine

1   Prepare T-cell depleted E⁻ cells from TMC or PBMC in RPMI with 5% FCS as described in *Protocol 3*.

2   Centrifuge at 200 g for 7 min and resuspend the pellet to 12.5×10^6 cells/ ml in EBV-containing B95–8 supernatant. Incubate at $37\,°C$ in 5% CO_2 for 1–2 h.

3   Wash the cells twice to remove unbound EBV by centrifuging at 200 g for 7 minutes at room temperature and resuspend to 2×10^6 cells/ml in IMDM culture medium with 5% FCS (Section 2.1).

4   Dispense 0.5 ml (10^6 cells) into each well of a 48-well Costar plate and add 0.5 ml of the cytokine to be tested.

5   Culture at $37\,°C$ in 5% CO_2 for 12–14 days.

6   Harvest the supernatant for Ig class or Ig subclass assay as described in Section 7.

6.4 T-cell replacing factors

In addition to stimulating B-cell growth and differentiation, some cytokines can also replace T cells in specific antibody responses *in vitro*. In man, these T-cell replacing factors (TRF) can be readily assayed on thoroughly T-cell depleted, E⁻ cell preparations obtained from blood, tonsil, or spleen (30, 31). In this assay, E⁻ cells are cultured with antigen (influenza virus in the example described below) in the presence and absence of TRF, and antibody production is determined by specific ELISA. Antibody responses obtained in the presence of TRF are usually comparable with those obtained in the presence of T (E^+) cells.

Protocol 14

Assay for T-cell replacing factors (TRF) in specific antibody responses

Equipment and reagents

- RPMI-1640 culture medium supplemented with 10% horse serum (Section 2.1)
- Holding medium (Section 2.2)
- Purified influenza virus antigen (Section 2.8)
- Sterile 12×75 mm Falcon culture tubes (cat. no. 2054), pipettes, pipette tips
- 5% CO_2 incubator
- Benchtop centrifuge

Method

1 Prepare T-cell depleted E– (B) cells from TMC or PBMC as described in *Protocol 3* and resuspend to $1–1.5 \times 10^6$/ml in RPMI-1640 culture medium supplemented with 10% horse serum and 50 µg/ml of gentamicin (Section 2.1). Dispense 0.5 ml ($0.5–0.75 \times 10^6$ cells) into 12×75 mm culture tubes. Note that the horse serum is stable for many months at $-20\,°C$, but loses activity after a few days at $4\,°C$.

2 Dilute the purified influenza virus (Section 2.8) to 10-times the final concentration (usually 0.2 µg/ml) in the same medium, and add 100 µl to each culture tube.

3 Add 0.5 ml of medium to three tubes for a negative control, and 10^6 E^+ (T_H) cells in 0.5 ml of medium to three tubes for a positive control.

4 Dispense the cytokine to be assayed into the remaining tubes, and make up the total volume of each culture to 1 ml with culture medium.

5 Loosely replace the caps and incubate for 7 days at $37\,°C$ in a dry incubator with an atmosphere of 5% CO_2 in air.

6 At the end of the 7-day culture period, wash the cells once by centrifuging at 200 g for 10 minutes at room temperature and resuspend in 0.5 ml of culture medium containing 5% FCS. Cover the tubes with aluminium foil rather than recap them, and incubate for a further 12–18 h at $37\,°C$. (This step minimizes background in the ELISA assay by removing free virus and horse serum present in the culture medium.)

Protocol 14 continued

7   Collect supernatants for the assay of specific antibody (Section 7.3). IgG subclass antibody can also be measured (Section 7.2). Supernatants for ELISA may be stored at −20 °C before assay.

Table 5 Specific antibody responses obtained with TRF

Antibody to X31 (ng/ml)

Responding cells	Antigen	TRF	Response IgM	IgG
PBM E[−a]	−	−	< 1	< 1
PBM E[−]	+	−	< 1	2
PBM E	−	+	< 1	< 1
PBM E[−]	+	+	2	220 ± 80[b]
PBM E[−] + E[+]	+	−	2	241 ± 41

[a] Depleted of T cells by two cycles of E-rosetting with AET–SRBC (Section 2.2).
[b] ± 1 SEM

A typical result from a TRF-induced antibody response to influenza virus is given in *Table 5*.

The antibody cultures are usually carried out in triplicate in 12 × 75 mm capped Falcon tubes, but a micromethod is also available using fivefold fewer cells in round-bottomed microtitre plates (32). In this case, the responses obtained are more variable, and more replicates (> 6) should be used. The micromethod is essentially the same, except that 10^5 E[−] cells in 200 μl are cultured in round-bottomed microtitre wells. Washing of the cells in microtitre wells (see step 6 above) is best carried out by sucking off the medium from each well using a 21-gauge needle attached to a suction pump. If the needle is slid down the side of the microtitre well as far as the top of the curvature, the cell pellet will not be disturbed. The cells can then be washed by resuspending them in medium and repelleted by centrifugation at 200 *g* for 5 min on a centrifuge with a microtitre tray adapter.

7   Enzyme immunoassays for immunoglobulin secreted by human B cells

All the assays we use for the detection of human Ig and specific antibody are based on solid-phase enzyme-linked immunosorbent assays (ELISA).

7.1   Measurement of Ig (IgM, IgG, IgA, and IgE) secretion

The effect of B-cell differentiation factors is easily monitored by measuring Ig production with an ELISA assay. The example that follows is for IgG, but the other isotypes or total Ig can be measured in the same way by substituting the appropriate antibodies for capture in step 1 and detection in step 8 as shown in *Table 6*. The assays for IgE and IgG subclasses have an extra step 10.

Table 6 Conditions for Ig class and IgG subclass assays

Assay	First layer (step 1)	Second layer (step 8)	Third layer (step 10)
IgM	Goat anti-human IgM (Sigma I-0759) 1 µg/ml	HPO–goat anti-human IgM (Sigma A-6907) 1 µg/ml	IgE and IgG subclass only
IgG	Goat anti-human IgG (Sigma I-3382) 1 µg/ml	HPO–goat anti-human IgG (Sigma A-6029) 1 µg/ml	
IgA	Goat anti-human IgA (Sigma I-0884) 1 µg/ml	HPO–goat anti-human IgA (Sigma A-7032) 1 µg/ml	
IgE	Goat anti-human IgE (Sigma I-0632) 2 µg/ml	Rabbit anti-human IgE (MIAB Ab 105) 0.1 µg/ml	HPO–goat anti-rabbit IgG (Sigma A-0545) 1 µg/ml
IgG1	Rabbit anti-human G (H+L) (Jackson 309–005–082) 1 µg/ml	Biotin mAb anti-IgG1 (Zymed 05–3340) 0.5 µg/ml	HPO (or AP) streptavidin (Amersham RPN-1231/1234) 1/1000
IgG2	Rabbit anti-human G (H+L) (Jackson 309–005–082) 1 µg/ml	Biotin mAb anti-IgG2 (Zymed 05–3540) 1 µg/ml	HPO (or AP)–streptavidin (Amersham RPN-1231/1234) 1/1000
IgG3	Rabbit anti-human G (H+L) (Jackson 309-005-082) 1 µg/ml	Biotin mAb anti-IgG3 (Zymed 05–3640) 2 µg/ml	HPO (or AP)–streptavidin (Amersham RPN-1231/1234) 1/1000
IgG4	Sheep anti-human IgG4 (Binding Site AB009) 2 µg/ml	Biotin mAb anti-IgG4 (Zymed 05–3840) 2 µg/ml	HPO (or AP)–streptavidin (Amersham RPN-1231/1234) 1/1000

Protocol 15

Measurement of Ig by ELISA

Equipment and reagents

- 4% normal goat serum
- PBS/BSA/Tween: PBS containing 1% BSA and 0.05% Tween-20
- 3 M NaOH
- PBS/Tween: PBS containing 0.05% Tween-20
- Bicarbonate coating buffer: 1.59 g Na_2CO_3, 2.93 g $NaHCO_3$, 0.2 g NaN_3. Make up to 1 litre in double-distilled water and adjust to pH 9.6.
- 2 M H_2SO_4
- 1 mg/ml p-nitrophenyl phosphate (e.g. Sigma 104–105) in alkaline phosphatase buffer: 1.59 g Na_2CO_3, 2.93 g $NaHCO_3$, 9.52 mg $MgCl_2$. Make up to 1 litre in double-distilled water and adjust to pH 9.6
- Affinity-purified goat anti-human IgG (Sigma cat. no. I-3382)
- ELISA plate reader

- Horseradish peroxidase (HPO)- or alkaline phosphatase (AP)-conjugated affinity-purified goat anti-human IgG (Sigma cat. no. A-6029)
- Rabbit anti-human IgE (MIAB cat. no. AB 105)
- HPO–goat anti-rabbit IgG (Sigma cat. no. A-0407) (For IgE assay only)
- Phosphate citrate buffer pH 5.0
- 0-phenyldiamine (OPD) (Sigma P-1526) in phosphate citrate buffer: 1 M Na_2HPO_4 (28.4 g/litre) and citric acid (21.0 g/litre) made separately. Mix equal volumes just prior to use and add 0.5 mg/ml OPD and 0.015% (v/v) H_2O_2.
- Non-sterile, flat-bottomed 96-well ELISA plates (Immunolon II and Dynatech M1298)
- Incubator

Protocol 15 continued

Method

1. Dispense 75 µl of affinity-purified goat anti-human IgG at 1 µg/ml in bicarbonate coating buffer and incubate at room temperature overnight. For other Ig classes use antibodies as shown in *Table 6*. Note that individual batches of antisera should be pre-titrated to determine the optimal signal-to-noise ratio with high, medium, and low concentrations of IgG.

2. Wash three times with PBS/Tween.

3. To block remaining protein binding sites, add 100 µl PBS/BSA/Tween to each well and leave at room temp. for 30–90 min. 4% normal goat serum (NGS) diluted in PBS can also be used in this step.

4. Wash three times with PBS/Tween.

5. Add 75 µl of the test supernatant and standards in duplicate. Set up an 11-point standard curve using doubling dilutions of either pooled normal human serum, or partially purified IgG at 1000 ng/ml in PBS/BSA/Tween, in duplicate on each plate along with a buffer-only zero standard.

6. Incubate at room temp. for 1–2 h. (When assaying for IgE, incubate overnight at room temp.)

7. Wash three times with PBS/Tween.

8. To each well, add 75 µl of horseradish peroxidase (HPO)- or alkaline phosphatase AP-conjugated, affinity-purified goat anti-human IgG diluted in PBS/BSA/Tween. For IgE, use rabbit anti-human IgE. Titrate individual batches of antisera to determine the optimal dilution.

9. Incubate at room temp. for 1–2 h (4 h for IgE) then wash three times with PBS/Tween and once with distilled water.

10. For IgE, add 75 µl of HPO–goat anti-rabbit IgG, incubate for 1–2 h at room temp., then wash twice with PBS/Tween and once with distilled water.

11. To each well, add 100 µl of OPD (HPO substrate) in phosphate/citrate buffer and incubate for 15–60 min at room temperature for colour development. Stop with 40 µl of H_2SO_4. If AP-conjugated antibodies are used, add 100 µl of *p*-nitrophenyl phosphate in alkaline phosphatase buffer and allow the colour to develop for about 1 h at 37 °C. Stop with 40 µl of 3 M NaOH.

12. Read absorbance on an automatic ELISA plate reader at 492 nm for OPD or 405 nm for AP. Express the results as ng/ml of Ig calculated from the standard curve. (Most automatic plate readers now come with computer software which will plot a standard curve obtained by one of several choices of curve-fitting methods and will calculate the sample concentrations. Alternatively, obtain a standard curve by plotting the logit OD against $\log_2$ of the antibody concentration:

$$\text{logit}_{OD} = \frac{\ln 1 - P}{P}$$

where $P = OD_{\text{sample}}/OD_{\text{max}}$ and OD_{max} is the optical density obtained when all the NPP is hydrolysed, usually about 11.0.

Protocol 15 continued

NB: The antisera can be stored undiluted in small aliquots at −70 °C, and frozen and thawed a maximum of three times. Immunoglobulin standards should be diluted in assay buffer to 10 μg/ml and stored frozen in small aliquots. By substituting class-specific antisera in steps (1) and (8) above, it is also possible to measure the levels of IgM, IgA, and IgE in culture supernatants. The different antisera and conditions for IgM, IgG, IgA, and IgE are shown in *Table 6*.

7.2 Measurement of IgG subclasses by ELISA

Measurement of IgG subclasses in tissue-culture supernatants by ELISA has proved quite difficult. A number of methods have been reported, but we have found that some of these are subject to high backgrounds and in some cases lack of specificity. In our experience some of these difficulties have arisen from the complex sandwich methods employed. To minimize this problem, a method was developed by Karolena Kotowicz in this laboratory which employs IgG subclass-specific polyclonal antibody as a capture antibody and biotinylated mouse monoclonal antibodies to the human IgG subclasses (Zymed), followed by HPO- or AP-conjugated streptavidin for detection. The different antibodies used for capture and detection are shown in *Table 6*. The individual steps of this assay are essentially the same as in Section 7.1 above, except for the use of these reagents and longer incubation times. In addition, PBS/Tween with 1% normal mouse serum (NMS) is used in blocking step 3, and PBS/Tween with 0.2% NMS is used as a diluent in steps 5, 8, and also 10 when streptavidin is used instead of second antibody. Note that BSA is never used as this causes serious cross-reactivity problems with mouse antibodies. Optimal incubation times and concentrations of reagents should be determined to suit individual circumstances.

7.3 ELISA for specific antibody production

Specific antibody production *in vitro* can be readily measured by solid-phase enzyme immunoassays (ELISA). In each assay, a standard curve is constructed to enable the results to be expressed in ng/ml. The standard is obtained by measuring the IgG concentration (Section 7.1) in pooled supernatants from influenza-stimulated PBM, which contain only specific antibody. Secondary standards from normal human serum can also be used after calibration. Specific antibody-containing supernatants are assayed as follows.

Protocol 16
ELISA assay for specific antibody production

Equipment and reagents
- Influenza virus (Section 2.8)
- PBS
- Sodium azide
- Alkaline phosphatase-conjugated, affinity-purified, goat anti-human IgG (Sigma cat. no. A-3150)

Protocol 16 continued

- 1 mg/ml *p*-nitrophenylphosphate (Sigma 104–105) in alkaline phosphatase buffer: 1.59 g Na_2CO_3, 2.93 g $NaHCO_3$, 9.52 mg $MgCl_2$. Make up to 1 litre in double-distilled water and adjust to pH 9.6
- PBS/BSA: PBS containing 1% BSA (Fraction V from Sigma)
- Non-sterile, flat-bottomed 96-well ELISA plates

- Alkaline phosphatase-conjugated streptavidin
- *p*-nitrophenylphosphate substrate (NPP) in bicarbonate buffer, pH 9.6, containing 10^{-4} M $MgCl_2$
- Incubator
- Multiskan automatic ELISA plate reader

A. ELISA assay for specific IgG

1 Prepare a suspension of influenza virus (same strain as used for stimulation *in vitro*) at 20–100 µg/ml in PBS containing 0.02% sodium azide, and dispense 75 µl into each well of a flat-bottomed, non-sterile, 96-well microtitre tray.

2 Incubate for 1 h at 37 °C.

3 Recover the virus (which may be used at least 20 times) and store at 4 °C.

4 Wash the plates twice with PBS and once with PBS 1% BSA.

5 Add 100 µl of 1% BSA in PBS to each well and incubate for 1 h at 37 °C to block the remaining non-specific binding sites.

6 Wash once with PBS containing 1% BSA.

7 Add 75 µl of the standard (serially diluted from 1:1 to 1:128) to eight consecutive wells for the standard curve, and 75 µl of medium or PBS containing 1% BSA to three wells for the negative control. Add 75 µl of test supernatant to each of the remaining wells.

8 Incubate for 1 h at 37 °C.

9 Wash the plate twice with PBS and once with PBS containing 1% BSA.

10 Add 75 µl of alkaline phosphatase-conjugated, affinity-purified, goat anti-human IgG, diluted in PBS containing 1% BSA. This particular antibody can normally be used at 1:1000, and stored at 4 °C. To detect specific IgM, IgA, or IgE, use the equivalent detection antibody of the desired specificity.

11 Incubate at 37 °C for 1 h.

12 Wash twice in PBS and twice in distilled water.

13 To each well, add 100 µl of *p*-nitrophenylphosphate substrate (NPP) in bicarbonate buffer pH 9.6 containing 10^{-4} M $MgCl_2$ and allow the colour to develop (approx. 1 h at 37 °C).

14 Read the absorbance on a Multiskan automatic ELISA plate reader at 405 nm. Express the results in ng/ml, obtained from the standard curve as described in Section 7.1 above.

B. ELISA assay for specific IgG subclasses

1 Coat non-sterile, flat-bottomed microtitre wells with 75 µl of purified influenza virus, block, then add standards and test supernatants as described in Part A, steps 1–9.

2   Puncture the vein using a needle connected to the collection bag, taking care not to puncture the opposite side of the vein.

3   Hold the needle in place with one hand and remove the clamp on the bleed line with the other hand. Collect until the free flow of blood has ceased. Throughout the collection, agitate the collection bag to prevent clotting of the blood.

4   When no further blood is flowing, clamp the bleed line and remove the needle.

5   Strip the bleed line three times to prevent the blood from clotting in the line. Seal the bleed line three times using a heat sealer.

6   Follow *Protocol 1* to separate the mononuclear cells.

In addition to using mononuclear cells from peripheral blood, a good source of haemopoietic stem cells, progenitor cells, and unprimed naïve cells has been the umbilical cord blood of newborns. In cord blood, the majority of T cells are either of the CD4CD45RA (45–50%) or CD8CD45RA (15–20%) naïve phenotype. Very few are of the CD4CD45RO (< 5%) or CD8CD45RO (< 1%) memory/effector phenotype.

Another possible source of lymphocytes is the cerebrospinal or synovial fluids from individuals with disease. Synovial fluid from persons with rheumatoid arthritis can contain neutrophils, macrophages, dendritic cells, and both CD4 and CD8 T cells. Cytokine secretion by these T cells *in vitro*, however, is less than that observed from T cells isolated from the peripheral blood or synovium of patients with rheumatoid arthritis (6).

Protocol 3

Separation of mononuclear cells from synovial fluid (SF)

Equipment and reagents
(In addition to *Protocol 1*)

- 25 ml heparinized Evans bottles
- Heparin

- HBSS with 2% fetal calf serum (FCS) (LabTech)

Method

1   Collect SF in 25 ml heparinized Evans bottles. Add extra heparin to SF to 5 U/ml to prevent clotting.

2   Centrifuge hard at 400 g for 15 min at RT to pellet the white cell infiltrate.

3   Aspirate the supernatant (which can either be stored at −20 °C or discarded).

4   Wash the cells by resuspending the pellet in the same tube in 20 ml of HBSS with 2% FCS

5   Centrifuge at 200 g for 10 min at RT.

6   Wash cells again by resuspending the pellet in 20 ml of HBSS with 2% FCS.

7   Centrifuge at 200 g for 10 min at RT.

8   Separate mononuclear cells from other cells using Lymphoprep as in *Protocol 1*.

Lymphocytes can also be isolated from a variety of different tissues from diseased individuals. For example, the synovial membrane of RA patients can contain a variety of cell types (7): T cells, B cells, and macrophages can all be recruited into the membrane. In the sublining tissue, lymphocytes can accumulate around the blood vessels or infiltrate into the stroma. T cells make up about 50% of the cells, while B cells constitute approximately 5% of the population. The majority of the T cells are of the CD4CD45RO phenotype. Despite this high number of T cells in the synovium, the concentrations of the T-cell cytokines IFN-γ and IL-4 are relatively low.

Protocol 4

Separation of mononuclear cells from solid tissue (synovial membrane)

Equipment and reagents
(In addition to *Protocol 1*)

- Enzymes: 5 mg/ml collagenase (Boehringer-Mannheim (now Roche)); 0.15 mg/ml DNase (Sigma)
- Dulbecco's MEM with 1% gentamicin (Gibco-BRL) and 1% FCS
- Sterile, sieve beaker (glass beaker with nylon mesh taped over)
- Conical flask
- 20 ml and 5 ml syringes (Becton Dickinson)
- Scissors/forceps
- 9 cm Petri dish (Nalge Nunc)
- 0.2 μM filter (Millipore)

Method

1   Wash the tissue with Dulbecco's minimal essential medium (MEM) to remove any contaminating blood and place in 10 ml of MEM in a Petri dish. Chop the tissue into approximately 0.5 mm pieces.

2   Transfer the tissue into the flask and filter the enzyme mixture over it using a 0.2 μM filter.

3   Incubate in a 37 °C waterbath and shake intermittently for 1–2 h depending on the consistency.

4   Remove the flask when the tissue is broken down and shake vigorously by hand for approximately 5 min to break up any remaining clumps. Add approximately 30 ml of MEM to the flask to prevent further enzyme activity.

5   Pipette the suspension in small volumes on to the sterile sieve beaker and wash through with MEM. (It is usually necessary to use the plunger of a 5 ml syringe to push the cells through the mesh.)

6   Pipette the suspension into a 50 ml conical tube, dilute further with MEM, and centrifuge at 200 g for 10 min at 4 °C.

7   Discard the supernatant and resuspend the cells in MEM. Centrifuge and wash twice as before.

8   Resuspend the cells in MEM and count.

9   If there is a sufficient cell yield,[a] separate mononuclear cells on Lymphoprep as in described in *Protocol 1*.

[a] *Expected yield*: cell numbers can vary enormously depending on the size, cellularity, and quality (e.g. freshness) of the tissue sample.

For a routine mitogen-induced or specific antigen-induced proliferation assay of T cells, PBMC can be used from fresh peripheral blood without further purification of the T-cell fraction. The benefit of using whole PBMC is that it provides autologous monocytes to act as antigen-presenting cells for the T cells. However, to determine the ability of T cells to produce cytokines within the PBMC population, the T cells should receive a specific stimulus such as anti-CD3, as cells other than T cells within this population can also produce cytokines. Alternatively, the T cells alone can be isolated from the PBMC population.

2.2 Positive selection of T cells

T cells alone can be isolated from peripheral blood, umbilical cord blood, fluids, or tissue of healthy individuals or patients with disease. T-cell lines and clones can be generated *in vitro* based on their antigen specificity and/or phenotype, and perpetuated in long-term culture by cytokine stimulation.

We recommend using the protocol provided by Dynal (UK) together with their reagents to positively select CD2 T cells. Essentially, this is a fast and reliable method that utilizes magnetizable polystyrene beads coated with a primary monoclonal antibody (mAb) to distinguish lymphocyte subsets. In this case, the CD2 T-cell subset can be isolated using a monoclonal primary antibody specific for the CD2 antigen (BMA 0111) that has been conjugated to a magnetic bead. The rosetted cells can then be washed and isolated using a powerful magnetic particle concentrator, and the magnetic bead removed using Dynal's Releasing buffer containing DNase. Use of immunomagnetic beads to isolate CD3-positive cells is not recommended because this protocol activates the T cells.

A variety of T-cell subsets can also be isolated using various techniques. In addition, CD4 or CD8 T cells can be induced to differentiate *in vitro* towards a TH1/TH2 or T_C1/T_C2 phenotype through the stimulation of the naïve T cell in a particular cytokine/anti-cytokine environment.

2.3 Isolation of naïve CD4 T cells (CD4+CD45RA+) and CD8 T cells (CD8+CD45RA+)

We also recommend using the protocol provided by Dynal with their reagents to positively select CD4 or CD8 T cells from umbilical cord blood. The anti-CD4 or anti-CD8 antibody and magnetic bead can then be removed using Dynal's DETACHaBEAD solution and the magnetic particle concentrator. The CD4CD45RA or CD8CD45RA T cells can then be negatively selected by depleting CD45RO cells using an anti-CD45RO antibody (UCHL1) and Dynal's sheep anti-mouse IgG conjugated to superparamagnetic beads. This protocol results in greater than 98% pure and viable CD4CD45RA or CD8CD45RA T cells.

3 Analysis of T-cell cytokine production

T cells produce an extensive assortment of cytokines as compared to other cell types (such as macrophages). In addition, T cells often produce cytokines at a lower concentration than most other cells. Therefore, a variety of assays have been developed to analyse cytokine production by T cells. Each method, of course, has its own advantages and disadvantages.

The most common method used to evaluate the concentrations of cytokines produced by T cells remains the enzyme-linked immunosorbent assay (ELISA). ELISA is highly specific and can be extremely sensitive (down to 10 pg/ml or less). ELISA makes use of the ability of purified anti-cytokine antibodies immobilized on to the plastic of microwell plates to specifically capture soluble cytokine proteins present in T-cell supernatants. After washing away unbound material, the captured cytokine proteins can be detected by first adding another purified anti-cytokine antibody that is conjugated to biotin. Next, an amplifying enzyme-labelled streptavidin complex is added which will bind to the biotin and which can be made to fluoresce following the addition of an appropriate substrate. The coloured product can then be measured spectrophotometrically at the appropriate optical density. By including a serial dilution of the cytokine at known concentrations in the assay, a standard curve can be developed in order to interpolate the concentration of the cytokine in the T-cell supernatant. Some of the drawbacks to using ELISA to measure T-cell cytokine secretion are that one can only measure cytokine production by the population as a whole, that the measured cytokine may not be biologically active, and that the measured cytokine concentration at a single timepoint may be an underestimate of true secretion due to uptake by cytokine receptor-bearing cells and/or cytokine degradation. For more on the ELISA protocol, see Chapter 12 in this volume.

Because of the inability of an ELISA to measure cytokine production by a single T cell, various other methods such as the enzyme-linked immunospot assay (ELISpot), the single-cell polymerase chain reaction (PCR), and *in situ* hybridization have been used in an attempt to solve this problem. Each is a valid method of accomplishing this. However, each requires a high degree of technical proficiency and can be difficult to reliably reproduce.

The ELISpot method of determining cytokine production is more qualitative than quantitative. It can detect the production of cytokine in the environment immediately surrounding a single T cell. Using two cytokine-specific antibodies directed against different epitopes on the same cytokine molecule, a coloured product or spot can be generated. The proportion of cells producing a particular cytokine in response to a stimulus can be determined by counting the number of spots on a plate. However, the number of spots will not tell you the concentration or amount of cytokine being produced.

Another method for studying cytokine mRNA in T cells uses the PCR. With PCR, only a small amount of RNA is needed, and therefore very few cells. In addition, the appropriate cytokine-specific oligonucleotide primers are easily obtainable and commercially available in kits that cover most of the cytokines produced by T cells (e.g. from Stratagene). A unique advantage to this technique is the possibility of storing cDNA obtained from different cell types for use in the cloning of as yet undefined cytokines, particularly when novel activities are described in supernatants or biological fluids. However, the extreme sensitivity of the PCR technique also creates disadvantages. A small contamination of the test sample will lead to false-positive results. Protocols for the RT-PCR measurement of cytokine mRNA are given in Vol. 1, Chapter 3.

Recently, a more useful method called intracellular cytokine staining (ICS) was developed to detect, via flow cytometry, the production of cytokines by a single T cell. Following fixation to preserve morphology, the T cells are permeabilized to allow the penetration of highly specific fluorescent anti-cytokine antibodies into the cytosol, endoplasmic reticulum, and Golgi complex. These antibodies can then be detected using routine flow cytometry. A major advantage to using ICS is that the T cells can first be labelled with fluorescent antibodies to cell-surface antigens before the detection of intracellular markers. This then allows the identification of individual cytokine-producing cells within a mixed population. For more on this protocol, see Chapter 10, this volume.

Another useful assay has been developed to allow the analysis of a number of different T cell-produced cytokines at the same time. The RNase protection assay (RPA) is a highly sensitive and specific method for the detection and quantitation of mRNA species. The RPA takes advantage of DNA-dependent RNA polymerases and their cognate promoter sequences from the bacteriophages SP6, T7, and T3 to synthesize high specific-activity RNA probes from DNA templates. This allows a cDNA fragment of interest to then be subcloned into a plasmid that contains the bacteriophage promoters, and the construct can then be used as a template for the synthesis of radiolabelled antisense RNA probes. Companies such as PharMingen have created multiprobe template sets that, with great specificity, allow the detection and quantification of up to 11 cytokine mRNA species and 2 housekeeping genes in a single sample of total RNA derived from standard methods. For details of this assay see Vol. 1, Chapter 3.

The most important cytokine assay remains the bioassay. By taking advantage of cell lines that specifically respond to a particular cytokine, the bioassay can evaluate the actual levels of functional and active cytokine. Unfortunately, bioassays have many limitations. The first limitation is the lack of molecular specificity. Some bioassays have been shown to be able to detect more cytokines than the intended one. For example, the well-known murine thymocyte co-stimulation assay was thought to be a specific bioassay for IL-1. However, this assay has been shown to be able to detect mouse IL-1α and IL-1β, IL-2, IL-4, IL-6, IL-7, and TNF-α, as well as many human cytokines. Specificity can be demonstrated with the use of neutralizing antibodies to the particular assayed cytokine. However, if multiple cytokines are present, accurate quantitation can be very difficult. Another drawback to the bioassay is the need to maintain a wide range of sensitive cells for different assays. These cell lines can often drift in sensitivity, which will necessitate time-consuming re-selection and re-cloning. In addition, if the secreted cytokine is denatured or neutralized by inhibitors, the bioassay will not be able to detect it. Further details of cytotoxic bioassays can be found in Chapter 13 of this volume.

Protocol 5

Bioassay for the detection of IL-2

Equipment and reagents

- Complete RPMI: RPMI-1640 with 10% FCS, 2 mM sodium pyruvate (Sigma), 50 U/ml IL-2, 2 mM L-glutamine, 100 U/ml penicillin/streptomycin
- CTLL-2 cells[a] (or HT2 cells) (both from American Type Culture Collection)
- Benchtop centrifuge
- [^{3}H]thymidine (2.6–3.2 Tbg/mmol 70–86 Ci/mmol) (Amersham)
- 96-well plates
- T-cell culture supernatant
- Humidified 5% CO_2 incubator
- Liquid scintillation counting system

Method

1 Grow CTLL-2 cells in complete RPMI with 10% FCS.

2 Grow cells to a concentration of 1×10^4 cells/well. Feed with fresh media every 3 days.

3 Two to three days after the last feeding, centrifuge at 400 g for 10 min at RT. Resuspend in fresh complete RPMI with 10% FCS. Repeat.

4 Centrifuge again at 400 g for 10 min at RT. Resuspend cells at a concentration of 4×10^5 cells/ml in fresh complete RPMI intron 10% FCS.

5 Place 100 μl aliquots of CTLL-2 cells into the wells of a 96-well plate (to give 4×10^4 cells/well).

6 Add 100 μl of the T-cell culture supernatant (neat or in serial dilution).

7 Incubate at 37 °C in a humidified CO_2 incubator for 24 h.

8 Pulse-label each well with 10 μl containing 0.5 μCi of [^{3}H]thymidine for 48 h.

9 Harvest the cells and measure the incorporation of [^{3}H]thymidine by liquid scintillation counting.

10 Compare the values obtained with a standard curve of CTLL-2 cells assayed with rIL-2 at concentrations ranging from 0.001 to 200 μg/ml.

[a] This cell line also responds to murine IL-4, but not human IL-4.

Ultimately, it is recommended that two or more of these protocols be used together to define the cytokine being produced by the T cell, and its concentration and bioactivity.

4 Cytokine production by T cells of different phenotypes

4.1 Cytokine production by CD4 T cells

In 1986, Mosmann *et al.* first described two types of mouse helper T-cell clones (TH1 and TH2), which were defined by their ability to secrete distinct patterns of cytokines (2). Subsequently, human TH1 cells were shown to secrete IL-2 and interferon (IFN)-γ, while human TH2 cells were shown to secrete IL-4, IL-5, IL-6, IL-10, and IL-13. A variety of markers have been proposed as being able to specifically identify TH1 and TH2 cells. In particular, the chemokine receptor CCR3 is selectively expressed on TH2, but not TH1, cells (8). These CD4 T-cell subsets also displayed functional differences that correlated with their cytokine production profiles. TH1 cells are involved in delayed-type hypersensitivity, induction of IgG2α, and defence against intracellular pathogens. TH2 cells, on the other hand, are involved in the induction of IgG1, IgG2β, and IgE, and defence against extracellular pathogens. Alternatively, dysregulation of TH1 cells may be involved in causing immunopathology and organ-specific autoimmune disease, while dysregulation of TH2 cells may be involved in atopy and allergy (9–11). Precursors to TH1/TH2 cells have also been described according to their cytokine profile. Termed TH0, these cells secrete all the above cytokines (12). Finally, T-regulatory 1 (T_R1) cells have recently been described (13). These cells secrete TGF-β and are thought to be able to downregulate an immune response.

To differentiate naïve CD4 T cells *in vitro* into either TH1 or TH2 cells, the T cells should receive an activation signal such as phytohaemagglutinin (PHA) or anti-CD3 in a particular cytokine environment. TH2 cells differentiate after priming in the presence of IL-4, while TH1 cells arise after priming in the presence of IL-12 and the absence of IL-4.

Protocol 6

Establishment of TH1 or TH2 T-cell subsets

Reagents

- IL-2, IL-4, IL-12, anti-IL-4, and anti-IL-12 (PharMingen)
- PHA, PMA, and calcium ionophore A23187 (Sigma)

Protocol 6 continued

Method

1 Isolate purified naïve CD4 T cells (isolated from peripheral blood or umbilical cord blood) (see *Protocols 1* and *2*).

2 Add the following on day 0:

For T_{H1}:

- 2 µg/ml PHA
- 2 ng/ml IL-12
- 200 ng/ml anti-IL-4

For T_{H2}:

- 2 µg/ml PHA
- 10 ng/ml IL-4
- 2 µg/ml anti-IL-12

3 Culture for 3 days in a 37 °C incubator.

4 Wash the cells, add fresh media and IL-2 (10 ng/ml) to each subset culture.

5 Culture for 4 days in a 37 °C incubator.

6 Wash the cells. Either re-stimulate under the same conditions to carry the T-cell line, *or* re-stimulate with anti-CD3 (10 µg/ml) and anti-CD28 (2 µg/ml) or with PMA (5 ng/ml) and the calcium ionophore A23187 (250 ng/ml) for 4–24 h to analyse the cytokine secretion profile.

4.2 Cytokine production by CD8 T cells

In 1994, Croft *et al.* described two CD8 T-cell subsets (T_C1 and T_C2) that were analogous to the CD4 (TH1 and TH2) subsets (3). T_C1 cells characteristically secrete IL-2, IFN-γ, and TNF-α, while T_C2 cells secrete IL-4, IL-5, and IL-10. These CD8 T-cell subsets may differ in their capacity to kill, may provide help for B-cell antibody production, and may be involved in the induction of inflammatory responses.

Protocol 7

Establishment of T_C1 or T_C2 T-cell subsets (14)

Reagents

- IL-2, IL-4, IL-12, IL-7, and TGF-β (PharMingen)
- PHA, PMA, and calcium ionophore A23187 (Sigma)
- Complete RPMI-1640 (*Protocol 1*) with 10 mmol/l N-acetylcyskine (pH adjusted to 7.2) NAC (Sigma)

Method

1 Isolate purified naïve CD8 T cells (isolated from peripheral blood or umbilical cord blood) (see *Protocols 1* and *2*).

Protocol 7 continued

2   Isolate bone marrow-derived stimulatory cells from an unrelated donor.

3   Irradiate allogeneic stimulatory cells with 600 cGy.

4   Mix together 2 CD8 T cells to 1 irradiated stimulator cell (for example, 2×10^6 CD8 T cells:1×10^6 irradiated stimulatory cells per well) in complete RPMI with NAC (10 mmol/l) added.

5   Add the following on day 0:

    For T_{C1}:
- 2.5 ng/ml IL-12
- 5 ng/ml TGF-β
- 40 U/ml IL-2
- 20 ng/ml IL-7

    For T_{C2}:
- 1000 U/ml IL-4
- 40 U/ml IL-2
- 20 ng/ml IL-7

6   Culture for 2 days in a 37 °C incubator.

7   Add fresh IL-2 (40 U/ml) and IL-7 (20 ng/ml) to both subset cultures.

8   Add fresh media containing IL-2 (40 U/ml), IL-7 (20 ng/ml), and NAC (10 mmol/l) to both subset cultures every 3–4 days.

9   On day 13, re-stimulate with allogeneic bone marrow-derived stimulator cells to carry the T-cell line *or* re stimulate with PMA (5 ng/ml) and Ca ionophore A23187 (375 ng/ml) for 24 h for cytokine secretion analysis.

To specifically differentiate naïve CD8 T cells *in vitro* into either T_C1 or T_C2 cells, the T cells should receive an activation signal such as allogeneic stimulator cells in a particular cytokine environment. T_C2 cells also differentiate after priming in the presence of IL-4, while T_C1 cells arise after priming in the presence of IL-12 and the absence of IL-4.

4.3 Cytokine production by double-negative (CD4–CD8–) αβ T cells

It has been shown that the majority of human CD4–CD8– αβ T cells have a T_H0-like phenotype, in that they can produce both IL-4 and IFN-γ. In addition, these cells can make IL-10 when given the appropriate stimulation (15).

4.4 Cytokine production by γδ T cells

The majority of T cells in the thymus and peripheral lymphoid organs express a T-cell receptor (TCR) composed of an α and β chain (αβ T cells). However, a minor population of T cells (1–5%) use a γ and a δ chain (γδ T cells) to form their TCR. In the mouse, γδ T cells can be found in the epidermis, lung, female reproductive tract, and epithelia of the small intestine. In humans, γδ T cells are solely found in the lymphoid organs. γδ T cells do not appear to act as effector T cells. However, they do seem to be involved in the regulation of an immune response (16, 17). As such, γδ T-cell functions are being studied as potential immuno-therapeutic tools/agents.

γδ T cells have been shown to produce IL-2, IL-3, and GM-CSF (18). More importantly, their ability to produce IFN-γ or IL-4 during early activation may provide a means of establishing a TH1 or TH2 αβ T-cell response. Mouse γδ T cells have been shown to respond to IL-15 by producing both IFN-γ and IL-4 (19). In addition, γδ T cells are particularly sensitive to stimulation by TNF-α (20). TNF-α increases their ability to proliferate and enhances their cytotoxicity.

4.5 Cytokine production by antigen-specific T cells

As mentioned previously, different subsets of T cells can vary in their cytokine production. Many factors can affect the type and amount of cytokine produced by the T cell. The type of accessory cell used to present antigen to a T cell can affect its cytokine production (21). TH2 clones secreted IL-4 in response to antigen presented by resting B cells, while TH1 clones secreted IL-2 in response to antigen presented by both B cells and macrophages. The dose of antigen that a T cell is exposed to or its density presented on MHC can be important (22). Differentiation into high IFN-γ-producing cells was seen with high antigen doses, while low doses of the same antigen led to high IL-4-producing cells. The affinity of interaction between MHC, peptide, and TCR can also influence T-cell cytokine secretion (23). Strong interactions lead to TH1-like responses, while weak interactions lead to TH2-like T cells. The type of co-stimulation present can also have an influence on the production of cytokines by T cells (24). The interaction of B7–1 and B7–2 on an antigen-presenting cell (APC) with their ligands CD28 and CTLA-4 on a T cell has been shown to be able to both positively and negatively regulate an immune response. Other factors such as antigen structure and genetic background can also influence the production of cytokines by T cells (25–27). In addition, cytokines (such as IL-4 and IL-12) present in the priming environment can have a dramatic effect on the production of other cytokines by T cells (see below).

Protocol 8
Establishment of tetanus antigen-specific T-cell lines

Equipment and reagents
(In addition to *Protocol 1*)

- Tetanus toxoid vaccine (TT, Wellcome). Dialyse for 24 h against PBS to remove the thiomersal Bp toxic preservative, filter to re-sterilize, and store at 4 °C.
- Humidified 5% CO_2 incubator

- [^{3}H]thymidine (2.6–3.2 Tbg/mmol 70–86 Ci/mmol) (Amersham), stock solution made to 50 μCi/ml
- Recombinant human interleukin-2 (rIL-2) (PharMingen)

Protocol 8 continued

- ^{137}Caesium (Cs) source
- 96-well (round-bottomed) microtitre plate (Nalge Nunc)
- 6- and 24-well tissue culture plate (Falcon)
- 20 Terasaki tissue culture plates (Nalge Nunc)
- 15 ml conical tube
- Scintillation counting system

A. Primary T-cell line

1 Adjust the concentration of PBMC (prepared as in *Protocol 1*) to 1×10^6 cells/ml in complete RPMI. (These PBMC can be either freshly prepared or thawed from liquid nitrogen storage.)

2 Pipette 2 ml of the cell suspension into each of five wells of the 24-well plate (i.e. 2×10^6 cells/well).

3 Add 3–3000 ng/ml TT to four of the five wells, using a 10-fold dilution for each. Leave the fifth well as a control (i.e. no tetanus). Note that these dilutions are necessary because individuals vary in their sensitivity to TT.

4 Incubate the cells at 37 °C in a humidified CO_2 incubator for 6 days.

5 Pipette the cells of each well gently to resuspend. Remove a 100 μl aliquot from each, including the fifth 'control' well, for measurement of T-cell proliferation.

6 Place each aliquot into one well of a 96-well microtitre plate.

7 Pulse-label each well with 10 μl of [^{3}H]thymidine (0.5 μCi) and incubate at 37 °C for 16 h.

8 Harvest and measure the incorporation of radioactivity by scintillation counting.

9 Select the well containing thosecells with the highest proliferation rate to establish a long-term cell line.

10 Add recombinant IL-2 to the selected culture to a final concentration of 10 ng/ml. This will promote the growth and expansion of T cells previously activated by tetanus antigen.

11 Return the cells to the incubator for a further 7 days.

The cells are now ready for secondary stimulation with antigen and feeder cells.

B. Preparation of autologous feeder cells for antigen presentation

1 Use PBMC from the same donor as the T-cell line as autologous feeder cells.[a] Irradiate the PBMC cell suspension (at 5×10^6 cells/ml) in complete RPMI with a sublethal dose of 4000 rads from a ^{137}Cs source to prevent feeder-cell growth and division, which would contaminate the T-cell line. Use a ratio of feeder cells to T cells of 2–5:1 (e.g. 2–5×10^6 feeder cells:1×10^6 T cells).

2 Adjust the feeder-cell suspension to the required concentration (i.e. 2×10^6 cells/ml).

3 Pipette 1 ml into each of four wells of a 24-well plate (i.e. 2×10^6 cells/well).

Protocol 8 continued

4 Add the appropriate concentration of tetanus antigen as determined from the proliferation assay.

C. Re-stimulation of the primary T-cell line

1 Suspend the two wells of the T-cell line by gentle pipetting. Transfer to a 15 ml conical tube and centrifuge at 400 g for 10 min at RT.

2 Resuspend the antigen-stimulated cells to 1×10^6 cells/ml in fresh complete RPMI. Add 1 ml of these cells to each of the four wells containing feeder cells and antigen. No IL-2 is added at this stage.

3 Incubate for 7 days.

4 Add rIL-2 (10 ng/ml).

D. Long- term maintenance of the T-cell line

1 Either analyse the cells for cytokine production or maintain the cell line by alternate weekly cycles as follows:
- *Week 1*: add antigen plus feeder cells prepared as above (Part B) together with rIL-2.
- *Week 2*: add IL-2 alone.

[a] JY cells (an EBV-transformed B-cell line) can also be used as feeder cells. This prolific cell line ensures a continuous supply of fresh feeder cells.

Protocol 9

Establishment of T-cell clones by limiting dilution

Equipment and reagents

- Complete RPMI medium with 7.5% of normal human AB serum (NHS)
- Round-bottomed, 96-well plates
- Irradiated feeder cells (*Protocol 8*)
- Tetanus antigen (*Protocol 8*)
- 10 mg/ml IL-2
- Humidified 37 °C, 5% CO_2 incubator
- Phase-contrast microscope
- 24-well tissue culture plate

Method

1 Using primary T-cell cultures selected for highest proliferation, prepare dilutions of 3000 cells/ml, 300 cells/ml, 100 cells/ml, 30 cells/ml, 10 cells/ml, 3 cells/ml in fresh complete RPMI with 7.5% NHS.

2 Pipette 100 μl of each dilution into the wells of a round-bottomed, 96-well plate (i.e. 300 cells/well, 30 cells/well, 10 cells/well, 3 cells/well, 1 cell/well, 0.3 cell/well).

3 Prepare irradiated feeder cells (as in *Protocol 8*) to a concentration of 2×10^6 cells/ml.

4 Add 50 µl of these feeder cells (1×10^5 cells) to each of the above wells.

5 Add tetanus antigen at an optimal concentration and IL-2 (10 ng/ml) in a volume of 50 µl to each of the above wells (final volume is 200 µl/well).

6 Incubate for 7–12 days in a humidified 37 °C, 5% CO_2 incubator.

7 Screen by phase-contrast microscopy from day 7 for growing colonies of cells.

8 Transfer growing cells to a 24-well plate for expansion.

9 Add complete RPMI, irradiated feeder cells at 2×10^6 cells/ml, and antigen at optimal concentration (no IL-2).

10 Incubate for 7 days.

11 Add complete RPMI, irradiated feeder cells at 2×10^6 cells/ml, and IL-2 (10 ng/ml).

12 Incubate for 7 days.

13 Continue with alternate weekly cycles of rest (irradiated feeder cells, no antigen) and re-stimulation (irradiated feeder cells plus antigen).

Note: Check these cells at each stage for antigen specificity. The starting frequency of tetanus-specific T cells in the PBMC population will greatly influence the number of positive colonies in the concentration range recommended. This can only be determined by trial and error with blood from individual donors. Primed donors (less than 1 year) are usually highly responsive.

5 Effect of cytokines on T cells

Cytokines have profound effects on the development, activation, differentiation, and proliferation of T cells. IL-2 is a potent proliferative factor for all subsets of T cells and acts by promoting progression through the G_1 phase of the cell cycle. It can also stimulate the cytolytic activity of CD8 T cells and increase T-cell motility. IL-2 shares many of its biological activities with other cytokines that use the common gamma-chain as part of their receptor (IL-4, IL-7, and IL-15) (28). IL-15 is a cytokine that has been shown to be able to stimulate the proliferation of T-cell lines, T-cell clones, activated double-negative T cells, double-positive T cells, and CD8 T cells. IL-15 is also thought to synergize with IL-12 to induce γδ T-cell proliferation of IFN-γ after culture with non-peptide antigen (29, 30). IL-7 is a stromal cell-derived cytokine that is absolutely necessary for the development of T cells. It acts as a growth and anti-apoptotic factor for T cells (31). As mentioned previously, IL-4 and IL-12 are most responsible for the differentiation of T cells into TH1/TH2 or T_C1/T_C2 subsets. IL-4 acts directly on the T cell by delivering a differentiation signal through STAT6 (32, 33). IL-12 also acts directly on the T cell by delivering a differentiation signal through STAT4 (34). The cytokine IFN-γ enhances the TH1 differentiating effects of IL-12. IFN-γ is thought to improve the responsiveness of T cells to IL-12 by inducing the expression of IL-12Rβ2, the signalling subunit of the IL-12 receptor (35). IL-18 is a recently dis-covered cytokine that has a potent effect on T-cell activation (36). IL-18 appears to function by inducing IFN-γ production by both T cells and NK cells. Thus, IL-18 is important in the TH1 differentiation pathway. IL-10, on the other hand, is an immunomodulatory cytokine produced by TH2 cells that is capable of inhibiting TH1 responses. IL-10 is thought to function by blocking the CD28 co-stimulation pathway in T cells, thus leading to anergy (37).

Activation, proliferation, and differentiation of CD8 T cells to generate effector cytotoxic T-lymphocyte responses can be augmented by cytokines produced by macrophages and/or dendritic cells (38). These cytokines include IL-1, IL-6, IL-12, and IFN-γ. It is unclear whether these cytokines act directly on the CD8 T-cell population or indirectly by enhancing antigen presentation or co-stimulation.

6 Conclusions

Cytokines have been shown to have powerful and wide-ranging effects on the immune system. Cytokines can also activate, mediate, amplify, and repress T-cell responses themselves. However, inappropriate differentiation into a TH1 or TH2 (or T_C1 or T_C2) response is thought to be a feature of many autoimmune and infectious diseases. Therefore, understanding the role that cytokines play in influencing a T-cell immune response and the influence T cell-produced cytokines have on an immune response is essential. This understanding may then lead to therapeutic manipulation of the immune response in chronic diseases and the development of better vaccination strategies.

References

1. Smith, K. A. (1984). *Annu. Rev. Immunol.*, **2**, 319.
2. Mosmann, T. R., Cherwinski, H., Bond, M. W., Giedlin, M. A., and Coffman, R. L. (1986). *J. Immunol.*, **136**, 2348.
3. Croft, M., Carter, L., Swain, S. L., and Dutton, R. W. (1994). *J. Exp. Med.*, **180**, 1715.
4. Swain, S. L., Weinberg, A. D., English, M., and Huston, G. (1990). *J. Immunol.*, **145**, 3796.
5. Hsieh, C. S., Macatonia, S. E., Tripp, C. S., Wolf, S. F., O'Garra, A., and Murphy, K. M. (1993). *Science*, **260**, 547.
6. Feldmann, M., Brennan, F. M., and Maini, R. N. (1996). *Annu. Rev. Immunol.*, **14**, 397.
7. Firestein, G. S. (1998). In *Textbook of Rheumatology* (ed. W. N. Kelley, S. Ruddy, E. D. Harris, Jr, and C. B. Sledge), p. 851. W. B. Saunders, Philadelphia, PA.
8. Sallusto, F., Mackay, C. R., and Lanzavecchia, A. (1997). *Science*, **277**, 2005.
9. Mosmann, T. R. and Coffman, R. L. (1989). *Annu. Rev. Immunol.*, **7**, 145.
10. Sher, A. and Coffman, R. L. (1992). *Annu. Rev. Immunol.*, **10**, 385.
11. Abbas, A. K., Murphy, K. M., and Sher, A. (1996). *Nature*, **383**, 787.
12. Firestein, G. S., Roeder, W. D., Laxer, J. A., Townsend, K. S., Weaver, C. T., Hom, J. T., Linton, J., Torbett, B. E., and Glasebrook, A. L. (1989). *J. Immunol.*, **143**, 518.
13. Groux, H., O'Garra, A., Bigler, M., Rouleau, M., Antonenko, S., de Vries, J. E., and Roncarolo, M. G. (1997). *Nature*, **389**, 737.
14. Halverson, D. C., Schwartz, G. N., Carter, C., Gress, R. E., and Fowler, D. H. (1997). *Blood*, **90**, 2089.
15. Katsikis, P. D., Cohen, S. B., Murison, J. G., Uren, J., Hibbart, L. M., Callard, R. E., Di Padova, F., Feldmann, M., and Londei, M. (1995). *Immunology*, **84**, 501.

16. Born, W., Cady, C., Jones-Carson, J., Mukasa, A., Lahn, M., and O'Brien, R. (1991). *Adv. Immunol.*, **71**, 77.

17. Salerno, A. and Dieli, F. (1998). *Crit. Rev. Immunol.*, **18**, 327.

18. Yokota, K., Ariizumi, K., Kitajima, T., Bergstresser, P. R., Street, N. E., and Takashima, A. (1996). *J. Immunol.*, **157**, 1529.

19. Ferrick, D. A., Schrenzel, M. D., Mulvania, T., Hsieh, B., Ferlin, W. G., and Lepper, H. (1995). *Nature*, **373**, 255.

20. Lahn, M., Kalataradi, H., Mittelstadt, P., Pflum, E., Vollmer, M., Cady, C., Mukasa, A., Vella, A. T., Ikle, D., Harbeck, R., O'Brien, R., and Born, W. (1998). *J. Immunol.*, **160**, 5221.

21. Chang, T. L., Shea, C. M., Urioste, S., Thompson, R. C., Boom, W. H., and Abbas, A. K. (1990). *J. Immunol.*, **145**, 2803.

22. Murray, J. S., Pfeiffer, C., Madri, J., and Bottomly, K. (1992). *Eur. J. Immunol.*, **22**, 559.

23. Murray, J. S. (1998). *Immunol. Today*, **19**, 157.

24. Kuchroo, V. K., Das, M. P., Brown, J. A., Ranger, A. M., Zamvil, S. S., Sobel, R. A., Weiner, H. L., Nabavi, N., and Glimcher, L. H. (1995). *Cell*, **80**, 707.

25. Murphy, E. E., Terres, G., Macatonia, S. E., Hsieh, C. S., Mattson, J., Lanier, L., Wysocka, M., Trinchieri, G., Murphy, K., and O'Garra, A. (1994). *J. Exp. Med.*, **180**, 223.

26. Kubin, M., Kamoun, M., and Trinchieri, G. (1994). *J. Exp. Med.*, **180**, 211.

27. Schountz, T., Kasselman, J. P., Martinson, F. A., Brown, L., and Murray, J. S. (1996). *J. Immunol.*, **157**, 3893.

28. Thorpe, R. (1998). In *Cytokines* (ed. A. R. Mire-Sluis and R. Thorpe), p. 19. Academic Press, San Diego, CA.

29. Garcia, V. E., Jullien, D., Song, M., Uyemura, K., Shuai, K., Morita, C. T., and Modlin, R. L. (1998). *J. Immunol.*, **160**, 4322.

30. Jullien, D., Sieling, P. A., Uyemura, K., Mar, N. D., Rea, T. H., and Modlin, R. L. (1997). *J. Immunol.*, **158**, 800.

31. Appasamy, P. M. (1999). *Cytokines Cell. Mol. Ther.*, **5**, 25.

32. Takeda, K., Tanaka, T., Shi, W., Matsumoto, M., Minami, M., Kashiwamura, S., Nakanishi, K., Yoshida, N., Kishimoto, T., and Akira, S. (1996). *Nature*, **380**, 627.

33. Hou, J., Schindler, U., Henzel, W. J., Ho, T. C., Brasseur, M., and McKnight, S. L. (1994). *Science*, **265**, 1701.

34. Thierfelder, W. E., van Deursen, J. M., Yamamoto, K., Tripp, R. A., Sarawar, S. R., Carson, R. T., Sangster, M. Y., Vignali, D. A., Doherty, P. C., Grosveld, G. C., and Ihle, J. N. (1996). *Nature*, **382**, 171.

35. Szabo, S. J., Dighe, A. S., Gubler, U., and Murphy, K. M. (1997). *J. Exp. Med.*, **185**, 817.

36. Dinarello, C. A. (1999). *J. Allergy Clin. Immunol.*, **103**, 11.

37. Ding, L., Linsley, P. S., Huang, L. Y., Germain, R. N., and Shevach, E. M. (1993). *J. Immunol.*, **151**, 1224.

38. Vizler, C., Bercovici, N., Cornet, A., Cambouris, C., and Liblau, R. S. (1999). *Immunol. Rev.*, **169**, 81.

Chapter 4

The generation and quantitation of cell-mediated cytotoxicity

Elizabeth Grimm

Department of Cancer Biology, UT M.D. Anderson Cancer Center, Box 79, 1515 Holcombe Blvd, Houston, TX 77030, USA

1 Introduction

Cell-mediated cytoxicity (CMC) is defined as the process by which a cell of the immune system directly kills another cell. CMC is composed of a specific series of events occurring between an effector cell (lymphocyte or monocyte) and a susceptible target cell, which ultimately results in the delivery of a 'lethal hit' by the effector to the target cell. An obligate event in CMC, which distinguishes it from other modes of immunologically mediated target-cell killing (e.g. complement-mediated cytolysis) is intimate cell membrane contact between the effector and the target, referred to as conjugate formation. This brief chapter will be restricted solely to the description of lymphocyte-mediated CMC systems. Many excellent reviews cover the complicated processes which encompass effector cell-mediated recognition, conjugate formation, triggering, and delivery of the lethal hit ultimately resulting in the death of the specific target (1, 2).

Lymphocyte populations capable of expressing CMC can be divided into two major categories based upon the target structures recognized by the effector population: major histocompatibility complex (MHC)-restricted and MHC-unrestricted killer cells.

Classical cytotoxic T lymphocytes (CTL) mediate antigen-specific, MHC-restricted cytolytic activity, presumably through the interaction of the T-cell receptor with a specific processed target antigen presented by the appropriate MHC structure. The generation of these MHC-restricted effector lymphocytes requires the coordinated assistance of accessory cell populations in order to educate and mature the T killer. In contrast, MHC-unrestricted cytotoxic effectors exhibit the inherent capacity to recognize an as yet undetermined characteristic(s) of certain 'abnormal' cell populations. As the name implies, the recognition process is independent of MHC, demands no prior antigen presentation, and requires no known interaction with accessory cells. Natural killer (NK) and lymphokine-activated killer (LAK) cells represent the major effector types expressing lymphocyte-mediated, MHC-unrestricted cytotoxicity. Considerable controversy remains surrounding attempts to unambiguously distinguish between NK and

LAK, based upon phenotypic or morphological criteria. We and others have proposed that a definition based solely upon activation requirements, and the resultant expression of differential susceptible target spectra, offers the most practical
distinctions (3). Natural killer cells are endowed with the inherent capacity to
spontaneously kill a defined target spectrum including some haematological
neoplasms (*Figure 1a*) (NK may play an additional role in inhibiting the vascular
spread of metastatic emboli), virally infected tissues, and may play a role in
controlling haemopoiesis (4). Although NK cells are not known to require any
activation prior to expression of their lytic activity, cytokine augmentation of
NK potency is well documented. In contrast, LAK manifest an absolute dependency upon activation prior to the induction of their unique capacity to recognize both NK-sensitive (*Figure 1a*), as well as a broad spectrum of NK-resistant
targets (*Figure 1b*), including both fresh and cultured tumours growing in sus-

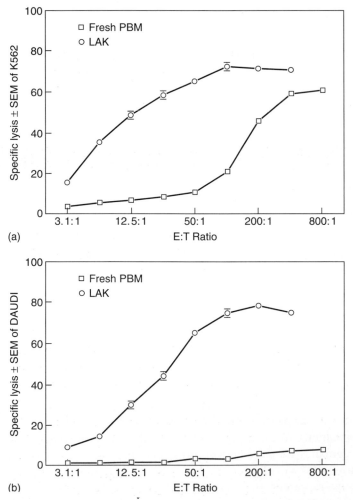

Figure 1 Killing (a) of the NK-sensitive target K562 and (b) the NK-resistant target Daudi
(PBL + IL-2, 4 days' activation) and by fresh PMBC from the same donor.

pension or adherently, embryonal tissues, virally infected tissues, tissue culture- and chemically-modified cells. Maintenance of this lytic potential as well as expansion of the lytic population is likewise dependent upon a continuing source of activation stimuli. We therefore hypothesize that LAK may represent one part of an inducible limb of the immune system, in which, when the local environment provides the appropriate quality and quantity of activation signals, prior effector functions may be overridden and a new, broad-spectrum target recognition system may be evoked. As such, even antigen-specific CTL and NK may be driven to acquire lytic activity against an entirely new, MHC-unrestricted target spectrum.

2 Techniques for the isolation of lymphocyte populations

2.1 Isolation of PBMC, PBL, or LGL

Peripheral blood mononuclear leucocytes (PBMC), derived from venepuncture or leucophoresis in the presence of anticoagulants (e.g. heparin, EDTA, etc.) can be isolated by sedimentation on gradients such as Histopaque 1077 for human (or rat) cells or Lympholyte-M for mouse blood (Sigma) (see also Chapters 2 and 3, this volume).

Protocol 1

Isolation of PBMC, PBL, or LGL

Equipment and reagents

- Anticoagulated blood
- Ca^{2+}/Mg^{2+} deficient Hank's balanced salt solution (HBSS)
- Cell centrifuge
- Sedimentation gradient (Histopaque 1077 for human or rat cells, Lympholyte-M for mouse blood; Sigma)

Method

1 Dilute the anticoagulated blood (1:2 blood to Ca^{2+}/Mg^{2+}-deficient HBSS for venepuncture-derived and 1:4 for leucophoresis-derived blood) and then layer over the gradient material as per manufacturer's instructions, and centrifuge at 400 g for 30 min at 18–20°C.

2 Aspirate the 'buffy coat' cellular interface and wash twice in HBSS suspending cells in 20 to 40 ml of HBSS used above. The wash is a 10 min centrifugation at 400 g at RT.

3 To eliminate contaminating platelets, the cell suspension may be subjected to slow-speed centrifuge runs until contaminating platelets are no longer evident microscopically (150 g for 10 min at RT; aspirate the supernatants to avoid losing the weakly packed pellet).

We find that platelet contamination can significantly inhibit lymphocyte activation, presumably through platelet-derived immunosuppressive agents such as the transforming growth factors. PBMC can be directly cultured or further enriched for effector cell precursors. Peripheral blood lymphocytes (PBL) are prepared from PBMC by plastic and nylon wool depletion of monocytes and B cells, respectively (5).

Protocol 2

Preparation of peripheral blood lymphocytes

Equipment and reagents

- Complete medium (complete defined serum-free medium and/or serum-containing complete medium)
- Cell centrifuge
- Tissue culture-grade plastic flasks (e.g. 175 cm^2)
- Sterile, pre-washed nylon wool

Method

1 Dilute PBMC to approximately 10^7 cells/ml in complete medium (either serum-supplemented growth medium or complete, defined serum-free medium) and incubate on tissue culture-grade plastic (e.g. 20 ml into a 175 cm^2 flask) for 1 h at 37 °C.

2 Aspirate non-adherent cells and gently wash adherent cells with warm medium to collect remaining non-adherent cells.

3 Pellet the non-adherent cells and resuspend to 5 × 10^7 cells/ml.

4 Incubate for 1 h at 37 °C on sterile, pre-washed nylon wool which has been pre-incubated with serum-containing complete medium (0.6 g of nylon wool per 10^8 cells).

5 Following incubation, aspirate the non-adherent cells, and gently wash the nylon wool with warm medium to recover residual non-adherent cells. (Plastic adherence followed by nylon-wool depletion significantly enriches for lymphocytes expressing T-cell and NK phenotypic markers.)

Protocol 3

Cell density purification

Equipment and reagents

- Percoll (Pharmacia) adjusted to 290 osmol/kg with 10 × PBS
- 50 ml conical, polystyrene centrifuge tubes
- Cell centrifuge
- RPMI-1640 medium containing 0.75% BSA
- Trypan Blue

Protocol 3 continued

Method

1 Layer PBL on to multistep, discontinuous Percoll gradients.[a]

2 Prepare a 4-step gradient in a 50 ml conical, polystyrene centrifuge tube by diluting the prepared Percoll with RPMI-1640 medium containing 0.75% BSA as follows. As an aid to monitoring the quality of layering as well as helping to identify the gradient interfaces, add a drop of Trypan Blue to alternating steps.

Fraction	% Percoll	Medium (ml)	Percoll (ml)
1	41.1	5.83	4.18
2	45.8	5.42	4.58
3	50.0	3.00	3.00
4	66.6	2.00	4.00

Up to 5×10^8 cells can be loaded per gradient.

3 Centrifuge the gradients at 500 g for 30 min, using slow acceleration and no breaking for deceleration.

4 Harvest individual fractions which collect at the interfaces, wash three times and resuspend for cell counting.[b]

[a] The choice of the densities and the number of steps composing the gradient will be determined by the cell populations desired, the purities desired, and by the total number of cells needing separation. As a general starting point, adjust Percoll (Pharmacia) to 290 osmol/kg with $10 \times$ phosphate buffered saline (PBS).

[b] Low-density cells (large granular lymphocytes) collect at the 41.1/45.8% interface, mixed granular and T cells at the high-density interface. NK cell activity can be greatly enriched by isolating the large granular lymphocyte (LGL) fraction. In contrast, LAK cells can be generated, albeit not at the same relative efficiency, from lymphoid cells of significantly disparate densities, indicating the profound heterogeneity of LAK precursors (7).

At this point, PBL can be further segregated into populations with differing morphologies based upon cell densities following the procedure of Timonen *et al.* (6).

2.2 Isolation of specific lymphoid populations based upon phenotypic markers or light-scatter characteristics

2.2.1 Fluorescence-activated cell sorting

An alternative approach to the isolation of either precursor or mature effector populations utilizes the technology of fluorescence-activated cell sorting (FACS). Cell sorting can provide a highly enriched population (> 95% purity) of moderate numbers of cells ($\leq 10^7$) within a few hours of sorting. The quality and quantity of the yield is dependent upon many factors including the condition of cells in the starting population, the relative frequency of the cell of interest within the starting population, the working condition of the sorter, and the skill of the operator. Many commercially available antibodies are available for analysing phenotypic markers expressed on lymphocyte subpopulations. Since the first description of T cells, NK, and LAK, phenotypic markers have been sought which could unambiguously describe the population of interest. It is important to remember that the vast majority of phenotypic markers describing lymphocyte populations recognize epitopes which are not uniquely relevant to the effector function. As a result, phenotypic markers have consistently proven to be shared by multiple cell types, and caution must be exercised in interpreting results based on phenotypic analysis (8, 9). Another concern of cell separation by phenotype involves the ability of many antibodies to directly modulate the activity of cell populations expressing the corresponding epitope (e.g. anti-CD2, anti-CD3, anti-CD16, etc.) (10). Because of the lack of functional specificity and the concerns of artefactual stimulation, we reported a method for cell sorting of a unique interleukin-2 (IL-2) responsive population based upon characteristic morphological alterations associated with IL-2 activation (11). These unique light-scatter and forward-scatter characteristics permit the isolation of all LAK activity as well as the cycling population involved in the maintenance and further expansion of LAK effector activity. This approach proved useful for human and mouse samples, and allows for the further phenotypic analyses of a population highly enriched for LAK cells.

2.2.2 Separation using antibody-coated magnetic beads

An alternative approach to lymphocyte separation based upon phenotypic markers utilizes magnetic beads coated with specific antibodies. Magnetic separation methodology represents a relatively simple and efficient means for generating moderate numbers of enriched cells (10^6–10^8), and the initial investment is considerably less than acquiring a FACS facility with a trained operator. After allowing the bead-anchored antibodies to attach to the appropriate cell-surface associated phenotypic epitope (or secondary antibody-labelled beads binding to primary antibody-labelled cells), the bead:cell conjugates are sedimented with a strong magnet, allowing the non-conjugated cells to be removed by pouring, and gentle washing. Both bound and unbound populations can be repeatedly absorbed by the antibody-bead preparation, rapidly generating purities greater than 80–90%. Prepared beads are commercially available, as well as starter beads which can then be coated with the antibody(ies) of interest. Since magnetic separation is based upon phenotypic markers, it suffers from the same potential pitfalls described above. Magnetic separation also presents unique problems, such as a possible difficulty in removing the antibody-anchored beads from positively selected cells. Overall, this technique is best suited for enrichment by negative selection. We have successfully used magnetic separation to remove B cells and monocytes (a rapid alternative to plastic and nylon wool depletion) from PBM suspensions, and for negative depletion of Leulla-presenting cells. We have also used magnetic beads to present anti-OKT3 for co-stimulation with IL-2 (see below) in macrophage-depleted lymphocyte populations. Rosenberg has described the use of antibody-conjugated magnetic beads to directly enrich for lymphocytes (12). Phenotypic analyses should always be performed to verify the resultant purities, as well as to control for unexpected alterations in the cell populations.

2.3 Isolation of tumour-infiltrating lymphocytes

With the hope of learning more about the dynamic interaction of the cellular immune response to cancer, methods for obtaining lymphocytes which have migrated into tumour tissues have been devised. Preliminary reports suggested that these tumour-infiltrating lymphocytes (TIL) might exhibit unique qualities which could prove beneficial for clinical applications (13). We routinely isolate TIL from a variety of tissues. A combination of mechanical and enzymatic disaggregation is used for tough, or firm, tissues (14). In contrast, for very soft, fragile tissues (e.g. CNS neoplasms), mechanical disaggregation alone often provides superior results.

Protocol 4

Isolation of tumour-infiltrating lymphocytes

Equipment and reagents

- Sterile complete medium
- Disaggregation medium: RPMI-1640 supplemented with 300 mg/ml L-glutamine, 100 mg/ml penicillin, 100 mg/ml streptomycin, 50 mg/ml gentamicin sulfate, 0.25 mg/ml amphotericin
- Sterile dissection scissors, forceps, and scalpels
- Sterile sealed containers
- Magnetic stirrer or shaker

- Enzymatic cocktail: 0.002% DNase (Sigma, type 1), 0.1% collagenase (Sigma, type IV), 0.01% hyaluronidase (Sigma, type V)
- Serum-containing complete medium
- Syringes fitted with 18- and 20-gauge needles
- Trypan Blue
- Sterile nu gauze
- Histopaque gradient (see *Protocol 1*)

Method

1. Transport tissue samples obtained during surgery or at autopsy, completely submerged in sterile, complete medium. As with all human-tissue manipulations, universal precautions should be employed by the person performing the transportation

2. Manipulate tissue samples in a disaggregation medium (serum is not included in the sample to be enzymatically disaggregated).

3. Disaggregate solid tissue to single-cell suspensions as soon as possible to achieve maximal viable recoveries. Use sterile dissection scissors, forceps, and scalpels to reduce the tissue into small cubes (approx. 1 mm^3).

4. Incubate the cubed tissue in an enzymatic cocktail in a sealed sterile container. Use either a magnetic stirrer or shaker to gently swirl the suspension. Treat the tissue until the majority of solid cubes have been digested (0.5–1 h at 37 °C or overnight at

room temp.) and then wash in serum-containing complete medium to remove residual enzyme.

5 For soft tissues, cut the sample likewise into the smallest possible pieces. Aspirate the tissue pieces through progressively smaller pipettes (25, 10, 5 ml pipettes). Allow the larger pieces in this crude suspension to settle at unit gravity for 5 min. Pass the remaining suspension through needle bores of decreasing diameter (i.e. 18- and then 20-gauge; smaller bore needles tend to significantly reduce viability) by drawing the tissue suspensions into the syringe, attaching the needle, and expressing the suspension. Repeat the entire process three times with each needle size. Check for cell viability.

6 Either directly culture this suspension under appropriate activation conditions to grow out the TIL, or process the sample further to enrich for TIL and/or for tumour cells.

7 Remove residual tissue clumps by passing the suspension through sterile Nytex gauze.

8 If desired, pass the resultant single-cell suspension over a Histopaque gradient to remove dead cells and debris.

9 Lymphocytes can often be enriched from the tumour population by preparing a discontinuous density gradient using diluted steps of Histopaque. Carefully layer 10 ml of cells (about 5×10^7) over three 10 ml steps of (25, 75, and 100%) Histopaque, and centrifuge at 400 g for 30 min at 18–20 °C. (Tumour cells usually collect at the 25–75% interface and lymphocytes collect at the 75–100% interface.)

NB: Even after enrichment procedures, the relative frequency of TIL may still be below the level of immediate detection, and may require significant expansion over an extended culture period before they become the predominant cell type.

3 Generation of lymphokine-activated killers

3.1 The generation of IL-2 activated killers

Lymphokine-activated killers (LAK) have been successfully cultured from virtually all lymphocyte compartments including peripheral blood, thoracic duct, skin, thymus, cerebrospinal fluid, and malignant tissues. LAK are readily generated by short-term tissue culture in the presence of exogenously added IL-2. Culture lymphocytes at a concentration of $5 \times 10^5 - 2 \times 10^6$ cells/ml, with a total volume of 10 ml in 25 cm², 25 ml in 75 cm², or 50 ml in 175 cm² flasks. Incubate upright at 37 °C, 5% CO_2 in 98% humidity. We have tested numerous media, sera, etc., for the optimization of LAK generation. Mouse, rat, and human LAK are readily generated in RPMI-1640 medium supplemented with glutamine (300 μg/ml), Hepes (10 mM), penicillin and streptomycin (100 μg/ml of each), and 5–10% serum. Fetal calf (FCS) and newborn calf serum (NCS) are generally equivalent, however, each new batch should be individually tested for its ability to generate LAK. After identifying a good batch, it should be reserved in order to use the same source throughout the course of a given series of experiments.

Although FCS or NCS work well, we prefer to use human AB serum for the generation of human LAK. Human serum batches should likewise be tested to identify good batches. All serum samples should be heat-inactivated (thawed serum heated to 55 °C for 30 min) and then aliquoted into single-use samples (e.g. 50 ml) and frozen at −20 °C until needed.

Motivated by potential clinical applications for the adoptive transfer of activated lymphocytes, several manufacturers have introduced serum-free, defined media for use in the activation of lymphocytes. Serum-free medium offers several advantages including reproducibility and the assurances of no risk of infectious agents. However, of all the products we have tested to date, only the Gibco product, AIM-V, has proved to be a suitable replacement for serum-supplemented medium. We consider AIMN the medium of choice, and use it exclusively for all clinical work. It is important to note that the ingredients in AIMN, as well as in other serum-free formulations, are generally not disclosed and may contain components which may have significant effects upon the system of study (e.g. indomethacin, insulin growth factors, steroid hormones, etc.). We suggest that data generated exclusively in serum-free mediums be reproduced in serum-supplemented complete medium.

We and others have published that IL-2 concentrations ranging from 22 pM to 22 nM induce LAK activity. Lower concentrations (< 2 pM) may satisfactorily activate lymphocytes in serum-supplemented medium. We have found no consistent differences between purified human and human recombinant forms of IL-2 obtained from several different producers, and routinely use recombinant products. As a general guide, lymphocytes are initially cultured in 2–10 nM IL-2. IL-2 induction of LAK activity can be detected within 24 h of culture, but we routinely culture for 4–6 days for the generation of a mature effector population. Cultures usually required feeding by day 6 with replacement of IL-2 for sustained growth and cytolytic activity. We have maintained potent lytic populations for more than 3 months, although many cultures lose much of their lytic activity after several weeks (> 28 days).

3.2 Anti-CD3/IL-2 activated 'T cell' killers

Ochoa *et al.* first reported the use of the T-cell activating antibody anti-OKT3 (anti-CD3) to augment IL-2 induction of effectors expressing LAK activity (10).

Activation with anti-CD3 presumably stimulates a transmembrane signalling structure associated with the T-cell antigen receptor. We and others have reported that when used in conjunction with IL-2, anti-CD3 generates a significantly increased yield (10–1000 ×) of cytolytic lymphocytes relative to IL-2 stimulation alone (15). By multiplying the lytic potency (expressed as lytic units) of the population by the increased total cellular yield, the anti-CD3/IL-2 activation scheme generated significantly increased lytic potential relative to IL-2 stimulation alone. We first used this activation method to generate large numbers of LAK (10^9–10^{10} total yield) from very small volumes (< 10 ml) of peripheral blood for use in adoptive immunotherapy protocols in which the patients could not afford to donate large numbers of fresh lymphocytes (15). We later applied the same activation scheme for the generation of TIL in which small numbers of lymphocytes were initially obtained or from tumours that proved highly immunosuppressive (i.e. glioblastoma) (16). This activation method involves the incubation of PBM plus monocytes or some other means of antibody presentation. The cells should be adjusted to 10^6/ml and incubated with anti-CD3 (e.g. Ortho-Clone OKT3, approved for clinical use) at 10 ng/ml for 48 h. The cells are then thoroughly washed and resuspended in complete medium supplemented with IL-2. Rapid cell growth requires cultures to be split often, frequently every other day. One pitfall of this activation mechanism is that cultures often begin to lose lytic activity after 3 weeks in culture. However, cell expansion in excess of 10^6-fold will often be achieved within this time, providing sufficient cell numbers for virtually any application.

3.3 Alternative cytokine activation strategies

Since the initial description of LAK, in which the obligate role for exogenously added IL-2 was determined, the involvement of several endogenously produced cytokines have been described (17). The cytokine tumour necrosis factor (TNF) has proven to play a central role in virtually all cell-mediated cytotoxicity (CMC) systems (18). The addition of anti-TNF neutralizing antibody during IL-2 activation eliminates $>90\%$ of LAK-mediated tumour lysis. Given the problematic toxicity associated with the high-dose, IL-2 administration protocols used in the first LAK clinical trials, alternative methods which might require less IL-2 were sought. We have reported that TNF-α, TNF-β, or interleukin-1 (IL-1) can all be used in conjunction with low-dose IL-2 to generate LAK of equivalent, or even augmented, lytic potency relative to high-dose, IL-2 stimulation alone (17, 19). There is preliminary evidence suggesting that TNF pre-stimulation prior to IL-2 activation, generates increased lytic potential at the population level, resulting from both increased effector-cell frequency and effector-cell efficiency (i.e. decreased recycling times). Preliminary data from our laboratory, confirming the report by Alderson (20), suggests that the exogenous addition of IL-7 is sufficient to stimulate LAK activity from both PBL and PBM cultures. Exogenously added IL-7 appears to be capable of inducing the endogenous production of IL-2 (Stephen Yang, personal communication). Yang also finds that neutralizing antibody against IL-2 inhibits LAK activity by IL-7-activated lymphocytes. Undoubtedly, many other stimulatory and inhibitory cytokine products serve to modulate LAK induction and potency. With a better understanding of the dynamic interplay occurring at the cellular level between these products, new approaches for the *in vitro* generation and maintenance of these effector populations should be defined.

4 Cryopreservation of lymphocytes and tumours

Precursor, as well as mature effector populations and tumour cells, may easily be stored frozen for later use. We find it useful to expand cultures of both stock

LAK and common tumour targets (i.e. Daudi, Raji), to be frozen in single-use aliquots (e.g. LAK at 10^7/tube, tumour targets at 10^6/tube). Samples can then be thawed and used when needed. Whenever possible, cultured cells should be harvested in early log phase with a viability greater than 90%.

Protocol 5

Cryopreservation

Equipment and reagents

- Complete medium
- Trypan Blue
- Cell centrifuge
- Freezing medium: 90% heat-inactivated serum, 10% dimethylsulfoxide (DMSO)

- Freezer vials
- Aluminium boxes
- 100% ethanol
- Liquid nitrogen freezer

Method

1 Wash the cells thoroughly in complete medium, and perform a viable cell count using Trypan Blue.

2 Pellet the cells and resuspend them in freezing medium to give a final concentration of 10^6–10^7 cells/ml.

3 Once the cells have been suspended in the freezing medium, they must be aliquoted into freezer vials and transferred to the freezer as rapidly as possible (about 1 min) to maintain maximal viability.

4 Place the freezer vials into aluminium boxes containing sufficient 100% ethanol to submerge the cell suspensions.

5 Transfer the freezer boxes into a $-80\,°C$ freezer overnight, and then into the vapour phase of a liquid-nitrogen freezer.

6 To use, rapidly thaw frozen samples by constant shaking in a $37\,°C$ waterbath, and then dilute 1/10 in warm, complete medium.

7 Wash cells extensively to remove the DMSO and use, e.g. plated as effectors or as ^{51}Cr-labelled targets.[a]

[a] Excellent viability can be maintained for at least 2 years if the cells are carefully frozen and thawed.

5 Cytotoxicity assays

In 1960, A. Govaerts transplanted a kidney from a donor dog X into a recipient dog Y. When the transplanted kidney was rejected, thoracic duct lymphocytes were obtained from the recipient dog X and added to a culture of kidney (epithelial) cells from dog Y. Some 48 h after the addition of the primed lymphocytes, lesions were noted in the confluent monolayer, indicating lymphocyte-mediated killing of the allogeneic cells (20). This represented one of the first reports of direct lymphocyte-mediated toxicity. This *in vitro* detection of CMC was adapted by several other investigators, including K. Theodor Brunner, Jean-Charles Cerrotini, and Borris D. Brondz into what have ultimately become the current methods for detecting killing.

5.1 ^{51}Cr-release cytotoxicity assay

Brunner *et al.* introduced two major changes to Govaerts' assay: they used tumour cells as targets for their sensitized effectors, and they adapted the ^{51}Cr-labelling technique to the study of target cell death (22). With minor modifications, this ^{51}Cr-release assay has remained the standard technique for measuring *in vitro* CMC, being relatively rapid, simple to perform, and reliable. The human Daudi (HLA class I-deficient), and Raji Burkitt's lymphoma cell lines are commonly used NK-resistant LAK targets, while the K562 erythroleukaemia line and the U937 lines are excellent NK targets. The use of fresh uncultured tumour cells (prepared as described above) as LAK targets may represent the closest approximation of *in vivo* interactions between LAK and tumour, and should be included in definitive studies, especially if autologous targets are available for clinical studies. We recommend that targets be stored in frozen aliquots rather than being maintained in long-term culture, to avoid the possibility of tissue culture induced changes in susceptibility to killer cells. Mycoplasma testing should also be routinely performed.

Protocol 6

^{51}Cr-release assay

Equipment and reagents

- Complete medium
- Appropriate pelleted target cells
- Effector cells
- Sodium ^{51}Cr in saline (11 mCi/ml at 650 mCi/mg)
- 5% CO_2 humidified incubator
- Round-bottomed, 96-well plates

- 0.1 M HCl
- Centrifuge fitted with multi-well plate rotor
- Katron filter-rack harvesting system (Skatron Inc.)
- Gamma counter windowed for ^{51}Cr

Method

1 Wash appropriate targets in complete medium and label the pelleted cells with 400 μCi sodium ^{51}chromate in saline per 10^7 targets. Label the targets for 1–2 h in a 37 °C, 5% CO_2, humidified incubator, with occasional shaking to inhibit pelleting.

2 Wash the targets three or four times in complete medium and then adjust to 5×10^4 cells/ml medium.

3 Wash the effector cells in complete medium, adjust to their final plating concentration, and aliquot into replicate wells.

Protocol 6 continued

4 Add effector cells at multiple ratios with a fixed number of targets, to obtain the characteristic sigmoidal killing curve. For example, a 0.6 ml suspension containing 3.84×10^6 total effector cells can be added in 0.1 ml aliquots to triplicate wells (96-well, round-bottom plates), and the remaining 0.3 ml repeatedly diluted with 0.3 ml medium, followed by adding 0.1 ml aliquots of targets at 5×10^4/ml in order to achieve effector-to-target ratios of 128:1, 64:1, 32:1, 16:1, 8:1, 4:1, 2:1, 1:1.

5 Determine spontaneous and maximal release by adding 0.1 ml aliquots of medium or 0.1 M HCl, respectively, on to replicate sets ($n = 3–6$) of 0.1 ml of targets alone.

6 Centrifuge the plates at 150 g for 5 min, and incubate in a humidified, 37 °C, 5% CO_2 incubator for 4 h.

7 At the end of the incubation period, centrifuge the plates again and harvest aliquots of the supernatants from each well.[a]

8 Count samples in a gamma counter, appropriately windowed for ^{51}Cr.[b]

[a] The Skatron filter-rack harvesting system represents a major improvement in both time and accuracy over manual harvesting.

[b] The entire sigmoidal killing curve can be described if sufficient E:T ratios, starting at a suitable high effector number, are assayed. We recommend that at least four and preferably more E:T ratios be assayed, whenever possible. Thorough characterization of this curve will greatly facilitate data interpretation.

5.1.1 Data analysis for the ^{51}Cr-release assay

^{51}Cr-release assays generate data expressed as c.p.m. By convention, this is transformed into per cent specific lysis (%SL) using the following equation:

$$\%SL = [(E - S)/(M - S)] \times 100;$$

where E refers to the mean of the experimental wells at a given E:T ratio, S is the mean of the spontaneous release wells in which targets were incubated with medium only, and M is the mean of the maximal release wells generated by targets incubated in 0.1 M HCl. We generally plate six spontaneous and six maximal wells, with experimental wells plated in triplicate.

Unfortunately, no standard method for data presentation has emerged. The simplest, and perhaps best, way is to provide the %SL ± SEM for each E:T ratio, either in a tabular format or graphically with %SL on the y axis vs. the log of E:T on the x axis (see *Figure 1a* and *b*). It is extremely important to present sufficient data to accurately describe the killing curve generated by a given effector/target combination. We attempt to plate at least eight E:T ratios starting at a sufficiently high effector-cell number to describe both the maximal killing plateau (abscissa) as well as the rest of the curve. Unfortunately, the effector-cell number often represents the limiting factor in an assay, significantly limiting the maximal achievable E:T ratio. In some cases, by decreasing the number of targets per well (e.g. from 5000 to 2000–2500), the assay can be modified to achieve the desired ratios. Presenting experiments in terms of %SL becomes problematic when large amounts of data must be presented and/or when several curves must be directly compared within one experiment. Lytic units have been used to avoid these problems by representing the potency of an effector population in terms of a single numerical value. Lytic units (LU) are generally defined as the inverse of the number of effector cells required to achieve a specific %SL against a given target (e.g. 30% SL for LAK and 15% for NK). Although the lytic unit, when applied correctly, may represent a useful means for data reduction, several potential problems can be associated with its use.

The first problem involves the types of data which can and cannot be presented in terms of lytic units. Lytic units should only be used as a means for comparing relative lytic efficiency of effector populations assayed in parallel, which are exhibiting similar potency against a given target. LU should not be used as a method of assigning absolute potencies, and should not be used to assess susceptibilities of differing relative targets to a given effector population. A second type of problem involves the mathematical model used to translate %SL data into lytic units. Since ^{51}Cr-release data describes a unique sigmoidal curve for each effector–target pair, attempting to describe the line with a linear regression fit can, at best, grossly approximate the curve. Curve fitting with a linear equation is further hampered if the point chosen for extrapolation (e.g. 15 or 30% SL) does not fall on the linear rise portion of the curve, or if too few points exist to accurately describe the linear rise portion. The sigmoidal curve is a better fit using non-linear models.

Pross *et al.* have published extensively on exponential fit models for describing NK killing data, and will generously provide investigators with ^{51}Cr-release cytotoxicity software for personal computer use (23) (Dr Hugh Pross, Dept of Radiation Oncology and Microscopy and Immunology, Queen's University, Kingston, Ontario, Canada; please include blank discs and stamped, self-addressed return envelope). However, significant controversy surrounds this approach as well, with several reports presenting extremely complicated arguments supporting specific non-linear models. A recent reappraisal of linear regression, exponential fit, and Von Krogh models for data analysis by Pollock *et al.* (24) encourages the reader to test the given models on data sets provided in order to better understand the associated problems. We highly recommend that investigators and their statistical support groups thoroughly review this and related literature, so as to better plan and process the ^{51}Cr-release cytotoxicity data for their unique applications.

5.2 Single-cell CMC assay

In contrast to the ^{51}Cr-release assay, which only describes the net lytic outcome of effector–target interactions, this simple approach provides additional information by directly measuring the frequency of effectors which can bind (binding frequency) as well as measuring specific killing (killing frequency) of a given target (25).

Protocol 7

Single-cell CMC assay

Equipment and reagents

- Effector and target cell populations
- Complete medium
- 30 °C waterbath
- Cell centrifuge
- Pasteur pipette
- 0.5% agarose
- Tissue culture receptacles
- 5% CO_2 humidified incubator
- 0.1% Trypan Blue
- 0.2% formaldehyde in saline
- Inverted microscope
- Fluorescein diacetate (FDA, Sigma)

Method

1 Mix equal numbers of effector and target cell populations in complete medium and place into a waterbath at 30 °C for 10 min.

2 Centrifuge the sample at 250 g at room temp. for 5 min. Prepare control tubes of target cells alone in parallel.

3 Discard the supernatants and resuspend the pellets in a minimum volume by six gentle aspirations with a Pasteur pipette (note that aspiration technique represents a crucial step for experimental accuracy and reproducibility).

4 Remove a small portion of this suspension and dilute for direct counting in order to measure the frequency of effector–target conjugates (the number of lymphocytes bound to target cells per 100 total lymphocytes).

5 Mix the remaining suspension with aliquots of 0.5% agarose (maintained liquefied just above its melting point) and pour as a thin layer (approx. 2 mm; note that thicker beds will require long focal length lenses) into tissue culture receptacles.

6 Overlay with complete medium to avoid dehydration, and place the cultures directly into 37 °C, 5% CO_2, humidified incubators for 1–4 h.

7 Assay samples for killing frequency by aspirating the medium overlay, adding a small volume of 0.1% Trypan Blue for 5 min at room temp., aspirating residual stain, and fixing with 0.2% formaldehyde in saline.

8 Count the conjugates, corrected for the spontaneous lysis of target cells plated alone, under normal light on an inverted microscope. If the effector and target cells are difficult to distinguish, pre-stain the effectors with agents such as the fluorescent dye fluorescein diacetate (FDA, Sigma), 1 μg/ml for 10 min at 37 °C in the dark, followed by three washes; this will allow easy discrimination without adversely affecting binding or killing frequencies.

5.3 Alternative approaches for measuring CMC, including non-radioactive assays

Many variables affect the ability of a given effector to specifically recognize, bind, and ultimately lyse a target cell. New and better ways of describing these complicated interactions are needed to expand our understanding of CMC. Alternative approaches already being studied include flow-cytometric assays for binding/killing frequency determinations, in which both the kinetics as well as the phenotypic profiles of effectors and targets can be simultaneously described (26).

Cytotoxicity assays without the use of radioactively labelled target cells have been developed (27, 28) and are identical to the chromium release assay in their performance, except that the targets are not pre-labelled and cytotoxicity is measured via a post-labelling step. One common approach is to measure lactate dehydrogenase (LDH) which is released upon cell lysis. The LDH is determined via the conversion of a tetrazolium salt into a red formazan product, with the amount of colour formed being proportional to the number of lysed cells. This method is available in kit form from Promega. As we continue to reduce radionuclide usage, such non-radioactive procedures are expected to gain in popularity. Our preliminary experience with the LDH method has been very favourable, and we intend to completely convert to such a method within the next few years.

References

1. Berke, G. (1989). In *Fundamental immunology* (2nd edn) (ed. W. Paul), p. 735. Raven Press, New York.
2. Henkart, P. A. (1985). *Annu. Rev. Immunol.*, **3**, 31.
3. Wolf, J. A. and Grimm, E. A. (1988). *Ann. Inst. Pasteur Immunol.*, **139**, 433.
4. Lotzova, E. and Ades, E. W. (1989). *Natural Immun. Cell Growth Regul.*, **8**, 1.
5. Julius, M. H., Simpson, E., and Herzenberg, L. A. (1973). *Eur. J. Immunol.*, **3**, 645.
6. Timonen, T., Ortaldo, J. R., and Herberman, R. B. (1981). *J. Exp. Med.*, **153**, 569.
7. Grimm, E. A. and Rosenberg, S. A. (1984). In *The lymphokines*, Vol. 9 (ed. E. Pick), p. 279. Academic Press, New York.
8. Ortaldo, J. R., Mason, A., and Overton, R. (1986). *J. Exp. Med.*, **164**, 1193.
9. Damle, N. K., Doyle, L. V., and Bradley, E. C. (1986). *J. Immunol.*, **134**, 2814.
10. Ochoa, A. C., Gromo, G., Alter, B. J., Sondel, P. M., and Bach, F. H. (1987). *J. of Immunol.*, **138**, 2728.
11. Loudon, W. G., Abraham, S. R., Owen-Scbaub, L. B., Hemingway, L. I., Hemstreet, G. P., and DeBault, L. E. (1988). *Cancer Res.*, **48**, 2184.
12. Topalian, S. L., Solomon, D., and Rosenberg, S. A. (1989). *J. Immunol.*, **142**, 3714.
13. Rosenberg, S. A., Spiess, P., and Lareniere, R. (1986). *Science*, **233**, 1318.
14. Rong, G. H., Grimm, E. A., and Sindelar, W. F. (1985). *J. Surg. Oncol.*, **28**, 131.
15. George, R. E., Loudon, W. G., Moser, R. P., Brunner, J. M., Steck, P. A., and Grimm, E. A. (1988). *J. Neurosurg.*, **69**, 403.
16. Grimm, E. A., Brunner, J. M., Carinhas, J., Koppen, J. A., Loudon, W. G., Owen-Schaub, L. B., Steck, P. A., and Moser, R. P. (1991). *Cancer Immunol. Immunother.*, **32**, 193.
17. Owen-Schaub, L. B., Gutterman, J. U., and Grimm, E. A. (1988). *Cancer Res.*, **48**, 788.
18. Shalaby, M. R., Espevik, T., Rice, G. C., Ammann, A. J., Figari, L. S., Ranges, G. E., and Palladino, M. A. (1988). *J. Immunol.*, **141**, 499.
19. Crump, W. L., III, Owen-Schaub, L. B., and Grimm, E. A. (1989). *Cancer Res.*, **49**, 149.
20. Alderson, M. R., Sassenfeld, H. M. and Widmer, M. B. (1990) *J. Exp. Med.*, **172**, 577–587.
21. Govaerts, A. (1960). *J. Immunol.*, **85**, 516.

22. Brunner, K. T., Mauel, J., Cerottini, J. C., and Chapuis, B. (1968). *Immunology*, **14**, 181.
23. Pross, H. F., Baines, M. G., Rubin, P., Shragge, P., and Patterson, M. S. (1981). *J. Clin. Immunol.*, **1**, 51.
24. Pollock, R. E., Zimmerman, S. O., Fuchshuber, P., and Lotzova, E. (1990). *J. Clin. Lab. Anal.*, **4**, 274.
25. Grimm, E. A. and Bonavida, B. (1979). *J. Immunol.*, **123**, 2861.
26. Wolf, J. A., Carinhas, J., and Grimm E. A. (1989). *Proc. Am.. Assoc. Cancer Res.*, **30**, 238.
27. Kolber, M. A. (1988). *J. Immunol. Meth.*, **108**, 255.
28. Decker, T. and Lohmann-Matthes, M.-H. (1988). *J. Immunol. Meth.*, **15**, 61.

Chapter 5

Cytokine regulation of endothelial cells

P. Allavena, G. Bianchi, M. Sironi, C. Garlanda, A. Vecchi,
Istituto di Ricerche Farmacologiche 'Mario Negri', Milano, Italy

A. Mantovani
Istituto di Ricerche Farmacologiche 'Mario Negri', Milano, Italy; Dept Biotechnology, Section of General Pathology, University of Brescia, Italy

1 Introduction

Endothelial cells (EC) have long been considered a 'passive' lining of blood vessels, endowed with negative properties, the most important one being that of representing a non-thrombogenic substrate for blood. As such, EC were thought to participate in tissue reactions essentially as targets for injurious agents. The possibility of isolating and culturing EC from various tissues permitted study of their complex reactions to a variety of activating stimuli. EC have, in this way, emerged as active participants in many physiological and pathological processes. It is now evident that haemostasis, inflammatory reactions, and immunity involve close interactions between immunocompetent cells and vascular endothelium. In particular, the ontogeny and function of white blood cells require an intimate relationship with vascular EC. Cytokines are mediators of these complex bidirectional interactions between leucocytes and vascular elements (for a review see refs 1 and 2).

EC represent both a source and a target of cytokines. Activation of EC by inflammatory stimuli or other modulatory peptides dramatically changes EC function and surface properties. Cytokine-induced EC functional reprogramming follows discrete patterns with limited overlapping. Typically IL-1 and TNF induce a programme related to inflammation and immunity, whereas IFN-γ activates accessory cell function (2).

In addition to responding to a variety of cytokines, EC are important producers of several of these polypeptide mediators, including IL-1, IL-6, colony-stimulating factors (G, M, and GM), and chemotactic cytokines (IL-8, monocyte chemotactic protein-1, MCP-1, Fractalkine).

In this chapter we will discuss selected aspects of the methodology involved in evaluating the interaction of cytokines with vascular cells. In particular, we will focus on methods and problems that are specifically related to the study of EC. These include the isolation, culture, and immortalization of EC; the measurement of their migratory activity in chemotaxis assays; the adhesive properties of EC evaluated as their interaction with leucocytes (adhesion and transmigration); finally, we will describe a recent, and feasible, *in vivo* assay for evaluating leucocyte recruitment.

Other functions, such as measuring the production of cytokines, present no EC-related specific problems and the reader is referred to other chapters in this book and elsewhere.

2 Endothelial cells

2.1 Human umbilical venous endothelial cells (HUVEC)

These cells have frequently been used for studies on cytokines. The method for culturing HUVEC has previously been described in detail (3, 4). It includes collagenase digestion of the vessels to isolate the cells. Collagenase has the advantage over other enzymes of selectively digesting the subendothelial basement leaving the cell membrane and most of the integral membrane glycoproteins intact. Isolation of EC from different tissues (i.e. aorta, brain, kidney, skin) has been described in detail (for a review see refs 4–8).

Protocol 1

Culture of endothelial cells

Equipment and reagents

NB: All culture reagents are from Gibco unless otherwise specified.

- Umbilical cords (at least 20 cm in length) collected in sterile plastic bags
- Ca^{2+} and Mg^{2+}-free PBS
- Collagenase solution: 0.1% in PBS containing Ca^{2+} and Mg^{2+} (CLS type I, Worthington Biochem.)
- Medium 199 (M199) and 20% fetal bovine or human serum
- Endothelial cell growth supplement (ECGS) (Collaborative Res.)
- Heparin—sodium salt (grade I-A from porcine intestinal mucosa, Sigma)
- 0.1% gelatin (Difco)-coated tissue culture flasks
- Trypsin (1.5 U/ml)–EDTA (0.02%)

Method

1 Collect umbilical cords from normal or Caesarean deliveries and excise any crushed area. Note that, under these conditions, cords can be maintained at 4 °C up to 1 week before processing.

2 Perfuse the umbilical vein with Ca^{2+}/Mg^{2+}-free PBS.

3 Remove HUVEC by short treatment at 37 °C with a collagenase solution.

Protocol 1 continued

4 Flush out the contents of the vein and wash the lumen with PBS.

5 Spin the cell suspensions at 300 g at 4 °C for 10 min.

6 Resuspend the EC pellet in tissue culture medium (most commonly M199 with 20% fetal bovine or human serum).

7 Seed cells in gelatin pre-coated (1 h at room temperature) culture flasks at a concentration not less than 20–40 $\times$ 10^3/cm^2.[a]

8 Passage the cells using trypsin–EDTA.[b]

[a] Note that cell counting is not easy, since cells detached from the vessel wall are not dispersed but are in sheets of 5–20 cells, the success of the culture being apparently related to the presence of such aggregates. In successful primary cultures the cells reach confluence in 7–10 days.

[b] After primary culture HUVEC can only be maintained for further passages in the presence of 50 µg/ml ECGS 100 µg/ml heparin and should always be grown on gelatin-coated culture flasks.

2.1.1 Comments

Studies on the influence of maternal variables on the success of EC cultures showed that if the mother habitually smoked more than 15 cigarettes per day this negatively influenced the success of the culture, whereas age, parity, use of oxytocin, and pathologies such as diabetes and hypertension had no significant effect.

It is of interest to consider how variables related to culture conditions can affect the HUVEC response to cytokines. When the cells are stimulated with cytokines, these peptides are added to complete culture medium in the presence of serum. During the time of cell activation by cytokines, serum can be substituted with 1% human or bovine serum albumin without any apparent change in cell response (9). The response of HUVEC to IL-1 and TNF declines with cell passage, in fact induction of membrane adhesive proteins for leucocytes gradually decrease with increased passage number; it is advisable therefore to test the HUVEC response to cytokines within the fifth passage. Cytokine activities are reversible and are not cytotoxic.

2.2 Mouse PmT-transformed lines

Normal EC of human and murine origin are cumbersome to obtain and culture. EC lines have been generated sporadically, and, in our experience, at least some of them lack important functions of normal EC. The polyoma middle T (PmT) oncogene transformed mouse EC (10) and can be used to generate immortalized EC cell lines, possibly representative of microvascular elements. These lines retain many properties of normal EC, including the production of and responsiveness to cytokines (11–13).

Protocol 2

Generation of endothelioma cell lines

Equipment and reagents

NB: All culture reagents are from Gibco unless otherwise specified.

- 15 days' gestation fetuses
- 0.05% trypsin + 0.02% EDTA
- DMEM medium + 20% FCS
- 6- and 12-well tissue culture plates

- Tetrovirus vector N-TKmT
- G418
- Ca^{2+}/Mg^{2+}-free PBS or saline
- Humidified, 5% CO_2 incubator

Method

NB: All procedures must be performed with sterile material under aseptic conditions.

1. Remove fetuses or organs of interest from six to eight fetuses of 15 days' gestation.
2. Cut the organ or fetus into small pieces and trypsinize (trypsin 0.05% + EDTA 0.02%) for 20 min at 37 °C.
3. Collect the supernatants and add the same volume of DMEM medium with 20% FCS.
4. Centrifuge at 300 g at 4 °C for 10 min.
5. Resuspend the pellet in 2–5 ml of DMEM + 10% FCS (complete medium) count and adjust to $0.5–1 \times 10^6$ cells/ml.
6. Add 2 ml of the cell suspensions into each well of 12-well plates and incubate at 37 °C, in a humidified 5% CO_2 incubator 5% CO_2.
7. After 24 h remove the medium and add about 10^5 neo-resistant CFU of the retrovirus vector N-TKmT per well in 1 ml of complete medium.[a]
8. After 2 h remove the medium and add fresh complete medium.
9. After 72 h select PmT infected–neomycin resistant cells with G418, 800 μg/ml.
10. Change the medium twice a week, keeping G418 at 800 μg/ml.
11. Check the wells for G418 resistant cells. (They usually are observed after 15–20 days.)
12. When the cells are confluent, wash the wells thoroughly (twice) with Ca^{2+}/Mg^{2+}-free PBS or with saline. Add 0.3 ml of 0.05% trypsin + 0.02% EDTA for 2–3 min. at 37 °C, resuspend the detached cells, and add 1 ml of complete medium. Transfer all the suspension to a well of a 6-well plate and bring to a final volume of 3 ml, with G418 at a final concentration of 800 μg/ml.
13. Check the cells for the growth every day.
14. When confluent, passage the cells 1:3.[b]

[a] Virus is produced by the GP+E cell line obtained through the courtesy of Dr E. Wagner (Wien, Austria).

[b] At this stage, cells should not be diluted too much, even if they are growing very well. Confluent monolayers can usually be kept for 1–2 days without damaging the cells. On the other hand, if cells are diluted too much, they stop growing and can either remain quiescent for some time and eventually grow again, or die. Maintain selection with G418.

Following this protocol, we have obtained stable cell lines from heart, brain, and whole embryos of C57BL mice. Cell lines show a cobblestone morphology at confluency and maintain a monolayer structure without overgrowth. Cells are positive for CD31/PECAM-1 antigen, show rapid uptake of fluoresceinated acetylated low-density lipoprotein, produce IL-6 constitutively, and are negative or weakly positive for factor VIII-related antigen. Transmission electron microscopy revealed that they were uniformly negative for the presence of Weibel–Palade bodies.

Transformed cells maintain many characteristics of normal endothelial cells, e.g. CD31 expression, modulation of adhesion molecules by cytokines, and cytokine production (12). They do not constitutively express ICAM-1, VCAM-1, E- and P-selectin, which can, however, be induced (with the exception of ICAM-1) by exposure to TNF-α and LPS, but not IL-1.

Endothelioma cells produce IL-6 and MCP-1/JE, whose production can be increased by IL-1 exposure and EDMF, an endothelial factor capable of inducing EC migration (13).

2.2.1 Comments

We have been growing lines originating from embryo tissues infected *in vitro* with the PmT oncogene of the polyoma virus since the early 1990s. They represent an easy and reliable source of endothelial cells of murine origin, suitable for studies on EC biology (11, 14). These lines do not need exogenous growth factors for proliferation.

All lines have been frozen, stored in liquid nitrogen, and put again into culture without problems.

PmT murine EC lines originating from haemangiomas (15, 16) have been used to generate mAbs against EC-specific antigens expressed constitutively, as CD31 or induced by cytokines, such as VCAM-1 and ELAM-1 (17).

EC lines from different organs can be useful to study the potential diversity of the microvasculature of different organs.

3 Chemotaxis

Chemotaxis is defined as the directional locomotion of cells sensing a gradient of the stimulus. Chemotaxis has been extensively studied with leucocytes that are 'professional migrants', but a variety of cell types including fibroblasts, melanoma cells, keratinocytes, and vascular endothelial cells exhibit directional locomotion *in vitro*. Migration, as well as proliferation, underlie the process of new blood vessel formation. Cytokines such as fibroblast growth factor (FGF), TNF-α, G- and GM-CSF induce endothelial cell migration *in vitro* and angiogenesis *in vivo*.

Two main techniques have been used to measure endothelial cell migration *in vitro*: repair of a wound inflicted on a cell monolayer; and chemotaxis across porous membranes. While the former approach may more closely resemble the *in vivo* endothelial monolayer that lines blood vessels, the latter is easier to quantitate and allows an analysis of directional vs. random locomotion. We will therefore focus on the description of endothelial cell migration through a porous membrane. Both a 'classic' modified Boyden chamber assay (18) and a micromethod (19, 20) will be described. Assays for chemotaxis and locomotion of polymorphonuclear leucocytes and monocytes are also discussed and described in Chapter 6, this volume.

3.1 Boyden chamber assay

Protocol 3

Boyden chamber assay

Equipment and reagents

- HUVEC (see *Protocol 1*)
- Boyden chambers (Neuroprobe)
- PVP-free polycarbonate filter (12 mm diameter, 5 μm pore, Sartorius)
- Clamps and forceps (Neuroprobe)
- Cytokines: 5 ng/ml FGF, 5 ng/ml GM-CSF, 500 U/ml TNF

- M199 medium containing 1% FBS
- Standard chemoattractants: e.g. 1 mg/ml human plasma fibrinogen
- Humidified 5% CO_2 incubator
- Glass slides
- Cotton wad
- Diff-Quick (Harleco)

Method

1 Detach confluent HUVEC by brief exposure of the cells to 1.5 U/ml trypsin–0.02% EDTA.

2 Centrifuge the cells and resuspend at a concentration of 2×10^6/ml in medium 199 containing 1% FBS.

3 Seed 200 μl of the stimulus (diluted in the same medium used for cell suspension) in the lower well of the chamber, carefully avoiding air-bubble formation.

4 Lay the filter on the surface of the stimulus with the opaque side up.

5 Tightly screw the upper part of the chamber to create an upper well in which 200–400 μl of the cell suspension is seeded.

6 Incubate the chamber at 37 °C in humidified air with 5% CO_2 for 6 h.

7 Absorb the liquid in the upper well with a cotton wad and carefully clean the upper side of the filter. Remove the remaining unmigrated cells.

8 Unscrew the upper part of the chamber, catch the filter with forceps, turn the filter over and put it on a glass slide so that the side that has contacted with the stimulus is now face-up.

9 Stain the filter with Diff-Quik following the manufacturers instructions.

3.1.1 Comments

Chemotactic activity of some cytokines is best observed after coating the filters with gelatin (or other extracellular matrix protein such as fibronectin). The filter should be soaked in 0.5 M acetic acid for 2 min, washed with PBS, incubated for 24 h in a 0.01% gelatin solution and air-dried.

Reading of the assay: chemotaxis is evaluated as the number of cells that migrate across the filter and adhere to its lower surface. For this reason, cells in a certain number (usually ten) of high-power fields (under oil immersion) are counted. The results are expressed as the mean number ($\pm$ SE) of migrated cells in three replicates. To compare the results from different experiments, it is important to count the same number of fields and to use the same microscope and magnification. Reading should be done in a blind fashion, after coding samples.

3.2 Microchemotaxis assay

The microchemotaxis method has the advantage of utilizing a minimal number of cells (1×10^5 cells/well compared to $4-8 \times 10^5$ /well in the Boyden chamber), and allows more samples to be evaluated in one experiment. The only difference from the Boyden chamber technique is that the micromethod uses a Plexiglas 48-well microchamber, each well has a volume of 25 μl. The cover piece, when it is mounted and screwed, forms 50-μl upper wells. One microchamber thus contains 48 replicates. The preparation of cells, filter, and chemoattractants is the same as described for the conventional method in *Protocol 3*.

A further discussion and description of this method can be found in Chapter 6, this volume.

Protocol 4

Microchemotaxis assay

Equipment and reagents

- As *Protocol 3*
- 48-well micro Boyden chamber, including filters (polycarbonate 25 $\times$ 85 mm, 5 μm pores), clamps, and special rubber policemen (Neuroprobe)
- Standard chemoattractants

Method

1 Aliquot 25 μl of an appropriate chemoattractant into the wells of the lower chamber.[a]

2 Put the filter on to the lower chamber leaving the opaque surface on top. Make a small nick in the filter (e.g. at the upper right edge) to avoid confusion concerning the order of the experimental groups in the same filter.

3 Mount the silicone trimming and then the upper chamber. Press and tightly screw the upper chamber to avoid air bubbles.

4 Seed 50 μl of the cell suspension (1.5×10^6/ ml) into the upper wells by leaning the pipette tip on the border of the well and quickly ejecting the cell suspension.

5 Incubate the chamber at 37 °C in 5% CO_2 for 1.5 h.

6 Remove the chamber from the incubator.

7 Unscrew and turn the chamber upside down.

8 Hold the upper chamber tightly and remove the lower chamber, keeping the silicone trimming and the filter in place. Note that at this point the migrated cells are on the upper surface (bright side) of the filter.

9 Remove the silicone trimming.

10 Lift the filter by placing a clamp on each end.

11 Wash the opaque surface of the filter, where the non-migrated cells remain, by gently washing this side with PBS. Do not completely immerse the filter in PBS otherwise the migrated cells will be lost.

12 Remove all non-migrated cells by scraping the opaque surface of the filter against the special rubber policeman.

13 Stain the filter with Diff-Quik according to manufacturer's instructions.

14 Place the filter on a glass slide and count the migrated cells present on the bright surface of the filter. Count 5–10 microscope fields at 1000 × magnification.

[a] Depending on the microchamber used, the 25 µl vol. may have to be varied by ± 2–3 µl. It is advisable to calibrate the lower wells in advance, so that, having seeded the chemoattractant, the liquid in the lower wells forms a small convex surface that guarantees a perfect adhesion of the filter thus avoiding the formation of air bubbles.

3.3.1 Comments

The methodology described above, with variations in filter type, incubation time, etc., could be utilized for evaluating the motility of haemopoietic cells, fibroblasts, smooth muscle cells, and tumour cells. For cells of non-haemopoietic origin, coating the filter with an extracellular matrix protein is often needed, although it increases background migration. Since the micromethod is technically more difficult, classical modified Boyden chambers may be a better choice for occasional use. It is important to define whether a cytokine that induces migration across filters induces random locomotion or chemotaxis. A checkerboard experimental design should be used whereby different concentrations of the cytokine are seeded in the upper and/or lower compartments of the chamber. For a chemotactic signal, maximal migration should occur in the presence of a positive concentration gradient between the lower and upper compartments, will little or no effect under negative gradient conditions (chemoattractant only in the upper well) or in the absence of a gradient (chemoattractant added to the upper and lower well) (18–20).

4 Leucocyte adhesion and transmigration

The emigration of leucocytes from blood to tissues is essential to mediate immune surveillance and to mount inflammatory responses. The interaction of leucocytes with EC can be divided into four sequential steps: tethering; triggering; strong adhesion; and migration. The selectin family of adhesion molecules mediates tethering; strong adhesion is mediated by the integrin family, which needs to be activated (triggering); and, finally, migration is induced by local pro-migratory factors including some cytokines and chemokines (21, 22). We have studied the adhesive properties and transendothelial migration of leucocytes, but this method may also be applied for the investigation of other cell types, for instance tumour cells. *Protocols 5* and *6* describe radioisotopic assays for monitoring adhesion and transendothelial migration, based on an assay described in ref. 23.

Some leucocytes (e.g. dendritic cells, lymphocytes) have a peculiar trafficking pattern from tissues into the lumen of blood or lymphatic vessels. To mimic this basal-to-apical process of migration *in vitro* we established a transmigration assay, schematically represented in *Figure 1* and described in ref. 24, that we named 'reverse transmigration assay'. *Protocol 7* describes the essential aspects of this assay.

4.1 Adhesion

Protocol 5

Adhesion assay

Equipment and reagents

- HUVEC (*Protocol 1*)
- Complete tissue culture medium: M199 with 20% FBS, 50 μg/ml endothelial cell growth supplement (ECGS, Collaborative Research), 100 μg/ml heparin (Sigma).
- Freshly isolated leucocytes
- 96-well plates (Falcon, Becton Dickinson)

- Cotton buds (Johnson and Johnson)
- ^{51}Cr (Amersham, 37 MBq, 1 μCi)
- Humidified 5% CO_2 incubator
- Gamma counter windowed for ^{51}Cr
- PBS (Biochrom KG)
- 1 M NaOH, 1% SDS

Method

1 Separate the various leucocyte subsets (neutrophils, monocytes, NK cells, or lymphocytes) from the buffy coats of normal blood donors, as described in refs 25 and 26.

2 Resuspend the cells at 10^7 cells/ml in RPMI-1640 medium + 10% FBS and label by incubating with 100 μCi ^{51}Cr for 1 h at 37 °C.

3 After labelling wash extensively and resuspend in RPMI-1640 + 10% FBS.

4 Culture EC in 96-well plates (1 $\times$ 10^4 cells/well) in order to reach a confluent monolayer in 36–48 h. Stimulate designated wells with 10 ng/ml of IL-1 during the last 18 h of culture.

5 Incubate EC with 100 μl of ^{51}Cr-labelled cells resuspended at 10^7 cells/ml and incubate at 37 °C for 30 min.

Protocol 5 continued

6   Carefully remove the supernatant and wash the cells twice to remove non-adherent cells.

7   Incubate the adherent cells with 100 μl of 1 M NaOH + 1% SDS for 5 min and count radioactivity using a gamma counter. Express cell adhesion as the percentage of input cells.

4.1.1 Comments

The spontaneous adhesion of resting leucocytes to unstimulated EC varies for different subsets. For instance, the adhesion of NK cells is usually 5–15%, a value intermediate between that of monocytes (20–40%) and the very low value of T cells and PMN (< 5%). With monocytes and NK cells there is usually a high degree of variability among different donors.

   The adhesive capacity of leucocytes to EC can be modulated by various signals. When EC are stimulated with IL-1, leucocyte adhesion increases, as EC express new adhesion molecules. Adhesion molecules involved in the interaction of leucocytes and EC are identified by the use of blocking mAb—most of which are commercially available—specific for the adhesion structures expressed by leucocytes or EC. Studies with specific mAb have demonstrated that adhesion through resting EC is mediated by the LFA-1/ICAM-1, -2 pathway, while IL-1 activated EC involves both LFA-1/ICAM-1 and VLA-4/VCAM-1 for monocytes and lymphoid cells. Neutrophils only use the first pathway, being VLA-4 negative. Cytokines can also affect leucocytes directly. IL-2 and IL-12, for instance, increase NK adhesion to EC, while IL-4 has inhibitory activity.

4.2 Transmigration (*Figure 1*)

Protocol 6

Transendothelial migration

Equipment and reagents

In addition to items needed for *Protocol 5*

- Single-well Boyden chambers (Neuroprobe)
- Nitrocellulose filter (12 mm diameter, 5 μm pore, Sartorius)
- Fibronectin (Sigma)
- PVP-free polycarbonate filter (12 mm diameter, 5 μm pore, Neuroprobe)
- 24-well plates (Falcon, Becton Dickinson)
- 3 ml vials

Method

1   Coat the PVP-free polycarbonate filters with 1 ml of 10 μg/ml fibronectin in PBS at room temperature for 2 h in 24-well plates.

Protocol 6 continued

2 Aspirate the fibronectin and add 10^5 EC in 2 ml of M199 complete medium and grow to confluence (5–6 days).

3 Place 0.2 ml of complete medium in the lower compartment of each Boyden chamber.

4 Mount a nitrocellulose filter (uncoated) into each chamber, then place a coated (step 2) PUP-free polycarbonate filter on top.

5 Immediately add 0.15 ml of complete medium. Do not allow the wells to dry out.

6 Assemble and screw the upper compartment of the chamber.

7 Label PBMC with 100 μCi of ^{51}Cr at 4 °C for 1 h, and seed cells (3–6 × 10^5 in 0.15 ml of complete medium) into the upper compartment of the chamber.

8 Incubate the chamber at 37 °C for 60 min.

9 Remove the chambers from the incubator.

10 Collect the medium containing non-adherent cells in a 3 ml vial (fraction A).

11 Gently wash the EC monolayers with 0.5 ml warm medium, collect the medium in 3 ml vials (fraction B).

12 Scrape (gently!) the EC monolayer and adherent leucocytes off with cotton buds and transfer to vials (fraction C).

13 Transfer the double filter system to vials, together with the medium from the lower compartment (fraction D).

14 Measure the radioactivity in each fraction. Fractions A+B represent non-adherent cells. Fraction D represents migrated cells. As migrated cells had first adhered to EC, the total number of adherent cells is calculated by summing the C+D fractions.

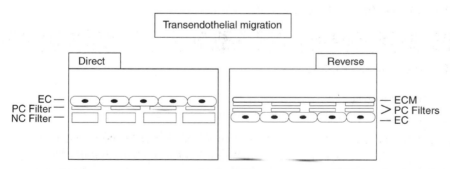

Figure 1 Schematic representation of a single-well Boyden chamber for the transendothelial migration assay. The set of filters is represented. EC, endothelial cells; ECM, extracellular matrix; PC, polycarbonate; NC, nitrocellulose.

4.2.1 Comments

The spontaneous transendothelial migration varies for different leucocyte subsets. Usually, only a proportion (about 30%) of EC-adherent leucocytes effectively transmigrate during the assay. When EC are activated with IL-1 a greater number of cells adhere and transmigrate, but the proportion of transmigrated cells over the input does not dramatically change (usually 30% of EC-adherent). It should be noted that IL-1 does not change the state of confluence of the mono-layer, as determined by staining.

The identification of the adhesion molecules involved in the transendothelial migration of leucocytes is performed with functional blocking mAbs specific for the adhesive structures. As transmigration first requires adhesion to EC, mAbs to the adhesive pathways LFA-1/ICAM-1, -2 and VLA-4/VCAM-1 eventually inhibit transmigration through resting and cytokine-activated EC, respectively. In addition, PECAM (CD31) is a molecule expressed both by leucocytes and EC, and plays a major role during transmigration (21). Chemoattractants can be seeded in the lower compartment to increase leucocyte transmigration.

4.3 Reverse transmigration

Protocol 7

Reverse transmigration *in vitro*

Equipment and reagents

In addition to items needed for *Protocols* 5 and 6
- Stripping buffer: 20 mM NH_4OH, 0.5% (v/v) Triton X-100

Method

1 Culture EC to confluent monolayers on fibronectin pre-coated PVP-free polycarbo-nate filters in 24 well-plates as described in *Protocol 6*.

2 Treat one-half of the filters with 1 ml of stripping buffer for 30 sec.

3 Quickly remove the stripping buffer and the digested EC monolayer (ECM) and wash twice with complete medium (*Protocol 6*). Cover the exposed ECM with 1 ml of complete medium. Do not allow the filters to dry out.

4 Place 0.2 ml of complete medium in the lower compartment of each Boyden chamber. Mount the first filter, coated with EC, upside down, and place the second filter coated with ECM on top.

5 Assemble and screw the upper compartment of the chamber.

6 Immediately add 0.15 ml of complete medium. Do not allow the filters to dry out.

7 Seed ^{51}Cr-labelled leucocytes (3–6 × 10^5 in 0.15 ml of complete medium) (*Protocol 6*) into the upper compartment of the chamber.

8 Incubate the chamber at 37 °C for 60 min.

9 Remove the chambers from the incubator.

10 Collect the medium present in the upper chamber (fraction A) and wash the ECM layer with 0.5 ml warm medium (fraction B).

11 Collect the ECM-adherent cells with cotton buds (fraction C), and the transmigrated cells in the lower compartment (fraction D).

Protocol 7 continued

12 Measure the radioactivity in each fraction. Fractions A+B represent the non-adherent cells. Fractions C+D represent the adherent cells. Fraction D represents the migrated cells. Please note that in the reverse assay the transmigrated cells comprise only the radioactivity present in the lower compartment.

5 The air-pouch model

The air-pouch model is an *in vivo* method for the evaluation of leucocyte recruitment at inflamed sites. It consists of a subcutaneous injection of air on the back of rodents (27). Recently, it has been used to study leucocyte recruitment in mice (28, 29) and has been also proposed as a method for studies of angiogenesis (30, 31). The methodology described here has been applied to mice and has been mainly used in studies of leucocyte recruitment, following the injection of appropriate stimuli into the pouch. The formation of an air sac on the back of the mouse allows a local injection of the agent under study and the evaluation of the local response. The response can be measured both at the cellular level, by counting the leucocytes recruited, and at the level of production of locally released soluble mediators into the fluid recovered from the pouch (28, 29). Staining the recovered cells can provide information on the selective recruitment of the different leucocyte populations (i.e. macrophages, granulocytes). Carrageenan was the stimulus originally described (32), but since then other agents, including inflammatory cytokines and chemokines, have been investigated in this model (28, 29, 33). Moreover, it has been used to evaluate the ability of various drugs to modulate *in vivo* leucocyte migration and cytokine and chemokine production (28, 29, 32).

Protocol 8

In vivo air pouch

Equipment and reagents

- Animals: CD1 mice, either sex
- Sterile, apirogen saline
- Iota carrageenan, 1% in sterile, pyrogen-free saline (Biochrome KG)
- 5 ml syringes fitted with 25-gauge needles
- 3 ml plastic Pasteur pipettes
- Haemocytometer
- Centrifuge
- Laminar-flow hood

Method

1 Inject mice subcutaneously on their back with 5 ml of sterile air (prepare syringes under a laminar-flow hood).

2 After 3 days re-inject the pouches with 3 ml of sterile air.

3 On day 6, inject 1 ml of 1% i carrageenan into the pouches. Inject controls with 1 ml of saline.

Protocol 8 continued

4   On day 7 (24 h later) kill the animals by carbondioxide inhalation. Incise the skin on the back and gently detach it to expose the surface of the air sac. Carefully inject the pouch with 1 ml of saline, then make a small incision in the upper part of the sac, recover the liquid with a plastic Pasteur pipette, and immediately put it in a test tube in ice.

5   Record the total amount of liquid collected; take an aliquot (usually 100 µl) for a cell count. If a differential count is needed, spin the cells in a cytocentrifuge and stain with Diff-Quick according to the manufacturer's instructions.

6   If the soluble factors are to be measured, centrifuge the remaining fluid at 600 g for 10 minutes at 4 °C, collect and store the supernatants at −20 °C until use.

5.1 Comments

The method described here uses carrageenan as a local stimulus for leucocyte recruitment. Other stimuli may also be used, basically following the same protocol. It must be noted, however, that water-soluble stimuli (for instance, proteins) must be prepared in 0.5% sterile carboxymethylcellulose to avoid the fast absorption of the agent from the local site of injection. The carrageenan injection causes a recruitment that lasts as long as 7 days (32), while other stimuli, e.g. IL-1β, recruit cells for shorter times (28)—4 h is the best time for evaluating IL-1β. Although the conditions reported above apply to the CD1 mouse (32), other strains can also be used. However, the best time for evaluating recruitment must be found for each strain.

References

1. Mantovani, A. and Dejana, E. (1989). *Immunol. Today*, **10**, 370.
2. Mantovani, A., Bussolino, F., and Dejana, E. (1992). *FASEB J.*, **6**, 2591.
3. Gimbrone, M. A., Cotran, R. S., and Folkman, J. (1974). *J. Cell Biol*, **60**, 673.
4. Balconi, G. and Dejana, E. (1986). *Med. Biol.*, **64**, 231.
5. Rayan, U. S., Ryan, W., Whitaker, C., and Chin, A. (19??). *Tissue Cell*, **8**, 125.
6. Schwartz, S. M. (1978). *In vitro*, **14**, 966.
7. Sherer, G. K., Fitzharris, T. P., Faulk, W. P., and LeRoy, E. C. (1980). *In vitro*, **16**, 675.
8. Spatz, M., Bembry, J., Dodson, R. F., Hervconen, H., and Murray, M. R. (1980). *Brain Res.*, **1941**, 577.
9. Bussolino, F. Breviario, F. Tetta, C., Aglietta, M., Mantovani, A., and Dejana, E. (1986). *J. Clin. Invest.*, **77**, 2027.
10. Williams, R. L., Courtneidge, S. A., and Wagner, E. F. (1988). *Cell*, **52**, 121.
11. Bussolino, F., De Rossi, M., Sica, A., Colotta, F., Wang, J. M., Bocchietto, E., Padura, I. M., Bosia, A., Dejana, E., and Mantovani, A. (1991). *J. Immunol.*, **147**, 2122.
12. Garlanda, C., Parravicini, C., Sironi, M., De Rossi, M., Wainstok de Calmanovici, R., Carozzi, F., Bussolino, F., Colotta, F., Mantovani, A., and Vecchi, A. (1994). *Proc. Natl Acad. Sci., USA*, **91**, 7291.
13. Taraboletti, G., Belotti, D., Dejana, E., Mantovani, A., and Giavazzi, R. (1993). *Cancer Res.*, **53**, 3812.

14. Bocchietto, E., Guglielmetti, A., Silvagno, F., Taraboletti, G., Pescarmona, G. P., Mantovani, A. Bussolino, F. (1993). *J. Cell Physiol.*, **155**, 89.

15. Vecchi, A., Garlanda, C., Lampugnani, M. G., Resnati, M., Matteucci, C., Stoppacciaro, A., Ruco, L., Mantovani, A., and Dejana, E. (1994). *Eur. J. Cell Biol.*, **63**, 247

16. Piali, L., Albelda, S. M., Baldwin, H. S., Hammel, P., Gisler, R. H., and Imhof, B. A. (1993). *Eur. J. Immunol.*, **23**, 2464.

17. Hahne, M., Jager, U., Isenmann, S., Hallmann, R., and Vestweber, D. (1993). *J. Cell Biol.*, **121**, 655.

18. Dejana, E., Languino, L. R., Polentarutti, N., Balconi, G., Ryckewaert, J. J., Larrieu, M. J., Donati, M. B., Mantovani, A., and Margurie, G. (1985). *J. Clin. Invest.*, **75**, 11.

19. Falk, W., Goodwin, R. H., Jr, and Leionard, E. J. (1980). *J. Immunol. Meth.*, **33**, 239.

20. Bussolino, F., Wang, J. M., Defilippi, P., Turrini, F., Sanavio, F., Edgell, C., Aglietta, M., Arese, P., and Mantovani, A. (1989). Nature, **337**, 471.

21. Springer, T. A. (1994). *Cell*, **76**, 301.

22. Adams, D. H. and Shaw, S. (1994). *Lancet*, **343**, 831.

23. Bianchi, G. Sironi, M., Ghibaudi, E., Selvaggini, C., Elices, M., Allavena, P., and Mantovani, A. (1993). *J. Immunol.*, **151**, 5135.

24. D'Amico, G., Bianchi, G., Bernasconi, S., Bersani, L., Piemonti, L., Sozzani, S., Mantovani, A., Allavena, P. (1998). *Blood*, **92**, 207.

25. Sozzani, S., Luini, W., Molino, M., Jilek, P., Bottazzi, B., Cerletti, C., Matsushima, K., Mantovani, A. (1991). *J. Immunol.*, **147**, 2215.

26. Allavena, P., Paganin, C., Martin Padura, I., Peri, G., Gaboli, M., Dejana, E., Marchisio, P. C., Mantovani, A. (1991). *J. Exp. Med.*, **173**, 439.

27. Sin, Y. M., Tan, C. H., and Chan, S. F. (1989). *Agents Actions*, **28**, 98.

28. Romano, M., Sironi, M., Toniatti, C., Polentarutti, N., Bussolino, F., Poli, V., Ciliberto, G., and Mantovani A. (1997), *Immunity*, **6**, 315.

29. Sironi, M., Guglielmotti, A., Polentarutti, N., Fioretti, F., Vecchi, A., Pinza, M., and Mantovani, A. (1999). *Eur. Cyt. Netw.* **10**, 437

30. Lichtenberg, J., Hansen, A., Skak-Nielsen, T., Bay, C., Mortensen, J. T., and Binderup, L. (1997). *Pharmacol. Toxicol.*, **81**, 280.

31. Lichtenberg, J., Vig Hjarnaa, P. J., Kristjansen, P. E., Hansen, D., and Binderup, L. (1999). *Pharmacol. Toxicol.*, **84**, 34.

32. Romano, M., Faggioni, R., Sironi, M., Sacco, S., Echtenacher, B., Di Santo, E., Salmona, M., and Ghezzi, P. (1997). *Mediat. Inflamm.*, **6**, 32.

33. Martin-Padura, I., Lostaglio, S., Schneemann, M., Villa, A., Simmons, D., and Dejana, E. (1998). **42**, 117.

Chapter 6
Assays for leucocyte migration

Jo Van Damme, Jean-Pierre Lenaerts, and
Sofie Struyf

Laboratory of Molecular Immunology, Rega Institute for Medical Research,
University of Leuven, Minderbroedersstraat 10, 3000 Leuven, Belgium

1 Introduction

In view of the recent developments in cytokine research, there has been a revived interest in chemotaxis assays. Indeed, within a short time a number of novel chemotactic cytokines (chemokines) have been identified. These low molecular weight proteins are different from other cytokines such as interleukin-1 (IL-1) and tumour necrosis factor (TNF), previously reported to be chemotactic for leukocytes. Chemokines belong to a large family of small proteins that exert their chemotactic activity different leucocytic cell types (1–4). Like several other chemotactic substances, such as formylmethionyl peptides (e.g. fMLP), the anaphylatoxin C5a, and leukotriene B4 (LTB4), chemokines bind to distinct serpentine-like receptors. Some chemokine receptors are essential for HIV-entry into monocytes or lymphocytes. Several chemokines, such as IL-8, have now been studied in detail with respect to leucocyte migration *in vitro* and *in vivo*. More recent members of the chemokine family have so far only been biochemically characterized and their role in cell migration has not yet been studied in great detail.

In part, the lack of sensitive and specific bioassays for measuring chemotaxis as well as the complexity of these tests can explain the late discovery and the initial slow progress in chemokine research. However, the assays that were used to detect their *in vitro* activity after production and purification were basically identical to well-established techniques, such as the Boyden chamber assay (5) and the agarose method (6) for chemotaxis described in this chapter. *In vivo* migration assays have also been successfully used to discover chemokines and to confirm the chemotactic activity of chemokines characterized by *in vitro* assays. Since many substances, including pro- and eukaryotic cell products, can exert chemotactic activity, chemokine identification had to wait for new techniques to be devised that could produce sufficient amounts of these proteins and to enable molecules to be purified to homogeneity. Today the limiting factor is the isolation of specific leucocyte types (such as haemopoietic precursor cells, dendritic cells, and T-lymphocyte subsets) in sufficient quantities to be used in chemotaxis assays. Assays for cell migration through endothelial cell mono-layers are described in Chapter 5, this volume.

2 Preparation of target cells and test samples

2.1 Isolation of leucocyte subsets for chemotaxis

Because chemokines are active on different types of leucocytes, isolation of these cells from fresh blood is an important step in the biological characterization of novel molecules by migration assays. In general, the isolation procedure used is a compromise between several parameters including viability, purity, and the number of isolated cells. To obtain a high cell viability, the speed of isolation is more crucial for granulocytes than for mononuclear cells, although the latter should not be activated during the isolation procedure. The low percentage of basophils, natural killer cells (NK), and dendritic cells in the peripheral blood from healthy volunteers necessitates a multistep isolation procedure based on the removal of irrelevant cells. Depending on the cell type of interest, a different combination of purification techniques is applied (*Table 1*).

During the initiation phase of leucocyte isolation, it is essential to keep the blood cells in a buffer containing an anticoagulant. If large volumes of blood need to be processed (> 1 litre), leucocyte-enriched fractions (buffy coats) are prepared by centrifugation. Furthermore, remaining red blood cells need to be removed by aggregation or lysis (*Table 1*). Erythrocytes can be lysed by treatment with NH_4Cl (8.3 g/litre) in phosphate-buffered saline (PBS) for 10 min, or by hypotonic shock in double-distilled water for 30 sec. Alternatively, red blood cells can be removed by aggregation and sedimentation with hydroxyethyl starch (see *Protocol 1*). To separate different leucocyte types, density gradient centrifugation is an essential tool (*Table 1*). Centrifugation of leukocytes on Lymphoprep (sodium diatrizoate–Ficoll solution, Nycomed Pharma) or Ficoll–Paque (Amersham Pharmacia Biotech) with a density of 1.077 g/ml permits the separation of mono-nuclear cells from granulocytes. If granulocytes are still contaminated with

Table 1 Overview of combined methods for peripheral blood leucocyte isolation

Isolation method	Cell type[a]				
	Neu	Eo	Ba	Mo	Ly
Erythrocyte removal:					
Aggregation (Plasmasteril)	+[b]	+	+	+	+
Lysis (hypotonic shock)	+	+			
Density gradient centrifugation:					
Lymphoprep	+	+		+	+
Percoll			+		
Magnetic sorting (MACS)		CD16[-c]		CD14[+b]	CD3[+]

[a] neu, neutrophils; eo, eosinophils; ba, basophils; mo, monocytes; ly, lymphocytes.

[b] Plus symbol (+) means enriched by positive selection with indicated method or marker.

[c] Minus symbol (−) means depleted by negative selection.

erythrocytes, further removal of the latter (e.g. by hypotonic shock) is mandatory. If only a small number of cells needs to be isolated, whole blood can be directly fractionated by density gradient centrifugation. Discontinuous or continuous (linear or non-linear) gradients generated with Percoll silica particles (Amersham Pharmacia Biotech) are used to separate leucocyte populations into layers with different densities. However, to obtain a higher cell purity or to isolate cell types that are present only at low percentages in peripheral blood (e.g. eosinophils), magnetic cell sorting is a powerful tool (*Table 1*). With respect to preparing cells for chemotaxis assays, any reaction that activates the cells needs to be avoided. Positive selection by labelling cells with magnetic microbeads (MACS, Miltenyi Biotec) via monoclonal antibodies against cell-specific membrane markers does not affect the migratory capacity of most cell types. Alternatively, cell populations can also be enriched by negative selection by retaining the labelled cells on the column with a strong magnetic field. Taken together, by using a combination of the different isolation techniques, the purity of individual cell populations is usually higher than 80% and may be higher than 95%. As an example, the isolation of peripheral blood neutrophils is outlined in *Protocol 1*.

Protocol 1

Isolation of granulocytes from human peripheral blood

Equipment and reagents

- Fresh human blood
- Heparinized tubes
- Phosphate-buffered saline (PBS)
- Hydroxyethyl starch (Plasmasteril, Fresenius)
- Double-distilled water
- 0.6 M NaCl
- Hank's balanced salt solution (HBSS)
- Human serum albumin (HSA)
- Ficoll–sodium diatrizoate (Lymphoprep, Nycomed Pharma)
- Trypan Blue
- 50 ml measuring cylinder
- Standard cooled laboratory centrifuge

Method

1 Collect 10 ml of fresh human blood in a heparinized tube and dilute 1:2 in PBS.

2 Mix 20 ml of the diluted blood with 10 ml of hydroxyethyl starch and place in a cylinder for 30 min at 37 °C to allow the erythrocytes to sediment.

3 Collect the supernatant and centrifuge at 500 g for 8 min at 4 °C.

4 Resuspend the cell pellet in 24 ml of double-distilled water for 30 sec to lyse the remaining erythrocytes, then add 8 ml of 0.6 M NaCl and centrifuge at 500 g for 8 min at 4 °C.

5 Resuspend the cell pellet with 5 ml of HBSS, supplemented with 1 mg/ml of HSA.

6 Load the leucocyte suspension carefully on to 30 ml of the Ficoll–sodium diatrizoate solution and centrifuge for 30 min at 400 g (without brake).

7   Remove the interphase layer of mononuclear cells completely, collect and wash the cell pellet (this contains the granulocytes and remaining erythrocytes) with 20 ml of HBSS + HSA (500 g, 8 min, 4 °C).

8   Discard the supernatant and resuspend the cell pellet in 1 ml of HBSS. Determine the cell number (using the haemocytometer) and the cell viability (by Trypan Blue staining), dilute to the appropriate cell concentration (1×10^6 cells/ml, see *Table 2*) and use immediately in the chemotaxis assay (under agarose or in microchamber).

2.2 Preparation of test samples and standards for chemotaxis

Test samples can be prepared during the isolation of the cells used to measure chemotaxis. Since chemotactic factors, including naturally occurring chemokine isoforms, have a variable specific activity, samples should be tested at multiple dilutions (e.g. 0.5 $\log_{10}$ steps) to obtain titration curves. Moreover, when chemo-tactic substances are applied at doses above their optimum, a reduction in migration efficacy normally occurs, resulting in a bell-shaped, dose-response curve. A purified standard preparation should be included in each chemotaxis assay, because the minimal effective concentration can be variable, depending on the origin and viability of the test cells. The chemotactic agent formylmethionyl-leucyl-phenylalanine (fMLP) can be used as a standard. If the optimal dose of fMLP (e.g. 10^{-7} M) yields reproducible results in the chemotaxis assay, it might be better to test just a single dose with multiple replicates (e.g. in each agarose plate or microchamber) to verify variability between different plates or chambers in the same assay. For testing chemokines, preference should be given to the use of a purified standard preparation of the chemokine under investigation (e.g. the neutrophil-activating protein IL-8), which allows a better calculation of the potency of the test samples (in units or ng/ml). The use of the corresponding chemokine standard might be essential when test samples are weak in potency. Indeed, if compared to an optimal dose of fMLP, such samples may be recorded as negative, since fMLP often induces a more pronounced migration than chemokines. To increase the reproducibility of the chemotaxis results, the test compounds need to be assayed in triplicate, preferably in different agarose plates or microchambers. If dilution series are used, duplicate measurements should suffice, especially when large numbers of fractions are to be assayed. With regard to column fractions obtained during cytokine purification, it is essential that these are made physiological before use in the assay. This can be achieved either by dialysis or by sufficient dilution (if possible) in control buffer (HBSS).

3 Chemotaxis under agarose

This method for chemotaxis originally described by Nelson *et al.* (6, 7), uses the migration distance of cells under agarose as a parameter for measuring the chemotactic effect of cytokines. Since the assay can be performed in tissue culture dishes, the technique allows a large number of samples to be handled (e.g. column fractions from purification runs) and a fast microscopic score of their chemotactic potency. The agarose assay for chemotaxis is applicable to different leucocyte types. In our laboratory this technique has been successfully used in isolating two novel chemotactic cytokines, specific for neutrophils (IL-8) and monocytes (MCP-1), respectively (8, 9). The purity of the test cells determines the specificity of the test system and allows discrimination between these two activities. Since the preparation of the test cells often involves a time-consuming isolation and purification procedure (e.g. granulocytes from peripheral blood, *Protocol 1*) the reader is advised to prepare the agarose plates (*Protocol 2*) the day before the actual chemotaxis assay is performed.

Protocol 2

Preparation of agarose plates

Equipment and reagents

- Fetal calf serum (FCS)
- 10 × concentrated Eagle's minimum essential medium (EMEM) with Earle's salts and sodium bicarbonate
- Pyrogen-free distilled water
- Solution A (per 10 ml): 2 ml FCS, 2 ml of 10 × concentrated EMEM with Earle's salts and sodium bicarbonate, and 6 ml of pyrogen-free distilled water
- Agarose (Indubiose, IBF)
- 6 cm (inner diameter) plastic tissue culture dishes (Nunc)
- Stainless-steel punch with inside bevel and template
- Vacuum system
- CO_2 incubator

Method

1 Pre-warm (50 °C) 10 ml of solution A.

2 Boil 0.18 g agarose in 10 ml of distilled water until completely dissolved (15 min), and subsequently cool to 50 °C (solution B).

3 Mix equal volumes of A and B at 50 °C (solution AB).

4 Pour 6 ml solution AB into 6 cm (i.d.) plastic tissue culture dishes and allow to cool (30 min). Transfer to the refrigerator (4 °C) until further processing.

5 Cut six series (per dish) of three wells (3 mm i.d., 3 mm interspace) in the gel using a stainless-steel punch with an inside bevel and use a template to align the wells as shown in *Figure 1*.

6 Remove the agarose cores with a pipette attached to a vacuum line, and incubate the plates at 37 °C (1 h) in a CO_2 incubator until the samples and cells are prepared.

The final step in the preparation of the agarose plates, i.e. punching out the wells, is best postponed until immediately before the chemotaxis assay, since leakage of fluid from the gel into the wells should be prevented. When cutting

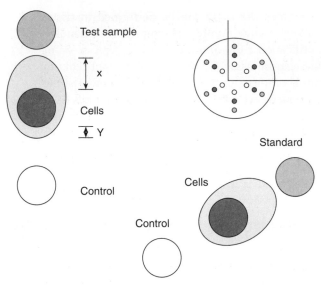

Figure 1 Chemotaxis under agarose. Well configuration: six series of three wells, each series containing a central well for cells and two surrounding wells for the test sample (or standard) and control medium, respectively. Cells migrate toward the chemotactic gradient of the test sample (distance X) and the control medium (random migration distance Y). $X - Y$ represents the effective migration toward the test sample.

the wells, care should be taken to avoid damaging the surface of the dish, because scratches in the plastic can inhibit cell migration. Also take care not to lift the gel or damage the wells when sucking out the punched cores. The configuration of cutting wells in an agarose plate (six series of three wells) allows six individual samples (standard included) to be tested in each plate according to the procedure described in *Protocol 3*.

Protocol 3

Chemotaxis assay under agarose

Equipment and reagents

- Agarose plates (see *Protocol 2* and *Figure 1*)
- Non-chemotactic medium (e.g. HBSS + 1 mg/ml HSA)
- Absolute methanol
- 37% formaldehyde
- May-Grünwald and Giemsa stains
- Humidified, 5% CO_2 incubator

Method

1   Fill the centre well of each series of three wells (see *Figure 1*) with 10 μl of cells, e.g. 3×10^5 neutrophils.

Protocol 3 continued

2   Add 10 μl of the control non-chemotactic medium and test-sample dilution to the inner and outer well, respectively.

3   Incubate the agarose plates for 2 h at 37 °C in a humidified CO_2 incubator.

4   Terminate the assay by adding absolute methanol (3 ml) to the agarose plates for 30 min at room temperature.

5   Fix the cells with 37% formaldehyde for 30 min.

6   Carefully remove the agarose (without rotating the gel) from the culture dish and stain the cells with May-Grünwald's and Giemsa's solutions.

7   Score the potency of the samples by counting the number of migrated cells or by measuring the effective migration distance (*Figure 1*).

The optimal incubation time needed to obtain a maximal migration distance under agarose depends on the cell type tested, monocytes requiring a longer period (3 h) than neutrophils (2 h). During incubation it is recommended that the actual migration distance is verified so that the assay can be stopped before the cells start to migrate into the well containing the test sample. A longer incubation time reduces the sensitivity of the assay, since further migration (towards the test-sample well) is stopped while spontaneous migration might still continue.

Quantifying the potency of the samples by microscopically measuring the migration distance is preferred, since counting the cells is more labour intensive. However, when single, supraoptimal doses are used, it should be kept in mind that the migration distance might remain suboptimal, whereas the number of migrated cells remains maximal. In addition, microscopic counting of cells might become essential when the cell isolation procedure did not provide a completely pure population. In practice, both the migration distance towards both the chemotactic sample (induced migration) and the control medium (random migration) are determined (*Figure 1*). The effective migration distance is calculated by subtracting the random migration (Y) from the induced migration distance (X). The potency of a sample tested at a single dilution can be expressed as percentage of the maximal effective migration distance of the internal standard. Preferably, the potency is expressed as a stimulation index, which is obtained by dividing the effective migration distance by the random migration distance $[(X - Y)/Y]$. If samples are tested at multiple dilutions, a titration endpoint can be calculated from the half-maximal effective migration distance or index. As a consequence, the potency of a chemotactic cytokine preparation can be expressed in biological units (U), 1 U/ml corresponding to the half-maximal effective migration distance or index obtained with an optimal dose of the internal chemokine standard. Alternatively, the specific activity and concentration of a sample containing a single chemokine can be expressed in ng/ml and U/mg, respectively, if assayed in direct comparison with a pure standard preparation of the same chemokine.

4 Chemotaxis through micropore filters

This method of chemotaxis is based upon the active migration of test cells through a filter with micropores of a precise size. The filter can be placed in a chamber to create two compartments as originally introduced by Boyden (5). Cells are added to the upper compartment, whereas the lower compartment is filled with the chemotactic substance. As a consequence, a chemotactic gradient is created and cells penetrate through the pores of the filter to the lower compartment. The number of migrated cells serves as a parameter to determine the potency of a chemotactic substance.

This assay system demands more sophisticated equipment than the agarose assay, but multiwell microchamber assemblies allowing rapid and accurate measurements can be obtained (10). A commercially available device commonly used to detect chemotactic cytokines is the 48-well chemotaxis chamber (*Figure 2*) from Neuroprobe. To increase the reproducibility of the assay it is recommended that samples are tested in triplicate wells within one chamber. The number of samples that can be tested per chamber therefore remains restricted, especially if dilution series are made.

The filter separating the two chamber compartments is the essential part of the test system. Depending on the cell type, different filter materials and pore sizes should be used (*Table 2*). Cellulose ester filters (150 μm thick) allow measurement of the migration depth of neutrophils (3–5 μm pores), monocytes (8 μm pores), or lymphocytes (8 μm pores) into the filter (11). Polycarbonate membranes are convenient when the number of migrated cells has to be determined (*Protocol 4*). For monocytes, polyvinyl pyrrolidone (PVP)-treated poly-

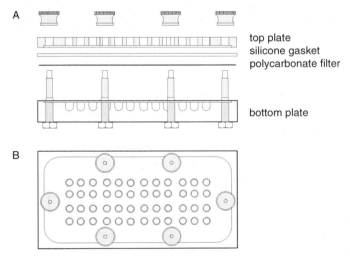

A

top plate
silicone gasket
polycarbonate filter

bottom plate

B

Figure 2 Schematic representation of the Neuroprobe 48-well chemotaxis chamber. The microchamber consists of a top and bottom acrylic plate, sealed by a silicone gasket. The upper wells (containing cells) are separated from the lower wells (containing chemoattractant) by the micropore membrane, in which the test cells migrate toward the chemotactic gradient. A, Side view; B, Top view.

Table 2 Conditions for the migration of various leucocyte cell types in the microchamber assay

Parameter	Cell population[a]					
	Neu	Eo	Ba	Mo	Ly	THP-1
Cell density (cells/ml)	10^6	10^6	2×10^6	2×10^6	10^7	2×10^6
Polycarbonate filter:						
Pore size (μm)	3–5	3–5	5	5–8	5	5
PVP treatment	—	—	—	+	—	+
Coating	—	—	—	—	+[b]	—
Incubation time (h)	0.75	1	1	2	4	2

[a] neu, neutrophils; eo, eosinophils; ba, basophils; mo, monocytes; ly, lymphocytes.

[b] Coating with fibronectin or collagen (type I or IV).

carbonate membranes with 5–8 μm pores are recommended, whereas PVP-free membranes (3–5 μm) should be used for neutrophils. To prevent migrated lymphocytes dropping through the pores to the bottom of the lower compartment, the lower surface of the PVP-free polycarbonate filter (5 μm) should be coated with collagen (type IV) or fibronectin (12). More recently, cultured cell lines such as monocytic THP-1 (*Table 2*) and lymphocytic SUP-T1 cells have successfully been used in the microchamber migration assay as an alternative to freshly isolated blood cells (13, 14). Although the response might be different from that of normal leukocytes (due to a different chemokine receptor expression pattern), these cell lines are very convenient in that the complicated leucocyte isolation procedure can be avoided and a higher reproducibility is usually obtained.

Protocol 4

Microchamber chemotaxis assay for monocytes

Equipment and reagents

- Fresh anticoagulated human peripheral blood
- Ficoll–sodium diatrizoate (Lymphoprep, Nycomed Pharma)
- PBS
- RPMI-1640
- HSA
- Trypan Blue
- Standard chemoattractant, e.g. monocyte chemotactic protein-1 (MCP-1)
- 48-well Neuro Probe microchamber *(Figure 2)*
- PVP-polycarbonate membrane (5 μm pore size, Nuclepore®, Corning)
- Hemacolor® solutions (Merck)
- Standard cooled laboratory centrifuge
- 5% CO_2 incubator

Method

1 Isolate mononuclear cells from fresh, anticoagulated human peripheral blood by centrifugation (400 g for 30 min at 4 °C, without break) on Ficoll–sodium diatrizoate (see *Protocol 1*).

2 Collect the mononuclear cells at the interphase and wash the cells twice with PBS, centrifuge at 200 g for 10 min at 4 °C.

3 Resuspend the cell pellet in HBSS plus 1 mg/ml HSA, determine the cell number and the viability with Trypan Blue, and dilute to 2×10^6 cells/ml.

4 Prepare serial dilutions of test samples and standard monocyte chemoattractant (e.g. MCP-1) in HBSS supplemented with 1 mg/ml of HSA.

5 Add 27 μl of the test samples to the lower compartments of the microchamber (*Figure 2*).

6 Put the PVP-polycarbonate membrane (5 μm pore size) on the bottom plate and reassemble the microchamber.

7 Add 50 μl of the mononuclear cell suspension to each well of the upper compartment.

8 Incubate the chamber for 2 h at 37 °C in a 5% CO_2 incubator to allow cell migration.

9 Undo the microchamber unit, wet the non-migrated cell side of the membrane with PBS, and wipe the cells off this filter side.

10 Fix and stain the cells which adhere to the lower surface of the membrane with Hemacolor® solutions, according to the manufacturer's instructions.

11 Rinse the membrane in water and place the membrane on a microscope slide to dry. Microscopically (400 × magnification) count the number of monocytes in 10 oil-immersion fields for each well.

If cellulose ester filters are used, the test samples can be evaluated by measuring the migration distance into the filter (leading-front assay), whereas with polycarbonate membranes the number of cells migrated through the pores has to be determined. The potency of a test sample is calculated from the average number of migrated cells (from triplicate wells for each dilution of the chemokine). Indeed, a variable and sharp, bell-shaped response curve is usually obtained for chemokines in this assay, resulting in a narrow optimal concentration range for each chemokine. The chemotactic activity can be expressed as a percentage of the maximal number of cells migrated to the optimal concentration of the reference chemoattractant, i.e. a pure preparation of a chemokine selectively attracting the leucocyte type under investigation. Alternatively, a chemotactic index can be calculated from the effective number of cells migrated to the test sample, divided by the number of cells migrated to the control medium. For the evaluation of the chemotactic potency of samples from stimulated cells, a supernatant of unstimulated cells should be run in parallel as a control.

5 *In vivo* leucocyte migration in response to cytokines

The biological relevance of chemotactic activities observed with cytokines *in vitro* can be demonstrated by their effect on cell mobilization *in vivo*. However, this approach involves specific expertise in, for example, histopathological techniques, radiolabelling of cells, or implantation of chambers (15). Although such *in vivo* techniques also suffer from low specificity and sensitivity they are a complementary adjunct to *in vitro* assays for unravelling the complexity of cytokine and chemokine interactions. An *in vivo* test designed to measure increased leucocyte infiltration in response to the intradermal injection of cytokines in rabbit skin has been successfully applied to chemokine research (16).

The sensitivity of this test for measuring the infiltration of neutrophils into skin can be increased by injecting the cytokine in combination with a vasodilator substance (e.g. PGE_2), allowing the detection of pmol amounts of IL-1, IL-8, and TNF. In addition, quantitation of this skin reactivity is facilitated by the use of radiolabelled neutrophils and albumin, resulting in the detection of cell accumulation and plasma protein extravasation. Such oedema formation serves as an additional parameter for local inflammation. Plasma leakage induced by certain cytokines (e.g. IL-8) is dependent on neutrophil emigration, since it is abolished when animals are made neutropenic (16). The specificity of the skin test can be enhanced by following the kinetics of the response to different cytokines. Indeed, it was observed that IL-8 elicited its skin reactivity faster than IL-1 (8). Similarly, upon intravenous injection, IL-1 causes a slower increase of the number of circulating granulocytes than IL-8 (8, 17).

Although previously reported to be chemotactic (18), pure IL-1 does not exert *in vitro* chemotactic activity for granulocytes (8). This discrepancy between the *in vivo* and *in vitro* effects of IL-1 on granulocytes can partly be explained by the finding that on cultured fibroblasts IL-1 is a potent inducer of granulocyte chemotactic proteins such as IL-8, and of monocyte chemotactic proteins, such as MCP-1 (*Table 3*). IL-8 and MCP-1 have been isolated from cell cultures with the help of the *in vitro* and *in vivo* chemotactic assays described here (8, 9). However, in view of the low specificity of these chemotactic assays it is essential to use purified test-cell populations and specific antibodies against each of these

Table 3 Induction of chemotactic factors by IL-1

Inducer		Production of chemotactic activity for[a]		
		Monocytes		Granulocytes
Type	Dose	Microchamber assay (%)[b]	Agarose test (%)[c]	Agarose test (%)[c]
IL-1β (U/ml)	100	70	59	51
	10	54	37	75
	1	62	15	24
	0.1	31	0	0
Unstimulated	—	15	0	0

[a] Monolayers of human fibroblasts were stimulated for 48 h with IL-1β.
[b] Percentage of the maximal number of effectively migrated monocytes to pure MCP-1 (*Protocol 4*).
[c] Percentage of effective maximal migration distance obtained with an optimal dose of pure MCP-1 or IL-8 (*Protocol 3*).

molecules in order to characterize the activity measured. The development of sensitive immunoassays in addition to bioassays is therefore crucial to detect these substances in body fluids.

Acknowledgements

The authors thank D. Brabants and C. Callebaut for excellent editorial help and R. Conings for the design of the figures. S. Struyf is a research assistant of the FWO-Vlaanderen.

References

1. Wuyts, A., Struyf, S., Proost, P., and Van Damme, J. (1999). In *The cytokine network and immune functions* (ed. J. Thèze), p. 125. Oxford University Press, Oxford.
2. Luster, A. D. (1998). *N. Engl. J. Med.*, **338**, 436.
3. Rollins, B. J. (1997). *Blood*, **90**, 909.
4. Zlotnik, A., Morales, J., and Hedrick, J. A. (1999). *Crit. Rev. Immunol.*, **19,** 1.
5. Boyden, S. (1962). *J. Exp. Med.*, **115**, 453.
6. Nelson, R. D., Quie, P. G., and Simmons, R. L. (1975). *J. Immunol.*, **115**, 1650.
7. Nelson, R. D. and Herron, M. J. (1988). In *Methods in enzymology*, Vol. 162 (ed. G. Di Sabato), p. 50. Academic Press, San Diego.
8. Van Damme, J., Van Beeumen, J., Opdenakker, G., and Billiau, A. (1988). *J. Exp. Med.*, **167**, 1364.
9. Van Damme, J., Decock, B., Lenaerts, J.-P., Conings, R., Bertini, R., Mantovani, A., and Billiau, A. (1989). *Eur. J. Immunol.*, **19**, 2367.
10. Falk, W., Goodwin, R. H., Jr, and Leonard, E. J. (1980). *J. Immunol. Meth.*, **33**, 239.
11. Wilkinson, P. C. (1988). In *Methods of enzymology*, Vol. 162 (ed. G. Di Sabato), p. 38. Academic Press, San Diego.
12. Larsen, C. G., Anderson, A. O., Appella, E., Oppenheim, J. J., and Matsushima, K. (1989). *Science*, **243**, 1464.
13. Struyf, S., De Meester, I., Scharpé, S., Lenaerts, J.-P., Menten, P., Wang, J. M., Proost, P., and Van Damme, J. (1998). *Eur. J. Immunol.*, **28**, 1262.
14. Proost, P., Struyf, S., Schols, D., Opdenakker, G., Sozzani, S., Allavena, P., Mantovani, A., Augustyns, K., Bal, G., Haemers, A., Lambeir, A.-M., Scharpé, S., Van Damme, J., and De Meester, I. (1999). *J. Biol. Chem.*, **274**, 3988.
15. Boyle, M. D. P., Lawman, M. J. P., Gee, A. P., and Young, M. (1988). In *Methods in enzymology*, Vol. 162 (ed. G. Di Sabato), p. 101. Academic Press, San Diego.
16. Rampart, M., Van Damme, J., Zonnekeyn, L., and Herman, A. G. (1989). *Am. J. Pathol.*, **135**, 21.
17. Van Damme, J., De Ley, M., Opdenakker, G., Billiau, A., and De Somer, P. (1985). *Nature*, **314**, 266.
18. Movat, H. Z. (1985). In *The inflammatory reaction* (ed. H.Z. Movat), p. 00. Elsevier, Amsterdam.

Chapter 7
Biological assays for haemopoietic growth factors

E. A. de Wynter, C. M. Heyworth, B. I. Lord, and
N. G. Testa
Paterson Institute for Cancer Research, Christie Hospital NHS Trust, Wilmslow Rd,
Manchester M20 4BX, UK

1 Introduction

The aim of this chapter is to summarize *in vitro* standard assays used to investigate the myeloid growth factors interleukin-3 (IL-3), granulocyte–macrophage colony-stimulating factor (GM-CSF), granulocyte colony-stimulating factor (G-CSF), macrophage colony-stimulating factor (M-CSF), and erythropoietin (Epo). Such methods are illustrated by experimental protocols using murine cells, and with selected examples using human bone-marrow cells.

Two primary approaches are used for the *in vitro* study of these factors. The first uses the clonal assays that first detected the CSFs, and then monitored their purification (1, 2). In these assays, in which cell proliferation is absolutely dependent on the continuous presence of CSFs, the progeny of single cells (colony-forming cells, CFC) are observed as colonies composed of haemopoietic cells (1). The second approach uses growth factor-dependent cell lines, which provide a quick method for their titration. Some of these are described here, while other cell line assays are described in Chapter 13, this volume.

The advantages of the clonal assays are:

(a) They are performed with freshly isolated haemopoietic cells, which are the physiological targets of these growth factors (1, 2).

(b) The CFC range from primitive multipotential cells, with extensive proliferation capacity (and some degree of self-renewal), to later cells committed to differentiation into one cell lineage, and which show a more restricted capacity for proliferation (1, 3, 4). Thus, the action of growth factors on a wide range of different populations of progenitor cells can be investigated (5, 6).

(c) They allow the study of the mature cells in the colonies and, thus, the influence of a given factor on the lineage along which CFC differentiate (1, 5–7).

(d) Purified subpopulations of CFC, and serum-free cultures, allow the distinction between the direct and indirect biological effects of the growth factor in primary cultures of haemopoietic cells (5, 8, 9). This type of information is particularly important for understanding the complex networks that regulate their proliferation and differentiation.

Factor-dependent cell lines provide quicker results than clonal assays for screening purposes (10). In addition, they offer the possibility of studying the mechanisms of action of the growth factor (11) in:

(a) promoting cell survival;

(b) stimulating proliferation;

(c) inducing differentiation; and

(d) inducing the functional activity of the mature cells.

Studies, similar to those performed with cell lines, are at present being undertaken using purified populations of CFC (9).

2 Preparation of cell suspensions

2.1 Murine bone marrow

Femora are the usual source of bone-marrow cells. For standard plating experiments, three femora are used to prepare a cell suspension as shown in *Protocol 1*.

Protocol 1

Preparation of a cell suspension from murine bone marrow

Equipment and reagents

- Mouse femora
- Sterile gauze
- Clean scissors
- Syringe
- 21-gauge and 25-gauge needles

- Culture medium
- Sterile container
- Microscope and haemocytometer or automatic cell counter

Method

1   Clean the dissected femora of muscle tissue by wiping with sterile gauze.

2   Cut the epyphysis with clean scissors.

3   Insert a 21-gauge needle attached to a syringe containing 1 ml of the culture medium, (preferably the same as to be used for culture) into the bone cavity.

4   Wash the bone cavity two or three times gently, but thoroughly, by flushing the medium up and down into a sterile container.

5   Change to a 25-gauge needle and aspirate gently to ensure breakdown to a single-cell suspension

6   Count the cells. Expect a yield of about $1.5–2.0 \times 10^7$ cells per femur.

2.1.1 Comments

For plating experiments, the cell suspension may be diluted to 5×10^5–10^6 cells/ml, or 10 × the cell concentration desired for plating. Although plating is usually performed as soon as the cells are ready, the cell suspensions can be kept on ice for 4–5 h without loss of cell viability of the CFC (3).

2.2 Human bone marrow

Protocol 2

Preparation of cell suspensions from human bone marrow

Equipment and reagents

- Human bone-marrow aspirates
- Sterile tubes
- Iscove's modified Dulbecco's medium (IMDM)
- Preservative-free heparin
- FCS
- Microscope and haemocytometer or automatic cell counter
- Centrifuge (MSE 3000I)

Method

1 Collect bone-marrow aspirates in sterile tubes containing 5–10 ml of Iscove's modified Dulbecco's medium (IMDM) plus 400 units of preservative-free heparin.

2 Centrifuge the cells at 800 g for 10 min RT. Discard the supernatant and resuspend the cells in IMDM plus 2% fetal calf serum (FCS), and mix gently by pipetting.

3 Count the cells and adjust the concentration as needed (see Protocol 1).[a]

4 Keep the cell suspensions on ice until plating.

[a] As the cellularity of bone-marrow aspirates varies with the pathology of the patient, and also with the aspiration technique, some judgement must be exercised about the volume used to resuspend the cells. Hypocellular marrow samples are resuspended in 1-2 ml, but usually 5-10 ml is used.

2.2.1 Comments

Sometimes the source of bone marrow is not a diagnostic aspirate, but marrow obtained from sections of ribs removed for access during surgery. Protocols for processing these samples may be found in ref. 12.

Caution: It is important to realize that **all** human bone-marrow samples are considered to be of potential risk (hepatitis virus, HIV, and other possible infective agents) and need to be handled with care. The use of appropriate laminar-flow cabinets, centrifuges which minimize aerosol contamination, the careful use (or avoidance when possible) of sharp instruments, the use of appropriate containers in transport, are essential precautions that **must** be undertaken. The legal requirements for safety at work are available in all laboratories. Careful reading of the required regulations and adequate instruction of the operators are essential requirements for working with clinical samples (3, 12).

2.3 Separation of excess red cells from human bone-marrow samples

This step is needed when it is judged that there is a large contamination with peripheral blood in the bone-marrow aspirate, or to separate the red cells in samples of peripheral blood and human umbilical cord blood.

Protocol 3

Separation of red cells from human bone marrow

Equipment and reagents

- Human bone-marrow aspirate
- Ficoll–Hypaque ($\rho = 1.077$ g/ml)
- Centrifuge
- Pipettes
- IMDM
- FCS

Method

1 Layer the bone-marrow aspirate on a volume ratio of 4 parts aspirate to 3 parts Ficoll–Hypaque slowly down the side of the tube (to avoid mixing) on top of a Ficoll–Hypaque preparation (density 1.077 g/ml).

2 Spin at 400 *g* for 30 minutes RT. Note that there should be a red pellet at the bottom of the tube, a clear layer of medium, a cloudy interface layer (with the cells to be harvested), and a plasma/medium layer on top.

3 Aspirate the interphase layer with a pipette (**never** mouth pipette, see Section 2.2.1) and discard the rest.

4 Suspend the cells in 10 ml of IMDM plus 2% FCS, and proceed as described in Section 2.2.

3 Standard clonal assays

3.1 Murine bone marrow

As an example, *Protocol 4* details the steps for the assay of Mix-CFC from murine bone marrow. This assay allows the growth of mixed colonies, which may contain several myeloid lineages (neutrophils, eosinophils. basophils, erythroid cells, monocytes–macrophages, and megakaryocytes), resulting from the clonal proliferation of Mix-CFC. In addition, pure erythroid colonies (progeny of burst-forming units—erythroid (BFU-E)) as well as colonies of neutrophilic granulocytes and macrophages (derived from GM-CFC), pure macrophage colonies (from M-CFC) or pure colonies of neutrophilic granulocytes (from G-CFC), eosinophils (from Eo-CFC), or megakaryocytes (from Meg-CFC) also grow. For further information, see ref. 13.

Protocol 4

Mix-CFC assay for murine bone marrow

Equipment and reagents

- Murine bone-marrow cells (see Protocol 1)
- 3 cm diameter Petri dishes (Falcon)
- 10% BSA (w/v) stock solution
- Growth factors or conditioned medium
- FCS (pre-tested, Flow or Gibco)
- 3.3% agar (w/v)

- Fully humidified gas incubator (5% CO_2 in air, or 5% CO_2 plus 5% O_2 in nitrogen)
- Microscope with zoom lens or an inverted microscope
- Pasteur pipettes
- Cytospin

Method

1 Using cells prepared in *Protocol 1*, adjust the cell concentration to 5×10^5/ml.

2 Make up the plating mixture as follows (this will give a final volume of 3.3 ml (to allow 0.3 ml for waste) when the agar is added in step 5):

	Volume (%)	For 3.3 ml
Cell suspension (10 × desired final cell concentration)	10	0.33
BSA (10% stock solution, see Sections 3.3.2(d))	10	0.33
Growth factors or conditioned medium	10	0.33
FCS (pre-tested, Flow or Gibco)	20	0.66
IMDM	40	1.32

3 Put the 3.3% agar into a boiling waterbath to melt, then allow to cool.

4 (Optional) While the agar is melting, warm the plating mixture to 37 °C in a water-bath to prevent the agar setting too quickly when added.

5 Add 0.33 ml of agar to the plating mixture, and mix thoroughly but gently. Plate 1-ml aliquots of this mixture (containing a total of 5×10^4 cells) into each of three 3-cm diameter Petri dishes.

6 Place the dishes on a tray and allow to set. Note that they will not set into a smooth gel at 37 °C, but they can be placed in a refrigerator for about 2 min to speed the process.

7 Put the plates into a fully humidified gas incubator at 37 °C. The gas mixture may be 5% CO_2 in air or 5% CO_2 plus 5% O_2 in nitrogen. (A low O_2 concentration may improve growth (3, 14).)

8 Incubate for 10 days.

9 Score the colonies under about 40 × magnification using a microscope with a zoom lens, or an inverted microscope.

10 Pick up individual colonies for cytological examination using a Pasteur pipette. Suspend the colonies in 0.1 ml of medium (plus a source of protein, either 1% serum or 0.1% BSA) for standard cytospin preparations.

Protocol 4 continued

11 Vary the conditions to select for the growth of discrete populations of murine CFC
   (13):
   - omit Epo if erythroid growth is not desired;
   - omit BSA when growing GM-CFC, G-CFC, and M-CFC (it is not an essential reagent);
   - score granulocytic colonies after 7 days for best results;
   - score colonies derived from relatively mature erythroid progenitors (CFU-E) after
     2 days' incubation—they may disappear later (3). Note that these colonies only
     need 0.2 units of Epo/ml.

3.2 Human bone marrow or peripheral blood

Basically similar conditions to those for murine bone marrow are used, but 7
days of incubation are required for CFU-E, 9–14 days for GM-CFC, and 14 days
for BFU-E and Mix-CFC. The main modification that may be needed is when the
cells are recovered for cytogenetic examination (14–16). Good chromosome
preparations have not been obtained when the matrix used for colony growth is
agar. Therefore, methylcellulose (viscosity 4000 c.p.s., Dow Chemicals) is used as
a 2.7% stock solution in IMDM (different batches may vary in viscosity, and concentrations should be tested for every batch). A detailed protocol for its preparation may be found in ref. 12. Volumes of the plating mixture in *Protocol 4*
are adjusted to allow a 50–50 mix of the stock methylcellulose preparation and
the rest of the culture components.

3.3 General comments

3.3.1 Factors and CFC

The CFU-E are the progenitor cell populations most sensitive to Epo, and therefore
are the choice population of CFC to study its effects (17). Earlier erythroid progenitors (BFU-E) need other factors (IL-3 or GM-CSF) to enable their proliferation
before Epo becomes essential for further progression and maturation along the
erythroid lineage. Multipotential Mix-CFC will proliferate in response to IL-3 and, to
a lesser extent, GM-CSF, while the bipotential GM-CFC will respond to GM-CSF. The
progenitors with the most restricted differentiation potential, G-CFC and M-CFC,
will respond preferentially to their respective lineage-specific stimulators, G- or M-
CSF (1, 2). These factors also interact to produce additive or potentiating effects on
colony growth (5, 6, 18). Other factors not covered in this chapter (e.g. stem-cell
factor (SCF), IL-1, IL-6, Tpo) also have additive or potentiating effects (12, 13).

3.3.2 Technical comments and possible problems

Possible problems may be encountered at each step in a culture protocol:

(a) Concentrated cell suspensions, or those with numerous red cells, may con-
    tain cell aggregates. To plate single-cell suspensions, cell aggregates must be
    dispersed by gentle pipetting.

(b) Two main precautions should be taken with synthetic culture medium. Even after preparing a stock according to the manufacturer's instructions, it should be checked that the osmolality is 280–300 mOsmol for murine cells (19) and 300 for human cells (3). Freshness of the medium is also essential. Storage at 4 °C for more than 2 weeks is discouraged (20).

(c) Every batch of serum should be pre-tested before use (see Section 4.1). Sometimes it is necessary to screen several batches to find one that supports adequate growth. Serum may be kept frozen at −20 °C for about a year. Thawed aliquots should be used within 2 weeks.

(d) BSA (Grade V, Sigma) also needs to be pre-tested. Deionized solutions should be used. Detailed protocols are found in ref. 3. Stock solutions may be kept frozen at –20 °C for about a year, aliquoted in convenient volumes to avoid repeated thawing and freezing.

(e) The main problems encountered in incubators are drying of cultures and temperature gradients. An increase in temperature of 0.1 °C over 37 °C may be critical, but decreases are better tolerated. Excessive opening of the incubator or excessive gas flow may contribute to dryness, resulting in poor growth.

4 Serum-free cultures

4.1 General comments

The assay of murine myeloid progenitor cells is usually performed in a soft-gel medium supplemented with either FCS or horse serum (HS). The variation in plating efficiencies achieved with different batches of sera can be enormous, and it is necessary to test each batch prior to the purchase of large quantities to maintain a consistent standard. This variation in batches of serum indicates that they contain varying levels of agents capable of modulating myeloid cell development. The development of a serum-free medium, which supports colony formation, overcomes the difficulties that the additions of unknown factors to colony-forming assays might cause, and eliminates the need for serum pre-testing. The use of serum-free media introduces a greater degree of certainty into experimental procedures employed to determine the relative effects of cytokines on myeloid progenitor-cell development (12, 13). Good commercial preparations of pre-tested serum-free media are now available (for example from StemCell Technologies and BioWhittaker).

4.2 Preparation of the reagents

The so-called serum-free medium (8) is generally prepared by adding a number of constituents to IMDM. A fully detailed protocol of the method is described elsewhere (13).

4.3 Preparation of serum-free medium

The solutions described in *Table 1* can be employed as substitutes for serum in the mixed colony-forming assay described above (*Protocol 4*). In these assays, serum-free medium constitutes 1 ml of the total volume of 3.3 ml.

Table 1 Supplements for serum-free cultures

Reagent	Volume (μl)	Final concentration
BSA	330	10 mg/ml
Soya bean lipids	42	25 μg/ml
Cholesterol	33	7.8 μg/ml
Linoleic-acid	33	5.6 μg/ml
Sodium pyruvate	33	1 mM
L-Glutamine	33	2 mM
α-thioglycerol	33	100 μM
Transferrin	33	300 μg/ml
Iscove's medium	430	

Further additions of other reagents such as haemin (final concentration 200 μM) can be made by adjusting the volume of Iscove's medium that is added to make the total volume up to 1 ml.

4.4 Comments

Highly purified natural or recombinant growth factors must be used for serum-free, colony-forming assays. This is because the crude conditioned-medium preparations of haemopoietic growth factors that are frequently employed in such assays will often contain serum or other impurities. Dose-response relationships for growth factor-stimulated colony formation are sometimes different from those seen in serum-containing assays, which must be accounted for in experimental design. Although colony formation may take slightly longer in serum-free cultures, the maximal plating efficiency achieved is generally equal to, if not greater than, that seen in serum-containing cultures.

5 Growth factor-dependent cell lines

A number of haemopoietic growth factor-dependent cell lines exist which can be employed to give an indication of the concentration and type of growth factor present in biological preparations (10). Some of those frequently used are listed in *Table 2*. Others are described in Chapter 13 (this volume). It should, however,

Table 2 Examples of cell lines dependent on haemopoietic growth factors for proliferation

Cell line	Growth factor-dependence
FDCP-1	IL-3, GM-CSF
FDCP-2	IL-3
32DCL23	IL-3, G-CSF
BAC1.2F5	M-CSF, GM-CSF
DAI	GM-CSF
NFS-60	GM-CSF
MI	G-CSF
J774	M-CSF

be noted that antibody-based assays are often available to unequivocally identify specific growth factors (see Chapter 12, this volume).

To establish whether a specific growth factor is present in a solution, and to determine its approximate concentration, follow *Protocol 5*.

Protocol 5

Biological assay for growth factors

Equipment and reagents

- Cells in suspension
- Benchtop centrifuge with swing-out rotor
- Culture medium
- Fischer's medium (Gibco)
- Horse serum
- Trypan Blue (Northumbria Biologicals)
- GF/C filters (Whatman)
- Isotonic [^{3}H] thymidine Sp Act 555 GBq/mmol concentration 3.7 MBq/ml
- Millipore cell harvester or similar apparatus
- 10% trichloroacetic acid (w/v)
- Liquid scintillation counter

Method

1   Culture cells in suspension until they reach an exponential growth rate.

2   Harvest by spinning at 800 g for 5 min in a bench centrifuge using a swing-out rotor.

3   Resuspend the cell pellet in the appropriate medium, centrifuge again. Repeat twice more.

4   Resuspend the cells at a concentration of 1–2×10^6/ml in Fischer's medium (Gibco-plus glutamine) plus horse serum (10% (v/v)) and plate out in a total volume of 100 μl. Seed the cells at trial concentrations of 1–2×10^5 cells/ml with either dilutions of the preparation under test or dilutions of a standard preparation of the appropriate growth factor. The final concentration of horse serum (or if the cells are normally cultured in it, fetal calf serum) should be 10–20% (v/v). Incubate the cells in a gassed CO_2 in air incubator at a temperature of 37 °C.

5   After 24 or 48 h assess the effects of the growth factors on survival and proliferation using the Trypan Blue assay, in which the cell suspension is mixed 1:1 with Trypan Blue solution and those (viable) cells excluding dye counted.

6   A second method for assessing proliferation (DNA synthesis) involves the measurement of [^{3}H] thymidine incorporation. After 24 or 48 h add 10 μl [^{3}H] thymidine to each well and continue the incubation for 4 h. Remove the cells from the incubator and serially transfer them to GF/C filters on a Millipore cell harvester or similar apparatus. Wash the cells three times with trichloroacetic acid (10% (w/v), 5 ml) and count the TCA-precipitable material retained on the filter in a liquid scintillation counter.

7   Compare the relative growth-promoting activities of the standard and the diluents of the preparation under test to quantify the growth-promoting activity in the sample.

6 Enrichment of progenitor-cell populations from murine bone marrow

6.1 General comments

Progenitor cells exist in very small numbers: the pluripotent cells representing about 0.4% of the total bone-marrow cells, and the more restricted committed progenitors being perhaps 2–3% of the population. Therefore to study the direct effects of growth factors on progenitor cells, it is desirable to enrich the concentration of the appropriate cells. Historically, cells are separated by physical parameters—density and size—and these properties are incorporated into modern techniques, which employ electronic sorting of cells tagged with fluorescent molecules or a process of continuous-flow centrifugal elutriation. It is these two processes that will be outlined. The numbers of animals and/or cells used will be stated merely as a guide to the convenient and practical handling of a sort. They may of necessity vary with specific practical requirements.

Protocol 6

Density gradient separation and FACS sorting of murine bone-marrow cells

Equipment and reagents

- Stock solutions of metrizamide (Nygaard, Oslo)
- High-density stock *Solution A* ($\rho_A \sim 1.10$ g/ml) and low-density stock *Solution B* ($\rho_B \sim$ 1.06 g/ml). Dissolve 21 g and 11 g of metrizamide powder, respectively, in 42 ml and 64 ml of Hanks' balanced salt solution, buffer with Hepes (pH 6.7). In each case, add 1 g BSA and make up the volumes to 100 ml with double-distilled water.
- Fluoresceinated wheat-germ agglutinin (WGA-FITC, Polysciences Inc.). Store at −20 °C in 15 μl aliquots (15 μg) aliquots.
- 1 mg/ml rhodamine-123 in double-distilled water. Use fresh.
- PBS

- Fischer's medium (Gibco, plus glutamine)
- FHS (Fischer's medium plus 10% horse serum)
- 0.2 M *N*-acetyl-D-glucosamine (NADG). Store frozen.
- Equipment and reagents for harvesting bone-marrow cells from murine femora (see Protocol 1)
- Laminar-flow hood
- 15 ml tubes
- 5 ml *glass* tubes
- Needles
- Centrifuge
- Pipettes or syringes and needles
- FACS system

A. Measurements and adjustments to stock metrizamide solutions

1 Adjust pH to 6.5 ± 0.1 osmolality.

2 Adjust to 300 ± 10 mOsmol of stock solutions A and B.

3 Measure the density (density meter or bottle) at 4 °C to 3 decimal places.

Protocol 6 continued

4 Filter-sterilize through 0.45 μm filtration units.

5 Store stock solutions A and B at −20 °C in 10–20 ml aliquots.

6 For 1-step density cut, mix solutions A and B to give a density of 1.080 ± 0.001 g/ml (maintain all solutions at 4 °C). Thus: to 10 ml of metrizamide solution B add x ml of metrizamide solution A:

$$x = \frac{1.080 - \rho_B}{\rho_A - 1.080} \times 10$$

B. FACS sorting

NB: All solutions and cell suspensions should be maintained at 4 °C.

1 Remove and clean the femora from 20 mice. Operating under a laminar-flow hood, flush the marrow into 7 ml of metrizamide solution B. (Yield $\geq 4 \times 10^8$ cells.)

2 Add 15 μl of WGA-FITC and mix thoroughly.

3 Place 3 ml of metrizamide ($\rho = 1.080$ g/ml) in a 15 ml tube. Holding the tube at 45°, carefully layer 1 ml of the cell suspension (max. of 5×10^7 cells) on to the surface of the metrizamide by trickling it down the wall of the tube. Run six tubes in this way.

4 Break the sharp partition between the cells and the metrizamide by stirring gently with a needle point.

5 Centrifuge at 1000 g for 15 min at 4 °C. Use minimum braking force on the centrifuge to minimize gradient disturbance.

6 Collect the band of low density ($\rho \sim 1.080$ g/ml) cells from the interface using a pipette or syringe and needle.

7 Wash once in Fischer's medium, centrifuging at 800 g for 10 minutes at 4 °C.

8 Resuspend the cell pellet in 4 ml of PBS and count the cells. (Yield: 2×10^7 cells.)

9 Transfer to the FACS. Note that the detailed running of this instrument is beyond the scope of this chapter. It is recommended that an experienced operator is available.

10 Set the pre-sterilized FACS to record forward-angle light-scatter (FSC: proportional to the cell size) and right-angle or side, light-scatter (SSC: proportional to the heterogeneity of the cellular contents). Run a few thousand cells through the instrument to establish their distribution as illustrated in Plate 1a (Gates 1, 2, and 3 illustrate the major cell groups delineated by the light-scatter characteristics of normal bone marrow).

11 Define a new window (gate G1 in Plate 1b) to exclude very small cells (residual erythrocytes and approximately 50% of the lymphocytes) and cells with high side-scatter (mainly maturing granulocytic cells and monocyte/macrophage cells).

12 Switch the FACS to record the fluorescence in the cells selected by step 11 above. Plate lc shows the distribution, together with a further window set to detect cells showing the greatest affinity for WGA (G2).

13 Put 4 ml of FHS into a 5 ml glass tube, wetting the inside of the tube to the top. This is to prevent the film of cells directed into the tube from drying. Place the tube

Protocol 6 continued

below one of the deflection plates of the sorter, start the flow (~ 3000 cells/sec) and collection of the cells in the window defined.

14 On completion of the sort (~ 2–3 h, yielding ~ 10^6 cells), centrifuge the cells (10 min at 800 g, 4 °C) and resuspend the pellet in 1 ml of PBS.

15 Re-sort the cells at 300 cells/sec using the same selection parameters. The final yield (~10^5 cells) can contain better than 90% of *in vivo* CFC and these are now ready for assay. WGA-FITC is not toxic to either the multipotent cells assayed by the spleen-colony technique (21) or to committed progenitor cells assayed as *in vitro* colony-forming cells (see above). For use in growth-factor assays, however, its presence may complicate interpretation and it can be removed as follows.

16 Centrifuge the collected cells and resuspend the pellet in 5 ml of NADG. Incubate for 15 min at 37 °C.

17 Centrifuge and resuspend as required for assays or further sorting. **NB:** To select the more primitive WGA$^+$, Rh-123 dull progenitors, it is necessary at step 12 to open the collection window to receive all WGA-positive cells.

18 Mix 0.1 ml of the Rh-123 solution with 1 ml of the cell suspension (at 10^7 cells/ml).

19 Incubate for 20 min at 37 °C then centrifuge (10 min at 800 g).

20 Resuspend the cell pellet in fresh medium and incubate for 15 min at 37 °C.

21 Wash twice by centrifugation in PBS and resuspend for further FACS analysis.

22 On the FACS instrument, set the fluorescence window to exclude the Rh-123 positive cells and collect those with dull labelling only.

6.2 Murine cells

6.2.1 FACS sorting for *in vivo* multipotent and *in vitro* committed CFC

The essence of this method is to label the appropriate cells with a fluorescent marker, to carry out a preliminary density selection, then to sort the cells using a flow cytometer on the basis of their size, cellular heterogeneity, and fluorescence intensity. The fluorescent markers generally used are fluoresceinated wheat-germ agglutinin (WGA-FITC), which binds selectively mainly to multipotent and some committed progenitors, and rhodamine-123 (Rh-123), which is incorporated by the more mature elements of the WGA-selected cells. Hence the more primitive (stem) progenitors are designated as WGA+ Rh-123 dull cells.

For further reading on this technique, including extended sorting with rhodamine-123, see refs 9 and 21–26. It is also possible to use immunological markers to select for early progenitors (27–29). For example, a commonly used combination of antibodies (CD5, CD45R, CD11b, Gr1, and TER 119) eliminates maturing cells by negative selection of cells labelled with a mixture of specific lineage markers (lin⁻) (see *Figure 1*). Further purification of primitive cells may be achieved by positive selection of cells labelled with specific markers, e.g. Sca 1

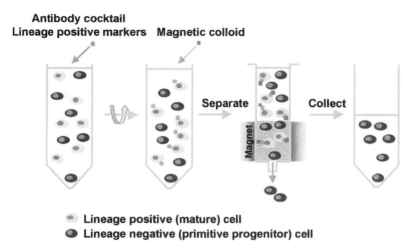

Figure 1 Enrichment of primitive progenitors using negative selection to isolate lineage-negative cells.

Table 3 Phenotype of mouse stem and progenitor cells

	LTRC	LTC-IC	Progenitors (late)
CD34	−	+	+
Sca-1	+	+	−
CD90 (Thy-1)	?	Low	Low
CD117 (*c-kit*)	Low	?	?
Lineage markers	−	−	+
WGA	+		
Rhodamine	Low		Low

LTRC, long-term repopulating cell (marrow repopulating ability); LTC-IC, long-term culture—initiating cell; Sca, stem-cell antigen; WGA, wheat-germ agglutinin.

antibody: to give a selection for the Sca 1^+Lin$^-$ population. The phenotype of mouse stem and progenitor cells is outlined in *Table 3*.

6.2.2 Centrifugal elutriation for *in vitro* committed CFC

The protocol outlined below is developed from that reported by Williams *et al.* (30) who obtained highly enriched populations of GM-CFC containing little contamination with other committed progenitors (BFU-E, Mix-CFC, Meg-CFC). A preliminary density selection is followed by elutriation according to cell size. A Beckman centrifuge with the JE-6B elutriation rotor is used. The reagents and density separation methods are as described in the FACS protocol above (*Protocol 6*).

6.2.3 Use of the elutriator for *in vivo* CFC

Multipotent progenitor cells may also be enriched using the elutriator (31). Animals must first be primed by thiamphenicol and bleeding, after which the spleen becomes highly enriched in these progenitors. The elutriation procedure is carried out as above, collecting fractions in the range of 12 to 16 ml/min flow rates. Low-density cells (≥ 1.079 g/ml) subsequently separated from this fraction contain spleen CFC at 50–100% purity. This method is particularly useful for high cell-number yields, but the CFC obtained are less primitive than those obtained by FACS analysis.

Protocol 7

Centrifugal elutriation

Equipment and reagents

- Reagents and density separation system as *Protocol 6*
- Fischer's medium (Gibco plus 2 mM glutamine)
- Cyclophosphamide dissolved in physiological saline (200 mg/ml dose)
- Mice
- Beckman centrifuge with a JE-6B elutriation rotor, chamber, and pumping system
- Horse serum
- 70% ethanol

Method

1 Inject 20 mice intraperitoneally (i.p.) with 200 mg/kg cyclophosphamide dissolved in physiological saline.

2 On the 4th day (e.g. Tuesday to Friday) post-injection, remove the femora and suspend the marrow in 10 ml of Fischer's medium with added glutamine. Centrifuge at 800 g for 10 min at 4 °C.

3 Remove 9 ml of the supernatant and resuspend the cell pellet in the remaining supernatant.

4 Add 1 ml of the low-density metrizamide (B solution) and mix.

5 Layer the cells on two tubes of metrizamide at $\rho = 1.080$ g/ml at 4 °C. (For the density separation procedure see under FACS Protocol 6, steps 3–8, above.) Collect low-density cells from the interface and wash once in Fischer's medium. Centrifuge for 10 min, 800 g, 4 °C.

6 Resuspend the cell pellet in 3 ml of Fischer's medium. (Starting with 20 mice this should yield $\sim 2 \times 10^7$ cells.)

NB: For the elutriation process from this stage, use FHS (Fischer's medium containing 5% HS) which should be at 4 °C at the start of elutriation. The elutriation rotor, chamber, and pumping system should be set up as described in the manual, sterilized with 70% ethyl alcohol, and thoroughly washed with sterile Fischer's medium prior to starting stage 2. After use it should again be cleaned and both the rotor and chamber dismantled and dried.

7 Load the 3 ml of cells directly into the 50 ml loading chamber (see the manufacturer's manual for details of the elutriator operating procedure) and flush the cells into the elutriator rotor with FHS at a flow rate of 10 ml/min. Collect 10 ml of effluent and switch the flow of FHS to bypass the loading chamber.

8 Increase the flow rate sequentially to 14, 16.5, 19.5 ml/min, collecting 100 ml for each fraction. (These fractions may be collected together and discarded.)

9 Collect further 100 ml fractions, sequentially increasing the flow rate to 22, 25.5, 29, 32 ml/minute. These may again be collected cumulatively and together represent the GM-CFC-rich fraction. Together this should yield $2-6 \times 10^6$ cells with a 7–14 day colony plating efficiency in agar with IL-3, CSF-1, or GM-CSF of 20–50%. **NB:** collecting the fractions sequentially and pooling gives a cleaner sort than collecting all four together at the highest flow rate.

10 Finally, maintaining the flow rate at 32 ml/min, switch off the centrifuge and collect the cells that have sedimented in the chamber. If sorting for GM-CFC, these also may be discarded.

6.3 Human cells

6.3.1 General comments

Like the murine stem cells, human haemopoietic progenitor cells exist in very small numbers. The CD34 antigen is expressed on haemopoietic colony-forming and stem cells, but is absent on more mature blood cells. These CD34+ progenitor cells occur at a frequency of 0.5–4% in bone marrow, 0.05–0.2% in steady-state peripheral blood, and 0.1–2% in cord blood. A number of techniques have been developed to enrich or purify the CD34 population utilizing either physical characteristics (centrifugal elutriation) or immunological characteristics (immunoadsorption) (see *Table 4*). Performance varies in terms of purity, yield, and enrichment of CFC. FACS sorting permits the separation of any population or subpopulation of cells by combining both physical and immunological parameters. As cells labelled with a fluorescent marker pass through a laser beam, they are examined individually and can be characterized based on fluorescence intensity, size, cell density, and the nucleocytoplasmic ratio. Highly purified populations are obtained with this method.

6.3.2 Immunoadsorption methods

These methods are commonly used as an alternative to FACS sorting. In negative-selection methods, cells are labelled with antibodies and the unlabelled cells

Table 4 Commercially available systems used for enrichment of CD34 cells

System	Supplier
Fluorescence-activated cell sorting (FACS)	
(a) Panning	AIS
(b) Affinity column chromatography	CellPro
(c) Adsorption on ferromagnetic beads	
– Large beads	Dynal and Baxter
– Middle-size beads	Immunotech
– Microbeads	MIltenyi Biotech
Negative selection with lineage markers	StemCell Technologies

Table 5 CD34+ cell enrichment using different separation techniques

Technique	Total MNC recovery (%)	Purity of CD34+ cells (%)	Yield of CD34+ cells (%)	CFC enrichment (*x*-fold)
FACS ($n = 23$)	1.4	71.2	38.3	30
CELLector ($n = 11$)	1.4	32.5	23.0	17
Dynabeads ($n = 11$)	0.6	28.4	4.9	14
CELL-PRO ($n = 5$)	1.1	76.8	36.8	45
MiniMACS ($n = 12$)	1.4	76.6	62.6	104

n, Number of experiments.

collected, whereas for positive selection the target cells are labelled and collected. For example, in a typical positive-selection procedure mononuclear cell (MNC) fractions may be labelled with a CD34 antibody and the labelled target cells then adsorbed to antibody-coated beads, flasks, or retained on columns. Unwanted cells are removed and target cells detached, collected, and assessed for purity. Results obtained in our laboratory using five of these positive selection methods are shown in *Table 5*. (For further reading on the use of these systems see ref. 32.)

6.3.3 Comments on the advantages and disadvantages of the systems

These are all procedures relying on the CD34 monoclonal antibody–antigen interaction. Different CD34 monoclonal antibodies are used in the different methods. With each system it is important to follow the manufacturer's directions, particularly concerning sample preparation. The preparation method may vary if human umbilical cord blood or cells from leukopheresis harvests are used.

- CELLector flasks (AIS uses clone ICH-3). Some progenitor cells are lost in the first stage of this process on the soya-bean agglutinin flasks. However, the flasks are sterile, tissue culture flasks and are easily manipulated. The capacity of the system is restricted to 2×10^7 cells/T25 flask unless the large-scale T150 flasks are used. In our hands MNC from cord blood do not perform well in this system.

- Immunomagnetic CD34-conjugated beads (DYNAL uses clone 561). Again sterility can be maintained in this system, but it does require some expertise to obtain good results. There have been problems with detaching the cells from the beads, although the use of the DETACHaBEAD reagent appears to have reduced this problem. Do not start with less than 5×10^7 MNC.

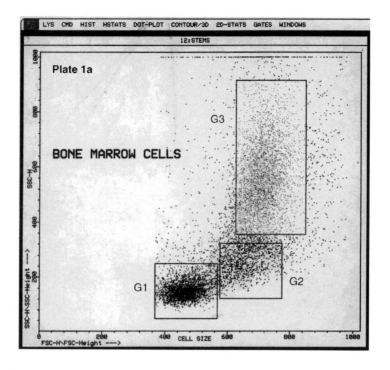

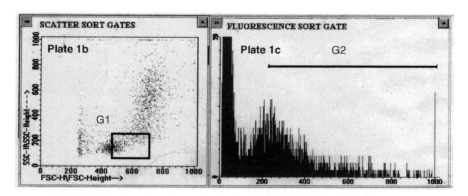

Plate 1 (a) Dot plot light-scatter analysis showing the major white blood cell types found in bone marrow. Gate 1 (G1) contains mainly granulocytes together with multipotent progenitor cells. Gate 2 (G2) contains mainly cells with distinctive developing cell-lineage characteristics together with the remaining multipotent progenitors. Gate 3 (G3) contains mainly the more mature granulocytic cells and the monocyte/macrophages. (b) Dot plot, light-scatter picture and some maturing cells. (c) Fluorescence histogram of cells selected in G1. The G2 gate includes cells with strong WGA affinity and is selected for collection as multipotent progenitor cells. It excludes virtually all of the lymphocyte population.

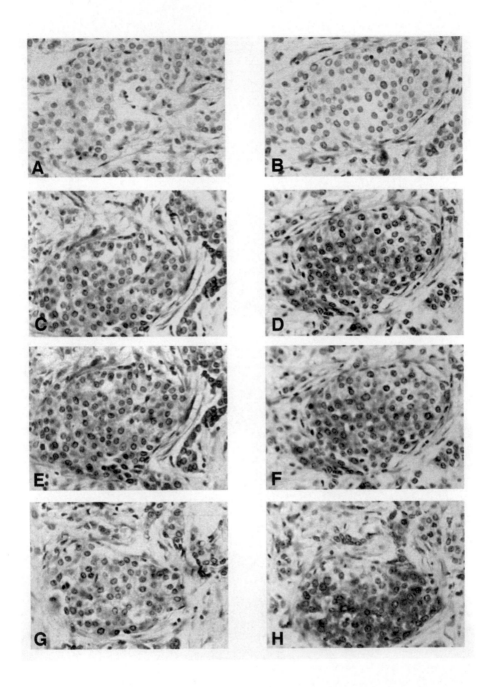

Plate 2 Comparison of the sensitivity of the standard peroxidase method (A, C, E, and G) and the high-sensitivity Catalyzed Signal Amplification System (CSA) system (B, D, F, and H) to detect VEGF protein (see here as a brown colour reaction) in sequential sections of a breast carcinoma exposed to no (A, B; negative controls), 20 µg/ml (C, D), I µg/ml (E, F), or 0.2 µg/ml (G, H) of monoclonal anti-VEGF antibody. At the lower end of the antibody concentration range (G, H), only the CSA method continues to clearly localize VEGF.

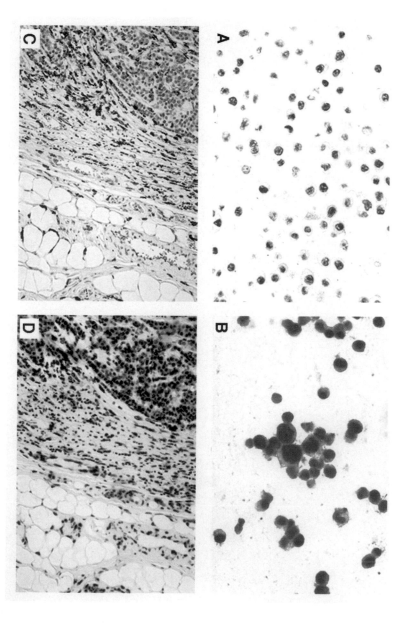

Plate 3 Localization (seen here as a brown colour reaction) of VFGF mRNA in a wax section of a breast carcinoma using non-isotopic, *in situ* hybridization (D). The specificity of this protocol was demonstrated using wax-embedded sections of MCF-7 cells stably transfected to express high levels of VEGF$_{165}$. These were exposed to either a negative control (i.e. sense probe) (A) or the corresponding anti-sense (B) oligo-probe for VEGF. CD68-positive macrophages were localized in a sequential section of the same breast carcinoma by immunohisto-chemistry (C). Both tumour cells and macrophages (and occasional endothelial cells in capillaries) were seen to express detectable levels of VEGF mRNA in such tissues.

- Immunomagnetic beads (MILTENYI-Isolation Kit uses QBEND 10). Good capacity and up to 2×10^8 cells can be processed on the MiniMACS column. Care must be exercised when preparing the sample as the column may become blocked if the sample contains large numbers of red cells or platelets. Aim for a good single-cell suspension. This system is easy to use, yields good enrichment of CFC with high purity of CD34+ cells (after two cycles). Highly purified populations of CD34 cells can be obtained in 1 h.

- Immunoaffinity columns (CELLPro-Kit uses clone 12.8). Excellent capacity and up to 5×10^8 cells can be processed with each column. However, the performance of this system is reduced if cord blood cells are used, probably due to the large numbers of red cells even after density gradient centrifugation. In addition, there may be problems associated with the biotinylated antibody, which, in our hands, loses affinity for the target cells after storage at 4 °C.

Note which antibody is used in the separation procedure as the same one *cannot* be used in the analysis. This is of particular importance if enzymatic methods have been used for detaching cells, as the antigen may be destroyed (see ref. 32).

6.3.4 FACS sorting of CD34-positive cells

Mononuclear cells are labelled with a CD34 antibody directly conjugated to a fluorochrome, and the cells sorted by flow cytometry. Generally, sorting speeds used are 4–5000 cells/sec. Nevertheless, if 5×10^7 cells are to be sorted, this can take up to 4 h. To reduce the time taken to sort cells, any of the systems outlined above may be used as a pre-enrichment step. We routinely use the MACS system that yields enriched populations in 1 h.

Protocol 8

Labelling cells for FACS sorting with the CD34 antibody

Equipment and reagents

- IMDM/2% FCS (Iscove's modified Dulbecco's medium plus 2% fetal calf serum)
- PBS/1% BSA
- 5 ml sterile tubes
- Screw-top 15 ml centrifuge tubes—conical bottom

Method

NB: Avoid capping of the antibody on the cell surface by working quickly and maintaining all solutions at 4 °C.

1   Prepare cell suspensions from bone marrow or other sources (using either *Protocol 2* or *3*) and enriched populations of CD34+ cells obtained using the MACS system or other enrichment protocols.

2   Decide the total number of cells in the suspension to be labelled with the CD34 antibody.

Protocol 8 continued

3 Suspend these cells in PBS/1% BSA at a concentration of 10^7 cells/ ml.

4 Remove a small aliquot of cells to serve as a control by labelling with a matched isotype-control antibody. Add the appropriate CD34 antibody to the remaining cells and incubate for 20 minutes at 4–12 °C. (The quantity of antibody to be used is predetermined by titration.) (See ref. 32.)

5 Wash the cells once with 3–4 ml of PBS/1% BSA and resuspend in the same buffer at a concentration not exceeding 5×10^6 cells/ml.

6 Prepare two 5 ml tubes containing IMDM/2% FCS for collection of the sorted cells.

7 Maintain on ice ready for cell sorting.

6.3.5 Comments

If MNC suspensions are to be sorted then proceed as outlined above, taking care to remove as many red cells as possible prior to labelling and to retain a portion of these cells as a negative control. If required, these cells can be labelled with an isotype-matched control antibody conjugated with the same fluorochrome.

If subpopulations are required, e.g. CD34/38/33, it is possible to label with more than one antibody simultaneously, providing they are all *directly* conjugated to different fluorochromes. *Table 6* illustrates the phenotype of human stem and progenitor cells.

6.3.6 Analysis of CD34+ cells on FACS

The set-up for the analysis of CD34+ cells will vary according to the instrument used, and it is essential to have the cooperation of a trained and competent operator. A number of methods have been previously described for analysis and there have been concerted efforts to standardize methods of analysis particularly for clinical samples. In this laboratory, the ISHAGE protocol is used for all

Table 6 Phenotype of human stem and progenitor cells

	LTRC	LTC-IC	Progenitors (early)	Progenitors (late)
CD34	+	+	+	+
CD33	–	–	–	+
CD38	–	–	–	+
CD45RA	?	–	Low	+
CD71	?	–	Low	+
CD90 (Thy 1)	Low	Low	Low	
CD117 (*c-kit*)	Low	?		+
Lineage markers	–	–		
HLA-DR	–	–		+
AC133	+	+	+ (some)	
Rhodamine	?	Low		

blood and bone-marrow samples and the reader is referred to ref. 33 for a detailed discussion of the method.

A quick method for analysing the purity of enriched CD34 populations is presented below.

Protocol 9

Analysis of CD34+ cells by FACS

Equipment and reagents

- CD34+ cells
- FACS Vantage system
- FITC- and PE-labelled Calibrite beads (Becton-Dickinson)
- Unlabelled 10 μm beads
- Control samples labelled with isotype-matched monoclonal antibodies

Method

1 Following the instructions provided by the manufacturer, use unlabelled 10 micron Calibrate beads to optimize the instrument settings and set the compensation parameters FITC- and/or PE-labelled beads.

2 Pass cells through the instrument, collect at least 20 000 events, and examine for the correct distribution of the populations, i.e. forward scatter vs. side scatter (FSC vs. SSC), see *Figure 2a*.

3 Set a 'gate' around blasts and small lymphocytes (*Figure 2a*, R1).

4 Examine control samples labelled with the isotype-matched monoclonal antibodies and adjust so that about 99% of the cells fall within the first decade (log scale FL1). Note that the negative cells fall in lower left quadrant. (Percentages and other statistics are automatically recorded.)

5 Pass CD34-FITC labelled cells through the machine and again collect 20 000 events.

6 Using the same 'gate' as for control samples, examine the cells for fluorescence— consider all cells outside the first decade to be positive (lower right and upper right quadrant). Again, percentages and other statistics are automatically recorded (*Figures 2b* and *c*).

By subtracting the values for the control sample from that of the CD34 labelled samples, the percentage of CD34$^+$ cells can be measured.

CD34-positive cells can be expressed either as a percentage of the lymphocyte population or as a percentage of the mononuclear cells. If the latter figure is required, omit step 3 in *Protocol 9* as there is no need to gate on the lymphocyte population. Values thus obtained for the ungated population correspond to the CD34+ cells in the total mononuclear fraction. The PC LYSYS program (Becton-Dickinson) provides information on both CD34 labelling as a percentage of the total cells and CD34 as a percentage of the gated populations.

For extensive details on FACS sorting the reader is referred to ref. 34.

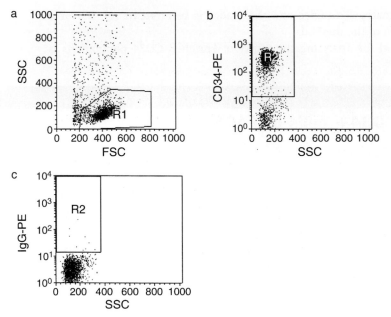

Figure 2 FACS analysis of CD34-positive labelled cells. Dot plot display of FSC vs. SSC of cells after isolation on MiniMACS columns. R1 designates the lymphocyte region (R1). Fluorescence of CD34 cells in the R1 region. Isotype control for CD34 labelled cells.

References

1. Metcalf, D. (1988). *The molecular control of blood cells*. Harvard University Press, Cambridge, MA.
2. Testa, N. G. and Dexter, T. M. (1990). In *Clinical endocrinology and metabolism*, Vol. 4 (ed. S. M. Shalet), p. 177. Baillière Tindall, London.
3. Testa, N. G. (1985). In *Cell clones* (ed. C. S. Potten and J. H. Hendry), p. 37. Churchill Livingstone, Edinburgh.
4. Humphries, R. K., Evans, A. C., and Eaves, C. J. (1981). *Proc. Natl. Acad. Sci.*, USA, **78**, 3629.
5. Heyworth, C. M., Ponting, I. L. O., and Dexter, T. M. (1988). *J. Cell Sci.*, **91**, 239.
6. Cook, N., Dexter, T. M., Lord, B. I., Cragoe, E. J., and Whetton, A. D. (1989). *EMBO J.*, **8**, 239.
7. Metcalf, D. (1980). *Proc. Natl. Acad. Sci.* USA, **77**, 5327.
8. Cormier, F., Ponting, I. L. O., Heyworth, C. M., and Dexter, T. M. (1991). *Growth Factors*, **4**, 157.
9. Lord, B. I. and Spooncer, E. (1986). *Lymphokine Res.*, **5**, 59.
10. Whetton, A. D. and Dexter, T. M. (1990). *Biochim. Biophys. Acta*, **989**, 111.
11. Whetton, A. D. and Dexter, T. M. (1985). *Nature*, **303**, 639.
12. Coutinho, L. H., Gilleece, M. H., De Wynter, E. A., Will, A., and Testa, N. G. (1993). In *Haemopoiesis: a practical approach* (ed. N. G. Testa and G. Molineux), pp. 75–106. IRL Press, Oxford University Press, Oxford.
13. Heyworth, C. M. and Spooncer, E. (1993). In *Haemopoiesis: a practical approach* (ed. N. G. Testa and G. Molineux), pp. 37–53. IRL Press, Oxford University Press, Oxford.
14. Bradley, T. R., Hodgson, G. S., and Rosendaal, M. (1978). *J. Cell Physiol.*, **97**, 517.
15. Duke, I. D., Eaves, C. J., Kalousek, D. K., and Eaves, A. C. (1981). *Cancer Genet. Cytogenet.*, **4**, 157.

16. Coutinho, L. H., Geary, C. G., Chang, J., Harrison, C., and Testa, N. G. (1990). *Br. J. Haematol.*, **75**, 16.

17. Testa, N. G. (1989). In *Critical reviews in hematology and oncology*, Vol. 9, p. 17. CRC Press, Boca Raton, FL.

18. Williams, D. F., Straneva, J. E., Cooper, S., Shadduck, R. K., Waheed, A., Gillis, S., Urdal, D., and Broxmeyer, H. E. (1987). *Exp. Hematol.*, **15**, 1007.

19. Iscove, N. N., Guilbert, L. S., and Wyman, C. (1980). *Exp. Cell Res.*, **126**, 121.

20. Testa, N. G. and Molineux, G. (ed.) (1993). *Haemopoiesis: a practical approach*, IRL Press, Oxford University Press, Oxford.

21. Till, J. E. and McCulloch, E. A. (1961). *Radiat. Res.*, **14**, 213.

22. Visser, J. W. M., Bauman, J. G. J., Mulder, A. H., Eliason, J. F., and Leeuw, A. M. (1984). *J. Exp. Med.*, **59**, 1576.

23. Bertoncello, I., Hodgson, G. S., and Bradley, T. R. (1985). *Exp. Hemat.*, **13**, 999.

24. Mulder, A. H. and Visser, J. W. M. (1987). *Exp. Hematol.*, **15**, 99.

25. Ploemacher, R. E. and Brons, N. H. C. (1988). *J. Cell Physiol.*, **136**, 531.

26. Visser, J. W. M. and van Bekkum, D. W. (1990). *Exp. Hematol.*, **18**, 248.

27. Spangrude, G. J., Heimfeld, S., and Weissman, I. L. (1988). *Science*, **241**, 58.

28. Spangrude, G. J. (1989). *Immunol. Today*, **10**, 344.

29. Baines, P., Mayani, H., Bains, M.. Fisher, I., Hoy, T., and Jacobs, A. (1988). *Exp. Hematol.*, **16**, 785.

30. Williams, D. E., Straneva, J. E., Shen, R. N., and Broxmeyer, H. E. (1987). *Exp. Hematol.*, **15**, 243.

31. Nijhof, W. and Wierenga, P. K. (1984). *Exp. Cell Res.*, **155**, 583.

32. de Wynter, E. A., Countinho, L. H., and Testa, N. G. (1993). *In Hematopoietic stem cells— the Mulhouse manual* (ed. E. Wunder, H. Sovolat, P. R. Henon, and S. Serke). Alpha Med. Press, Dayton, OH.

33. Sutherland, D. R., Anderson, L., Keeney, M., Nayar, R., and Chin-Yee, I. (1996). *J. Hematother.*, **5**, 213.

34. Hoy, T. G. (1990). In *Flow cytometry: a practical approach* (ed. M. C. Ormerod), pp. 125–36. IRL Press, Oxford University Press, Oxford.

Chapter 8

Assays for macrophage activation by cytokines

Anthony Doyle, Michael Stein, Satish Keshav, and Siamon Gordon
University of Oxford, Sir William Dunn School of Pathology, South Parks Rd, Oxford OX1 3RE, UK

1 Introduction

The circulating monocyte may undergo a wide spectrum of functional changes during its further differentiation. In the absence of inflammatory stimuli monocytes enter the tissues constitutively to become resident macrophages (1). These cells are relatively quiescent with respect to secretory or microbicidal activity and may have as yet uncharacterized trophic functions. In contrast, inflammatory recruitment causes monocytes to rapidly induce their secretory activity. These cells produce a large variety of enzymes, growth factors, and cytokines when appropriately triggered. Lymphokines produced at the site of inflammation regulate the fate of elicited macrophages determining whether they are further stimulated to a heightened state of activation with maximal host-defence function, e.g. by IFN-γ, or whether their secretory and defence activity is held in check (e.g. by IL-4 and IL-10).

Previously, macrophage activation has been defined in terms of an increased killing capacity for microorganisms or tumour cells, and respiratory-burst activity has often been used as a measure of cytocidal activation. As our understanding of the repertoire and regulation of macrophage activity expands, the concepts of priming and activation have become highly complex. However, by applying a small number of carefully selected assays it is possible to distinguish macrophages at a number of points on the activation spectrum (2). Our purpose here is to describe a panel of well-characterized assays that do not involve interactions between macrophages and a living target cell, but nevertheless readily discriminate between resident and elicited macrophages, and immunologically activated macrophages with enhanced microbicidal and tumoricidal potential. All the assays have been used in our laboratory on murine macrophage cultures and can be applied to human cells, with the caveat that detection of nitric oxide (NO) is highly variable.

In vitro culture of monocytes and macrophages modulates the activity of the cells even in the most-defined and controlled culture systems. Therefore, the assays described herein are best performed on freshly isolated primary cells, although, in our experience, the assays are also useful in comparing various longer term stimuli under the same culture conditions. Monocytes and macrophages adhere to tissue culture plastic, glass, and bacterial plastic in the presence of 10% fetal calf serum (FCS). This makes the isolation of almost pure monolayers a simple procedure when using elicited or resident cells where most other contaminating immune-cell populations are non-adherent in the presence of FCS. Adherence to serum-coated, tissue culture plastic can profoundly modulate macrophage activation.

2 Assay for respiratory-burst activity

The superoxide anion-release assay measures the change in colour of cytochrome *c* when it is reduced by superoxide anion released from the stimulated macrophage (3).

Protocol 1

Superoxide anion release assay

Equipment and reagents

- Hanks' buffered saline solution (HBSS, phenol red-free)
- Ferricytochrome C (Sigma, type IV) 8 mM stock
- Sodium azide (this is a cytochrome oxidase inhibitor and prevents the reoxidation of cytochrome *c*) 1 M stock
- Macrophages
- RPMI-1640 + 10% FCS
- 24-well plates
- Superoxide dismutase (Sigma, type 1)
- Phorbol myristic acid (PMA)
- Zymosan
- PBS
- Centrifuge (Beckman G5–6R)

Method

1 Plate macrophages at $1–5 \times 10^5$/well in RPMI-1640, 10% FCS in a 24-well tissue culture plate. This density ensures that oxygen anion release is proportional to the cell number.

2 Set up negative and positive controls:
   (a) a cell blank as a negative control;
   (b) wells in which 30 μg/ml superoxide dismutase should be added as a negative control;
   (c) elicited macrophages stimulated with a known trigger of respiratory burst, such as PMA at 10–100 ng/ml or zymosan at 100 μg/ml.

3 Wash adherent macrophages once with PBS and pre-incubate with 0.45 ml of the reaction mixture (HBSS with 80 μM ferricytochrome C and 2 mM sodium azide) for 5 min at 37 °C.

4 Add 0.05 ml of HBSS and stimulant.

5   After 60 min dilute a portion of the reaction mixture threefold with cold HBSS. Remove cell debris by centrifugation at 200 g for 5 min at 4°C.

6   The cytochrome c becomes a darker red in colour after reduction. Calculate super-oxide release from the difference in absorbance at 550 nm in the absence and presence of superoxide dismutase, using an extinction coefficient of 21.1/mM/cm (reduced minus oxidized).

2.1 Comments

This assay is easy to perform and provides a relatively direct estimate of micro-bicidal and cytocidal potential. Several other assays of respiratory-burst activity have been described elsewhere. These include H_2O_2 release (4) and chemilumin-escence (5) assays for monolayers and the nitrobluetetrazolium (NBT) reduction assay for single-cell analysis (6). FACS-based assays are likely to gain increasing application, but they do need further characterization. In assays where a cyto-kine or other modulatory compound being tested may also alter cell numbers or mass, it is best to determine total cell protein, e.g. Lowry or BCA method (Pierce), and express the results as per mg cell protein.

3 Assay for the secretion of nitric oxide

Nitric oxide is an extremely reactive molecule that mediates cytotoxic effects on microbes and tumour cells (7). Because it is rapidly converted to NO_2^- in the pres-ence of oxygen, the NO secretory activity of cells in culture can be estimated by determining NO_2^- concentrations by the colorimetric Griess reaction.

Protocol 2

NO_2^- accumulation assay

Equipment and reagents

- 24-well plates
- Peritoneal macrophages
- IFN-γ
- LPS (e.g. from *E. coli* 055:B5, Difco)
- N^G-monomethylarginine (NMMA, Sigma)

- Griess reagent: within 12 h of use, mix 1% (w/v) naphthylethylenediamine dihydrochloride with an equal volume of 1% (v/v) H_3PO_4 (all reagents from Sigma). Component solutions can be stored for up to 2 months at 4°C.

Method

1   Plate macrophages in 24-well plates as per *Protocol 1*. Note that the sensitivity of the assay is enhanced by culturing the cells in a relatively small volume of medium, e.g. 300–500 μl/well.

2   Prime macrophages for NO burst by adding IFN-γ (50–100 U/ml final concentration). Incubate for at least 2 h at 37°C.

Protocol 2 continued

3 Add LPS (20 ng/ml) to trigger NO burst. Incubate for 16 h at 37 °C. For each different cell type or stimulus include a negative control in which NO synthesis is inhibited by N^G-monomethylarginine (this is essential), add at a final concentration of 250 μg/ml at the same time as the LPS.

4 Remove the supernatant from the cultures, mix with an equal volume of Griess reagent, incubate at room temperature for 10 min and read absorbance at 550 nm.

5 Based on an expected yield of 0–50 nmol $NO_2^-/10^6$ peritoneal macrophages, prepare an appropriate series of NO_2^- standards diluted in culture medium, perform the Griess reaction and construct a standard curve for calculating the NO_2^- concentration in test samples. Express the results as the NMMA-inhibitable accumulation of $NO_2^-/10^6$ cells (or per mg cell protein).

3.1 Comments

This assay (*Protocol 2*) will reflect the cytocidal activation state of the cells. It can be modified to determine the effect of other compounds or cytokines on activation by pre-treating the cells with the above compounds.

4 MHC class II expression

Resident tissue macrophages not exposed to immunogen and specific T-cell cytokines express low levels of MHC class II molecules (2). Expression is upregulated by T cell-derived cytokines such as IFN-γ and IL-4 (8, 9). Flow cytometric analysis of fluorescently stained cells is the method of choice for comparing class II expression in different cell populations (standardization of cell numbers is easily achieved). Immunocytochemical analysis for class II expression has the additional advantage of single-cell analysis.

Protocol 3

Assay for MHC class II expression

Equipment and reagents

- Bacterial plastic Petri dishes
- Macrophages
- PBS
- Narrow-bore pipette (e.g. 5 ml)
- PBA: PBS, 0.1% (w/v) BSA, 10 mM NaN_3
- PBA containing 2% serum (from same species as secondary antibody)
- EDTA
- Eppendorf tubes
- Microcentrifuge
- Anti-MHC class II antibody or isotype-matched, negative control antibody
- Fluorochrome-conjugated secondary antibody
- Flow-cytometry system
- Tissue culture medium: RPMI (Gibco) supplemented with 10% heat-inactivated FCS, 10 mM L-glutamine, 50 U/ml penicillin and 50 μg/ml streptomycin

Method

1. Culture macrophages at a density of 5×10^5 cells/ml of tissue culture medium in bacterial plastic Petri dishes. Incubate at 37°C in a humidified 5% CO_2 atmosphere. Bacteriology-grade Plastics are used because macrophages can be readily detached without trypsin.

2. Detach cells and harvest: wash the monolayer three times with PBS to remove the tissue culture medium, add PBS containing 5 mM EDTA, incubate at room temperature for 5 min. Ensure the cells have rounded up and flush them from the surface using a narrow-bore pipette (e.g. 5 ml). Trypsin is avoided in order to prevent cleavage of cell surface receptors.

3. Pellet the cells by centrifugation at 200 g for 10 min at 4°C, resuspend in PBA, and transfer to an Eppendorf tube. Wash the cells three times with PBA to remove the EDTA. For each wash, pellet the cells by centrifugation: 20-sec pulse at low speed (approx. 6500 r.p.m.) in a microcentrifuge, aspirate and discard the supernatant, then resuspend in PBA (10^6 cells/ml).

4. After the last spin, resuspend the cells in anti-MHC class II antibody or the isotype-matched negative control antibody diluted in PBA containing 2% serum (from the same species as the secondary antibody) to saturate Fc receptors—approximately 1 μg of the antibody in 100 μl of PBA per 10^6 cells is usually appropriate. Incubate on ice for 30–60 min. Gently mix the cells occasionally.

5. Wash cells three times in PBA to remove excess primary antibody.

6. Resuspend pellet in the fluorochrome-conjugated secondary antibody. Incubate on ice for 30–60 min, protected from light to avoid quenching of fluorochrome. Shake occasionally. Secondary antibodies should be pre-titrated: optimal concentration is generally in the range between 1/50 and 1/200 dilution.

7. Wash the cells once to remove the free secondary antibody, resuspend the cells in PBA and analyse by flow cytometry. Relative antigen expression can be calculated by:

$$\frac{\text{geometric mean (sample 1)} - \text{geometric mean (isotype control 1)}}{\text{geometric mean (sample 2)} - \text{geometric mean (isotype control 2)}} \times 100$$

4.1 Comments

It is essential that antibodies are present at saturating concentrations and that they reach equilibrium. In general, a concentration of 1 μg/10^6 cells is optimal. The second antibody must be a $F(ab')_2$ since macrophages have abundant Fc receptors. Cells can be fixed before immunostaining by resuspending them in a freshly made solution of 2% (v/v) paraformaldehyde/PBS (do not use glutaraldehyde as a fixative as this is autofluorescent). Incubate for 15 min on ice and wash away the excess paraformaldehyde with PBS (three times). Incubate the cells in 10% FCS/PBS to block the remaining fixation sites, and wash three times with PBS. The advantage of fixation is that cells can be analysed up to 24 h later

5 Macrophage mannosyl receptor (MMR) assays

MMR is a cell-surface receptor that binds mannosylated or fucosylated proteins (10). MMR activity is downregulated on exposure to IFN-γ. We have found the degradation assay described below to be a very reliable and reproducible assay for discriminating between resident or elicited macrophages (high MMR activity) and IFN-γ activated cells (low MMR activity) (11).

Mannosylated-BSA (23 mol mannose/mol BSA; EY Labs), a glycoconjugate of mannose-bovine serum albumin, serves as a good ligand for the MMR. It is trace-labelled with Na[^{125}I]iodide by a modified chloramine T method.

Protocol 4

Labelling mannosylated BSA

Equipment and reagents

- Mannosylated BSA (2 mg/ml stock solution)
- Na[^{125}I]iodide (Amersham IMS 30, 100 mCi/ml)
- Chloramine T (10 mg/ml stock solution)
- Sodium metabisulfite (2.3 mg/ml)
- Potassium iodide (10 mg/ml stock solution)
- 0.1 M sodium phosphate buffer pH 7.6
- PD-10 column (Sephadex G-10, Pharmacia)
- DMEM, 5% FCS
- 10% TCA (v/v)

Method

1 Prepare stock solutions of mannosylated BSA, Chloramine T, sodium metabisulfite and potassium iodide in 0.1 M sodium phosphate buffer at pH 7.6.

2 Incubate 50 μl of mannosylated BSA stock with 1 mCi of Na[^{125}I]iodide and 30 μl of freshly prepared chloramine T on ice for 10 min.

3 Add 436 μg of sodium metabisulfite (190 μl) and 1.9 mg potassium iodide (190 μl) to terminate the reaction.

4 Pass the reaction products down a PD-10 column, pre-washed with 0.1 M phosphate buffer, pH 7.6.

5 Collect 300 μl aliquots, pool the first labelled peak and dilute in 5 ml of DMEM + 5% FCS.

6 Test the ligand for trichloroacetic acid (TC) precipitability (10% (v/v)) and screen by an uptake or degradation assay using macrophages which express MMR activity (resident peritoneal macrophages or elicited but not IFN-γ-activated macrophages).

Protocol 5

Binding and uptake of mannose-specific ligands

These assays are less time consuming than the degradation assays (described below) but not as sensitive, with potentially higher backgrounds. Binding and uptake are assayed at saturating concentrations of ligand using trace-labelled mannosylated BSA (120 ng/ml ligand per 5×10^5 macrophages) or β_2 glucuronidase (300 µg/ml per 5×10^5 macrophages) in the presence or absence of mannan. Binding is assayed at 4 °C, uptake at 37 °C. The reaction mixture contains FCS which does not inhibit mannose-specific binding. MMR-ligand binding is divalent cation-dependent.

Equipment and reagents

- Macrophages/monocytes
- 24-well plates
- PBS
- DMEM
- FBS
- Hepes buffer pH 7.0
- Mannan (Sigma)

- ^{125}I-labelled mannosylated BSA (as prepared in *Protocol 4*; 3×10^6 c.p.m./µg, 1.7 Ci/µg)
- 10 mM sodium azide
- 1 M NaOH
- Gamma counter and accessories

Method

1   Adhere macrophages/monocytes (5×10^5) for at least 1 h in 24-well plates.

2   Wash in PBS and incubate in 300 µl DMEM + 5% FBS, with Hepes buffer pH 7.0 and 40 ng ^{125}I-labelled mannosylated BSA (3×10^6 c.p.m./µg), with or without 1.25–2.5 mg/ml of mannan (Sigma).

3   Incubate the cells in duplicate for 60 min at 4 °C, or for 20–30 min at 37 °C.

4   Wash three times in ice-cold PBS with 10 mM sodium azide. Add 200 µl of 1 M NaOH to dissolve the cells, and measure cell-associated radioactivity in a gamma counter. Express the results as ng of mannosylated BSA specifically bound or taken up per 5×10^5 macrophages plated or per mg of cell protein.

NB: Degradation of ^{125}I-labelled mannosylated BSA by macrophages can be measured by the appearance of TCA-soluble labelled material in the medium. Degradation of ^{125}I-labelled mannosylated BSA is detectable after about a 40-min incubation at 37 °C and continues at a linear rate for several days if the macrophages are maintained in the continuous presence of ligand. We have found overnight culture to be convenient.

Protocol 6
^{125}I-labelled mannosylated-BSA degradation assay

Equipment and reagents

- Adherent macrophage monolayers
- Sterile labelled ligand
- 96- or 24-well plates
- Culture medium (see *Protocol 3*)
- Mannan (Sigma)
- 10% TCA (v/v)

- 30% (v/v) H_2O_2
- 4 M KI
- Chloroform
- Vortex mixer
- Microcentrifuge
- Gamma counter and accessories

Protocol 6 continued

Method

1   Add trace amounts of sterile ligand (approximately 10^6 c.p.m. in 10 μl) to mono-layers of adherent macrophage populations (5×10^5–1×10^6 macrophages/well) in 96- or 24-well plates, in culture media (0.2–1.0 ml) with FCS, in the absence or presence of mannan (1–2 mg/ml).

2   Include cell-free blanks, with and without mannan.

3   Incubate for 16 h to 2 days and then remove an aliquot of medium. Determine the TCA-soluble radioactivity.

4   If the supernatant following TCA precipitation is not clear or if there is a high background, remove contaminating protein and/or free iodine by incubating a 0.25-ml aliquot of the supernatant with 10 μl of 30% (v/v) H_2O_2 followed by excess potassium iodide (5 μl of 4 M KI). Leave the mixture to react for 10 min at room temp. Thereafter, add 0.7 ml chloroform (to extract protein), vortex the tube vigor-ously for 20 sec, centrifuge (microcentrifuge, high speed, 5 min), and measure the amount of radioactivity in an aliquot of the clear aqueous phase in a gamma counter. Calculate cell-dependent, mannan-inhibitable degradation per unit time as a function of macrophage number or protein.

5.1 Single-cell assays

The uptake of ^{125}I-labelled mannose–BSA or ^{125}I-labelled β-glucuronidase by macrophages can be detected at the single-cell level by autoradiography. To increase the cell-associated radioactivity a higher specific activity ligand should be used (5×10^6 c.p.m./μg) at saturation. Establish macrophage cultures in 24 well plates containing circular coverslips. Add ligand as above, incubate for 20–30 min at 37 °C, wash well by immersing coverslip in fresh medium, and fix. Radioactivity associated with the coverslips can be determined directly before processing.

5.1.1 Comments

Optimal culture conditions are essential. Note that pH variations in crowded cultures may perturb MMR activity. In prolonged degradation assays, cell viability should be monitored by phase-contrast microscopy. β-Glucuronidase is a more stable ligand than mannosylated BSA.

Kinetic parameters of specific binding and ligand uptake can be determined. The degradation assay is not saturable, but it is sensitive and linear for prolonged periods of incubation. Specificity is established using unlabelled competitive inhibitors of MMR-binding, such as mannan or unlabelled ligand. Cell-free blanks are essential and provide a measure of background activity in binding, uptake, and degradation assays.

Mannosylated BSA–FITC (Sigma, cat. no. A7790) and galactosylated BSA–FITC (Sigma cat. no. A2420) are now available for fluorescent assays of MMR-specific and -independent activity. An antibody against human MMR (mAb MR 15–2–2, product number GB 996152) is available from Dr R. Bos, TNO Prevention and Health, PO Box 2215, 2301 CE Leiden, The Netherlands. Monoclonal antibodies against murine MMR are under development in several laboratories, but are not yet commercially available. For a recent review on MMR see ref. 15.

6 Macrophage cytokine assays

Following exposure to bacterial products such as LPS, macrophages are a major source of cytokines including IL-1, IL-6, and TNF-α. Secreted cytokine levels reflect the state of macrophage activation. For instance, resident peritoneal macrophages produce about 100-fold less TNF-α following LPS challenge than do macrophages primed by lymphokines (e.g. IFN-γ) and phagocytic stimuli such as uptake of the yeast cell wall product zymosan (12). Quantitation of protein is usually more amenable than the measurement of mRNA. Secreted protein can be measured by bioassay or more directly by ELISA (see Chapters 12 and 13). Many ELISA kits or pairs of monoclonal antibodies suitable for ELISA are now commercially available (e.g. Genzyme, Pharmingen). See Chapters 12 and 13 (this volume) for more details of cytokine ELISAs and bioassays. Chapter 3, Vol. 1, describes assays for the detection of cytokine mRNA.

7 Conclusions

The markers described here provide a basis for correlating the activation state with functional phenotype of macrophages recovered from experimental animals. From *Table 1* it is evident that activated macrophages, which express high levels of MHC class II molecules and produce large amounts of reactive oxygen and nitrogen intermediates and cytokines, are the opposite extreme in the activation spectrum to resident macrophages with their low secretory capacity, low MHC class II, and high MMR expression. Elicited populations are best distinguished by high MMR expression and significant cytokine secretion. It is important to emphasize that the macrophage population exposed to cytokines

Table 1 Activation profiles of resident, elicited, and activated macrophage populations

| | Macrophage population | | |
	Resident	Elicited	IFN-γ activated
Respiratory burst	low	low/high[a]	high
NO burst	low	low	high
MHC class II	low	low	high
MMR	high	high	low
TNF-α secretion	low	high	high

[a] Thioglycollate broth-elicited peritoneal macrophages can produce high levels of superoxide anion, but low H_2O_2 is detected, possibly as a result of scavengers in the cells.

produced by antigen-responsive lymphocytes at the site of an response will not necessarily become activated. In contrast to IFN-γ, the cytokines IL-10, IL-4, and IL-13 are known to downgrade or temper macrophage activation, such that if these are the dominant cytokines produced at the site, macrophages are likely to be maintained in a non-activated state (high MMR, reduced pro-inflammatory cytokine secretory ability) (13). Indeed, IL-4 has been shown to greatly enhance MMR activity, in contrast to IFN-γ (14). IL-10 is a potent antagonist of macrophage immune activation by IFN-γ, whereas immunomodulation by IL-4 and IL-13 give rise to an alternative activation state (1).

The recent development of PCR-based assays for known and novel gene expression by macrophages, including microarray techniques, provides a powerful method to expand the range of markers which can eventually be used to define the macrophage phenotype. Further studies concentrating on *in vivo* events, the cytokine network, and the control of gene expression will hopefully enhance our understanding and characterization of macrophage activation.

References

1. Gordon, S. (1998). In *Fundamental immunology* (4th edn) (ed. W. Paul), pp. 533–45. Lippincott Raven, PA.
2. Gordon, S. (Section ed.) (1997). *Weir's handbook of experimental immunology* (5th edn) (ed. L. A. Herzenberg, D. M. Weir, L. A. Herzenberg, and C. Blackwell), Vol. IV, pp. 153–175.12. Blackwell Scientific, Oxford.
3. Babior, B. M., Kipnes, R. S., and Curnutte, J. T. (1973). *J. Clin. Invest.*, **52**, 741.
4. Nathan, C. and Root, R. K. (1980). *J. Exp. Med.*, **146**, 1648.
5. Trush, M. A., Wilson, M. E., and Van Dyke, K. (1978). In *Methods in Enzymology*, Vol. 57 (ed. M. Deluca), p. 462. Academic Press, San Diego.
6. Murray, H. W. and Cohn, Z. A. (1980). *J. Exp. Med.*, **152**, 1596.
7. Ding, A. H., Nathan, C. F., and Stuehr, D. J. (1988). *J. Immunol.*, **141**, 2407.
8. Basham, T. Y. and Merigan, T. C. (1983). *J. Immunol.*, **130**, 1492.
9. Crawford, R. M., Finbloom, D. M., Ohara, J., Paul, W. E., and Meltzer, M. S. (1987). *J. Immunol.*, **139**, 135.
10. Pontow, S. E., Kery, V., and Stahl, P. D. (1992). *Int. Rev. Cytol.*, **137B**, 221.
11. Ezekowitz, R. A. B., Austyn, J. M., Stahl, P. D., and Gordon, S. (1981). *J. Exp. Med.*, **154**, 60.
12. Stein, M. L. and Gordon, S. (1990). *Eur. J. Immunol.*, **21**, 431.
13. Doyle, A. G., Herbein, G., Montaner, L. J., Minty, A. J., Caput, D., Ferrara, P., and Gordon, S. (1994). *Eur. J. Immunol.*, **24**, 1441.
14. Stein, M., Keshav, S., Harris, N., and Gordon, S. (1992). *J. Exp. Med.*, **176**, 287.
15. Martinez-Pomares, L. and Gordon, S. (1999). *The Immunologist*, **7**, 119.

Chapter 9

Cytokine production by individual cells

B. Burke, J. S. Lewis, and C. E. Lewis

Section of Pathology, Division of Genomic Medicine, University of Sheffield, Beech Hill Rd, Sheffield S10 2RX, UK

1 Introduction

In recent years, fundamental problems have emerged in the analysis of cytokine production. Aspects of cytokine biology such as their overlapping biological effects, association with carrier proteins, competition with inhibitors, rapid induction, transient storage, and ability to bind to surface sites on producer cells, have meant that considerable care has to be taken in the selection of appropriate and meaningful techniques for their accurate detection.

Cytokines are not produced in isolation but usually together with enzymes, hormones, inhibitors, and other cytokines. This has led to problems of specificity in the use of bioassays to quantify their release, and subsequently to the development of other strategies for the study of cytokine production. One such approach has been to employ various immunostaining techniques in order to both highlight the intracellular production of cytokines and to identify the immunophenotype of producer cells. However, to date, few definitive studies have been performed to show that the synthesis and intracellular storage of cytokines correlates with their subsequent release. With this in mind, attention has focused mainly on the measurement of the secreted product by radio- and enzyme-linked immunoassays which quantify the accumulated level of cytokine released into the culture supernatant by entire cell populations.

More recently, this technology has been extended to visualize cytokine release by *individual* cells. This has yielded important information about the frequency of cytokine-producing cells in a population at any one time. In some instances, these sensitive immunoassays have also been adapted to (a) measure the amount of cytokine released per cell, and/or (b) identify producer cells. A further advantage of their application has been to demonstrate marked heterogeneity in cytokine secretion by cells of the same phenotype.

This chapter outlines various methods currently available for immunolabelling cytokines in producer cells, as well as a non-isotopic method for labelling cytokine mRNA in tissue sections. In addition, several sensitive assays for measuring cytokine release at the single-cell level are described. These include the reverse haemolytic plaque assay, the cell-blot assay, and a modification of the ELISA assay, now commonly known as ELISpot.

2 Immunolocalization of cytokines

2.1 Immunostaining techniques for the localization of cytokines in cytocentrifuge preparations of human or murine cells

2.1.1 Indirect labelled avidin-biotin (LAB) technique

It may be important, when applying immunocytochemical techniques in the investigation of cytokine production, to note reports indicating the presence of both cytoplasmic and membrane-bound (integral membrane protein or cyto-

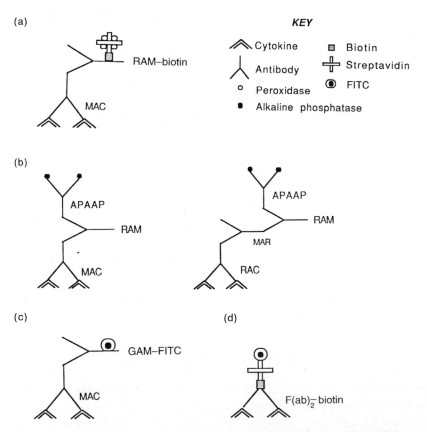

Figure 1 Immunolocalization of cytokines by the following techniques: (a) labelled avidin–biotin (LAB); (b) alkaline phosphatase antialkaline phosphatase (APAAP); and (c, d) indirect immunofluorescent techniques. Abbreviations: RAM, rabbit anti-mouse IgG; MAC, monoclonal anticytokine; APAAP, alkaline phosphatase antialkaline phosphatase; RAC, rabbit anticytokine; GAM, goat anti-mouse IgG; FITC, fluorescein isothiocyanate; F(ab)₂, Fab fragments (anticytokine).

kine bound to its receptor) forms of such cytokines as IL-1 (1) and TNF-alpha (TNF-α) (2). The LAB technique outlined below has previously been used to distinguish between TNF-α and -β at these two cellular sites (3). Additionally, this sensitive method has also been modified to label TNF-α/β (4) and IL-6 (5) in cryostat sections of human tissue.

Protocol 1

Indirect labelled avidin-biotin (LAB) technique (see *Figure 1a*)

Equipment and reagents

- Cytocentrifuge preparations
- Phosphate-buffered saline (PBS): 150 mM NaCl, 2 mM KH_2PO_4, 8 mM K_2HPO_4, pH 7.6
- 4% paraformaldehyde in PBS
- Humidity chamber
- 3% hydrogen peroxide in methanol
- Methanol
- Primary antibody: anticytokine antibody (rabbit polyclonal or mouse monoclonal) (DAKO)
- Normal goat serum in PBS (1/50) (DAKO)
- Biotinylated secondary antibody: goat anti-rabbit IgG or rabbit anti-mouse IgG (depending on which primary antibody is used) (DAKO)
- Peroxidase-labelled streptavidin (1/200)
- 3-amino-9-ethylcarbazole
- *N,N*-dimethylformamide.
- 0.1 M sodium acetate pH 5.2
- Kaiser's jelly mountant (BDH)

Method

1 Fix cytocentrifuge preparations in 4% paraformaldehyde in PBS for 5 min at room temperature.[a] Protect cells from the deleterious effects of desiccation by the use of humidity chambers during subsequent incubation periods.

2 Rinse slides twice in PBS for 2 min each time. (All remaining steps are followed by such rinses).

3 Fix in 100% methanol for 3 min (this helps to preserve membrane integrity but strips away membrane-bound cytokines, e.g. TNF-α).[b, c]

4 Inactive endogenous peroxidase activity in cells with 3% hydrogen peroxide solution in methanol for 10 min at room temp.

5 Incubate slides in 1/50 normal goat serum in PBS for 10 min at 37 °C.

6 Tap off the serum and incubate the slides in 1/50–1/1000 dilutions of the primary antibody (depending upon antibody titre) in PBS for 1–2 h at 37 °C.

7 Incubate the slides in 1/50–1/200 dilutions of the biotinylated secondary antibody in PBS for 1 h at 37 °C.

8 Incubate the slides in 1/200 peroxidase-labelled streptavidin for 1 h at 37 °C.

9 Incubate the slides in substrate to facilitate colour development (red):

(a) Dissolve 4 mg of 3-amino-9-ethylcarbazole in 1 ml of *N,N*-dimethylformamide.

(b) Add to 14 ml of 0.1 M sodium acetate buffer pH 5.2 and 0.15 ml 3% hydrogen peroxide in methanol and filter.

Protocol 1 continued

    (c) Add this solution to the slides for 5–15 min at room temp.

    (d) Rinse in double-distilled water, counterstain with haematoxylin, and mount in aqueous-based medium, such as Kaiser's jelly.

[a] The optimal type of fixative will vary for different cytokines. Cross-linking of proteins by aldehyde-based fixatives yields good preservation and cellular detail, but can also diminish the antigenicity of some cellular proteins. Where little or no staining is achieved after formaldehyde exposure, other less stringent fixatives such as 100% methanol, 100% acetone, or 50% methanol/50% acetone should be tried, as described in *Protocols 2* and *3*.

[b] Exposure of cells to methanol (i.e. step 3) in this procedure largely strips away membrane-bound cytokine, leaving mainly a diffuse, cytoplasmic pattern of staining. Membrane staining can be completely abolished by omitting step 3, and then blocking surface binding sites with avidin bound to 20 nm gold particles prior to step 8. The attachment of large gold particles to the avidin molecules greatly reduces their ability to penetrate the membrane. Thus, only binding sites on the membrane are taken up by this first avidin layer, leaving cytoplasmic binding sites available for the second (peroxidase-labelled) avidin layer.

[c] When the methanol step is omitted, predominantly membrane-bound cytokine may be visualized in the form of cytoplasmic halos. To reveal both cytoplasmic and membrane staining in this procedure, cells are first permeabilized with a 0.03% Triton X-100 solution for 15 min (3).

2.1.2 Enhanced alkaline phosphatase antialkaline phosphatase (APAAP) technique

This immunocytochemical procedure employs a soluble complex of alkaline phosphatase and a monoclonal antibody for this enzyme linked to the primary antibody (directly or indirectly) by an anti-mouse IgG (6). The advantage of this method compared to the more commonly used peroxidase-based alternatives is the lack of interference posed by endogenous peroxidase activity. This technique has been used to localize IFN-γ, TNF-α, IL-β, and IL-6 in peripheral blood mononuclear cells (PBMC) (C. E. Lewis, unpublished observations; see *Figure 2*).

Protocol 2

Enhanced APAAP techniques (see *Figures 1b* and *2*)

Equipment and reagents

- Cytocentrifuge preparations
- 50% acetone/50% methanol mixture
- Tris-buffered saline (TBS): 0.05 M Tris–HCl, 0.15 M NaC1 pH 7.6
- Human γ Fc fragments (DAKO)
- 10% normal human AB serum (NHS) in TBS
- Primary anticytokine antibody (mouse or rabbit)
- APAAP complex (DAKO)
- Secondary (sheep or goat) anti-primary antibody
- Naphthol AS/MX phosphate
- *N,N*-dimethyl-formamide
- 0.1 M Tris pH 8.2
- 1 M levamisole
- Fast Red TR salt
- Haematoxylin
- Kaiser's jelly mounting medium (BDH)

Method

1 Fix cytocentrifuge preparations in 50% acetone/50% methanol at room temp. for 2 min (*or* 4% paraformaldehyde in PBS for 5 min). Carry out the remaining steps at room temp. (unless otherwise specified), with slides protected from desiccation in a humidity chamber.

2 Directly immerse slides in Tris-buffered saline (TBS) for 5–10 min.

3 Incubate slides in 20 μg/ml human Fc fragments in TBS for 30 min (to block endogenous Fc receptors or other potential IgG binding sites on target cells).

4 Rinse the slides twice in TBS for 2 min each time.

5 Incubate in 10% normal human AB serum (NHS, filtered and heat-inactivated for 1 h at 56 °C) in TBS for 45 min.

6 Tap off the serum and incubate the cells for 1–3 h at room temperature (*or* 1–24 h at 4 °C) in the optimal concentration of antibody raised against the purified, native, or recombinant cytokine. (This is usually in the range 1/50 to 1/5000, although this will vary with different antibodies. Check this with preliminary titrations for each antibody.)

7 Rinse the slides twice in TBS for 2 min each time. Wash between all remaining steps in this way.

8 *Either*:
   • If the primary antibody was raised in rabbit, apply 1/50 mouse anti-rabbit IgG in TBS/10% NHS for 60 min, followed by 1/50 rabbit anti-mouse IgG in TBS/10% NHS for 30 min.

Or:
   • If the primary antibody was raised in mouse, apply 1/50 rabbit anti-mouse alone in TBS/10% NHS for 30 min.

9 Incubate the slides in 1/50 of the APAAP complex in TBS for 30 min.

10 Repeat steps 8 and 9, but incubate for a maximum of 10 min each time.

11 Incubate the slides with Fast Red substrate solution for 10–30 min at room temperature, after which immunoreactive cells will be red in colour. This solution is prepared as follows:
   (a) Dissolve 2 mg of naphthol AS/MX phosphate in 0.2 ml of *N,N*-dimethylformamide in a glass tube.
   (b) Add 9.8 ml of 0.1 M Tris buffer pH 8.2.
   (c) Add 0.01 ml of 1 M levamisole to block endogenous alkaline phosphatase.
   (d) Immediately before staining, dissolve 10 mg of the Fast Red TR salt in the above solution and filter.
   (e) Incubate for 50–60 min (monitor colour development using a light microscope).
   (f) Rinse with double-distilled water.

B. BURKE *ET AL.*

Protocol 2 continued

12 Counterstain nuclei (blue) with haematoxylin for 10–30 sec and rinse in tap water for 1 min. Mount preparations in an aqueous-based medium (such as Kaiser's mounting medium).

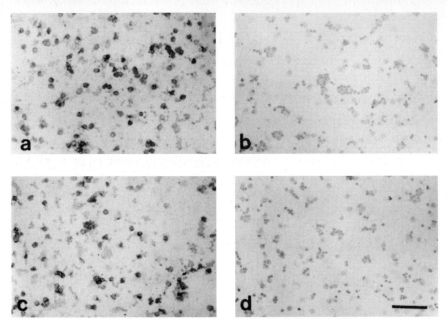

Figure 2 Photomicrographs of monocyte-enriched human PBMC stimulated for 12 h with 10 μg/ml lipopolysaccharide and immunostained by the APAAP technique using either a) 1/200 purified rabbit IgG against human IL-1β or (C) 1/100 purified rabbit IgG against human IG6. No staining was seen with the corresponding concentrations of purified pre-immune rabbit IgG (b, d). All preparations are lightly counterstained with haematoxylin to highlight nuclei. Bar = 100 μM

2.1.3 Indirect immunofluorescence

This technique was originally used to label the alpha and beta forms of IL-1 in human monocytes (7).

Protocol 3

Indirect immunofluorescence (see *Figure 1c*)

Equipment and reagents

- 50% methanol/50% acetone mixture
- PBS (*Protocol 1*)
- 1/5 normal goat serum (NGS) in PBS
- 1/50–1/200 monoclonal anticytokine in PBS

- 1/50 goat anti-mouse IgG–FITC (fluorescein isothiocyanate) conjugate in 2% NGS in PBS
- 9:1 glycerol/PBS containing 1 mg/ml *p*-phenylene diamine

152

Protocol 3 continued

Method

1 Fix cells in 50% methanol/50% acetone for 10 min at $-20\,°C$ or $-70\,°C$ and air-dry. Note that this form of fixation works well for IL-1 but may not be ideal for other cytokines. Carry out the remaining steps at room temperature (unless otherwise specified).

2 Rinse in PBS for 10 min.

3 Block non-specific staining by incubating the slides in 1/5 normal goat serum (NGS) in PBS for 30 min.

4 Tap off the serum and incubate the slides in 1/50–1/200 monoclonal anticytokine in PBS for 1 h.

5 Wash the slides three times in PBS for 2 min each time.

6 Incubate the slides in 1/50 goat anti-mouse IgG–FITC (fluorescein isothiocyanate) conjugate in 2% NGS in PBS for 30 min.

7 Wash the slides three times in PBS for 2 min each time.

8 Wash the slides twice in double-distilled water.

9 Mount the slides in 9:1 glycerol/PBS containing 1 mg/ml p-phenylene diamine to inhibit fading of the fluorescent signal.

An alternative immunofluorescent method to the procedure outlined above has been described by Feldmann and co-workers (8), in which specific staining was enhanced by the use of the biotinylated form of the F(ab)$_2$ portion (rather than the entire antibody molecule) of polyclonal anticytokines followed by FITC-conjugated streptavidin (see *Figure 1d*).

The reader is also directed to a study by Andersson and his co-workers (9), which describes the application of indirect immunofluorescence to detect the simultaneous production of two cytokines by single cells. Indirect immunofluorescence can also be used to localize, at a subcellular level, transcription factors responsible for upregulating cytokine gene expression (10).

2.1.4 Amplified detection method for use on formalin-fixed tissue sections

Using this method (in combination with appropriate isotype-matched, negative control antibodies) it is possible to detect cytokine (e.g. VEGF) in paraffin-embedded tissues and cell clots (J. S. Lewis and C. E. Lewis, unpublished observations). Cellular and secreted protein may be detected depending on the antibody used, and staining with this method is approximately 50 times more sensitive than conventional peroxidase staining methods.

Protocol 4

Amplified avidin–biotin staining method for formalin-fixed, paraffin-embedded tissue sections (using the Dako Catalyzed Signal Amplification System kit®; see Plate 2)

Equipment and reagents

- Xylene
- Absolute alcohol, 95% alcohol, 70% alcohol
- Primary monoclonal anticytokine
- Dako Catalyzed Signal Amplification System kit®
- Silane-coated slides (Sigma)
- 3% hydrogen peroxide in water
- TBS (*Protocol 2*)
- TBST: TBS (*Protocol 2*) with 0.1% Tween-20
- 10% human AB serum (Sigma) in PBS
- Biotinyl tyramide in hydrogen peroxide/PBS (DAKO CSA kit)
- Diaminobenzidine tetrahydrochloride (DAKO CSA kit)
- Gill's haematoxylin
- Scott's tap water (Tap water with 41 mM sodium bicarbonate and 166 mM magnesium sulphate)
- Piccolyte organic mounting medium (DAKO)

Method

1 De-wax and rehydrate sections (2×5 min in xylene, 2×5 min in absolute alcohol, 1×5 min in 95% alcohol, 1×5 min in 70% alcohol, and 10 min in distilled water). Use silane-coated slides to increase tissue adherence.

2 In a humidified chamber, incubate sections for 5 min in 3% hydrogen peroxide in water to block endogenous peroxidase activity.

3 Rinse sections in distilled water and quench in fresh TBST for 5 min.

4 Wipe the slides dry, avoid direct contact with the sections, and incubate in the protein block solution (included in the Dako CSA kit) for 5 min. (Where excessive non-specific staining occurs incubation in 10% human AB serum in PBS may aid specificity.)

5 Tap off excess fluid and apply the primary monoclonal antibody. For VEGF the optimal dilution was found to be 5 µg/ml (in TBS without added Tween-20) for 45 min at room temperature. Determine the optimal antibody titre and duration of incubation for individual cytokine protocols.

6 Rinse with TBST and place sections in a bath of TBST over a magnetic stirrer bar for 1 h at room temperature.

7 Dry the slides as described in step 4 and incubate in biotinylated rabbit anti-mouse IgG in Tris–HCl (provided with the Dako CSA kit) for 15 min.

8 Rinse and quench the sections as described in step 3, then incubate for 15 min in the streptavidin–biotin complex (provided with the Dako CSA kit) in PBS.

9 Repeat the wash step. Incubate the sections in biotinyl tyramide in hydrogen peroxide/PBS for 7 min.

10 Repeat the wash step. Incubate the sections in streptavidin–HRP (provided with the Dako CSA kit) for 15 min.

11 Develop the substrate-chromogen with diaminobenzidine tetrahydrochloride exposure for 5 min.

12 Wash the slides in distilled water, counterstain in Gill's haematoxylin, incubate in Scott's tap-water to give a blue background, and dehydrate (5 min in 70% alcohol, 5 min in 95% alcohol, 2 × 5 min in absolute alcohol, 2 × 5 min in xylene), before mounting in a permanent organic mounting medium such as piccolyte.

2.2 Non-isotopic *in situ* hybridization for the detection of cytokine mRNA in wax-embedded tissue sections

This method will detect mRNA transcripts for some cytokines (e.g. those expressed in abundance such as VEGF by tumour cells; see Plate 3) in appropriately fixed and embedded tissue specimens and cell clots. It is used in preference to isotopic methods for its ease of visualization of the bound probe, identification of surrounding tissue structure, and lack of any specialized training and facilities; although it is less sensitive than isotopic (radioactive) methods. The reader is directed to the protocols for the latter outlined elsewhere in this volume.

Protocol 5

Detection of cytokine mRNA in paraffin-embedded, formalin-fixed tissue sections using FITC-labelled antisense oligonucleotide probes for non-isotopic, *in situ* hybridization (with the Hybriprobe kit from Biognostik) (see Plate 3)

Equipment and reagents

- Xylene
- Absolute alcohol, 95% alcohol, 70% alcohol
- DEPC-treated water
- RNase-free water (DEPC-treated; Sigma)
- Pepsin HCl: 12.5 mg/ml pepsin, 0.2 M HCl
- Sealable humidity chamber
- FITC-labelled oligonucleotide probe
- 1 × SSC: 0.15 M NaCl, 0.15 M sodium citrate ($Na_3C_6H_5O_7$), pH 7
- Magnetic stirrer

- TBS: 0.05 M Tris–HCl, 0.3 M NaCl pH 7.5, containing 0.1% Triton X-100, 3% bovine serum albumin (BSA), and 20% normal sheep serum
- BCIP/NBT/INT 5-Bromo-4-chloro-Indoxyl Phosphate, Nitro Blue Tetrazolium chloride Indonitrotetrazolium violet (DAKO)
- Scott's tap water
- Aqueous mountant (e.g. Improved aquamount from BDH)

Method

1 De-wax sections and rehydrate (2 × 5 min in xylene, 2 × 5 min in absolute alcohol, 1 × 5 min in 95% alcohol, 1 × 5 min in 70% alcohol, 10 min in RNase-free, DEPC-treated, distilled water)

2 Incubate the sections in pepsin/HCl for 10 min.

3 Wash the slides in DEPC-treated water for 5 min.

4 Heat the Hybribuffer (in the Biognostik kit) (*or* similar buffer containing salmon sperm DNA, RNA fractions, and formamide) to 95 °C for 10 min, then cool rapidly on ice for 5 min. Immediately add the buffer to the sections and incubate for 4 h at 37 °C in a sealed humidity chamber.

5 Remove the excess fluid and incubate the sections for 16 h in 100 pmol/ml of the FITC-labelled oligonucleotide probe (included in the Biognostic kit) in hybridization buffer (included in the Biognostic kit) at 37 °C in a sealed humidity chamber. (This concentration and incubation length is optimal for VEGF mRNA.) Cover the sections with a clean glass coverslip to greatly aid this stage of the procedure.

6 Wash the hybridized sections briefly in 1 × SSC to remove the coverslips, then in fresh 1 × SSC buffer for 5 min at room temperature. Wash again with 0.1 × SSC buffer for 15 min at 37 °C to minimize background due to mismatched probe hybrids.

7 Block non-specific antibody staining by incubating the sections in TBS containing 0.1% Triton X-100, 3% BSA, and 20% normal sheep serum for 30 min at room temperature.

8 Remove the excess fluid without rinsing the sections and expose the tissue to anti-fluorescein Fab fragments conjugated to alkaline phosphatase (included in the Biognostic kit) (diluted 1/200 in TBS containing 3% BSA and 0.1% Triton X-100) for 90 min.

9 Wash the slides in TBS over a magnetic stirrer bar for up to 1 h depending on the degree of background staining.

10 Develop the substrate-chromogen with BCIP/NBT/INT or similar for 2–3 h to yield a brown reaction, counterstain in Gill's haematoxylin, incubate in Scott's tap water to give a blue background. Dehydrate and mount in a permanent aqueous mountant.

Care must be taken to control for non-specific staining in the above immuno-staining procedures (i.e. *Protocols 1–4*), especially the high-sensitivity, CSA method described in *Protocol 4*. Controls must be included to ascertain whether the primary and secondary antibodies are specific for their target antigens. This can be done by replacing the cytokine antibody with either diluent alone or pre-immune serum (or the IgG fraction of pre-immune serum, whichever is more appropriate) of the same species as the donor of the antibody. Alternatively, an inappropriate antibody (i.e. of irrelevant specificity) can be used. Such control preparations should be substituted at the same immunoglobulin concentration as that of the original (i.e. specific cytokine) antibody used. It is also recommended that antibodies and their control solutions be of comparable age, and thus contain similar quantities of protein aggregates, since the presence of such contaminants may contribute to non-specific staining. To ensure the removal of protein aggregates, all antibody and control preparations should be spun down at 14 000 g for 10 min at their final working concentrations, and the super-natants used in the staining procedure. If possible, abolition of staining by pre-absorption of the primary antibody with either a highly purified preparation of the native form of the cytokine or its recombinant analogue (10–100 μg/ml for 24 h at 4 °C) prior to use in these procedures is the ideal way of checking the specificity of the staining achieved. In addition, the specificity of secondary and/or tertiary antibodies in the above techniques can be checked by their omission and substitution with the appropriate buffer.

3 Detection of cytokine release by individual cells

3.1 Reverse haemolytic plaque assay (RHPA)

This is a variant of the plaque assay established by Jerne *et al.* (11) to detect and enumerate immunoglobulin-secreting B cells, which has been adapted to detect antigen secretion (12, 13). Studies have indicated the lower level of sensitivity of this immunoassay to be 10^{-18} M of secreted product. Secretory cells in a purified or heterogeneous cell population form plaques (zones of haemolysis around secretory cells) when incubated in a monolayer with protein A-coated ovine erythrocytes in the presence of a specific antiserum and complement. Since the size of plaques is directly proportional to the amount of product secreted per cell (13, 14), this technique can be used to measure the amount secreted by single cells, as well as providing an estimate of the frequency of cytokine-secreting cells in a given population. Producer cells can then be identified by routine immuno-cytochemistry of cells in the monolayer (15). In cytokine biology, the RHPA has been adapted for numerous purposes, including: the enumeration of murine T cells secreting IFN-γ (16); quantification of the release of various cytokines by human blood and tumour-infiltrating leucocytes (17, 18); IL-6 release by mega-karyocytes (19); and, in combination with TUNEL (terminal transferase dUTP nick end labelling), an investigation of the link between IL-1β release and apoptosis in anterior pituitary cells (20).

Protocol 6

Conjugation of protein A to red blood cells[a]

Equipment and reagents

- Sheep erythrocytes, in Alsever's solution
- 0.9% NaCl
- Protein A (PrA) from *Staphylococcus aureus*; Cowan Strain diluted to 0.5 mg/ml in 0.9% NaCl
- Dulbecco's modified essential medium (DMEM) supplemented with 0.1% BSA and 100 U/ml penicillin, 100 μg/ml streptomycin

- Ficoll–Hypaque
- 0.2 mg/ml chromium chloride hexahydrate ($CrCl_3 \cdot 6H_2O$). This solution of $CrCl_3$ must be made up and stored at 4 °C for at least 1 week before use in the conjugation procedure. It can be stored at 4 °C wrapped in foil, and used repeatedly for up to 6 months.
- Glass pipettes

Protocol 6 continued

Method

1 Dilute two 4-ml aliquots of sheep erythrocytes (sRBC; supplied in Alsever's solution. Do not store for longer than 2 weeks at 4 °C before use) 1:1 with a solution of 0.9% NaC1. Remove any sheep leucocytes present in this preparation by layering each 8 ml of diluted sheep blood over 4-ml aliquots of Ficoll–Hypaque in a centrifuge tube. Spin these tubes at 444 g for 25 min.

2 Discard the supernatant from each gradient and harvest the sRBC pellet at the base of each tube. Wash each pellet several times by repeated suspension with a glass pipette in 0.9% NaC1 solution and centrifugation at 444 g for 5–10 min.

3 Dilute each 1-ml pellet of sRBC in 5 ml of 0.9% NaC1 and add 1 ml of protein A ('PrA', from *Staphylococcus aureus*; previously diluted to 0.5 mg/ml in 0.9% NaC1) and 5 ml of 0.2 mg/ml chromium chloride hexahydrate. Gently resuspend the sRBC pellet in this solution using a glass pipette and incubate tubes at 30 °C for 1 h.

4 Harvest each 1 ml of PrA-conjugated sRBC (PrA–sRBC) by centrifugation at 300 g for 6 min and washed several times by repeated suspension and centrifugation steps in either 0.9% NaC1 (first wash) or DMEM supplemented with 0.1% BSA and penicillin–streptomycin (for subsequent washes). If considerable lysis of the cells is visible after the first centrifugation, or if the pellet does not resuspend readily in 0.9% NaC1, discard the preparation and repeat the procedure using a different batch of sRBC.

5 Resuspend and store the PrA–sRBC in 100 ml of DMEM (i.e. as a 2% solution (v/v) supplemented with 0.1% BSA and antibiotics, for a maximum of 3 weeks at 4 °C.

[a] The best monolayers in the RHPA are achieved using cells conjugated 1–5 days before use in the assay.

Protocol 7

Reverse haemolytic plaque assay (see *Figures 3* and *4*)[a]

Equipment and reagents

- Glass slides
- Acid alcohol
- 1% DMSO (dimethyl sulfoxide)
- 0.05 mg/ml poly-L-lysine
- Double-sided sticky tape
- Coverslips (22 mm²)
- 2% (v/v) suspension of PrA–sRBC (*Protocol 6*)
- Humidity chamber
- Cell culture (5% CO_2 in air) incubator
- 2% glutaraldehyde in PBS

- RPMI-1640 cell culture medium, supplemented with 0.1% BSA and 100 U/ml penicillin, 100 µg/ml streptomycin
- 1/50–1/100 dilution of polyclonal anticytokine antibody in supplemented RPMI-1640 as above
- 1/50 dilution of guinea-pig complement in supplemented RPMI-1640 as above
- Trypan Blue solution
- Haemocytometer

Method

1 Clean glass slides by immersion in acid alcohol for 5 min, followed by several rinses in double-distilled water, and then immersion in 1% DMSO for 5 min. Wash the slides several times in double-distilled water and then leave to air-dry in a clean environment.

2 Coat the slides with poly-L-lysine (0.05 mg/ml in double-distilled water) for 10 min. Rinse several times in double-distilled water and air-dry at room temperature or with a warm air current. Do not heat the coated slides above 40 °C during drying.

3 Construct Cunningham chambers in the following way. Attach two pieces of double-sided sticky tape, separated by a distance of 15–20 mm, to each dry, polylysine-coated slide. Then lower a 22 mm^2 coverslip on to the slide so that it sits on the edge of each strip of tape, this forms the roof of the chamber. Gently press down on the coverslip to make sure it adheres to the tape on both sides of the chamber.

4 For a 10-slide assay, spin down 10 ml of a 2% (v/v) suspension of PrA–sRBC at 300 g for 5–10 min. Decant and discard all but 0.5 ml of the supernatant. Resuspend the pellet of PrA–sRBC in this supernatant, to yield a 40% solution (v/v).

5 Add test cells (at a final working cell density of $1–10 \times 10^6$ cells/ml) to PrA–sRBC at a 1:1 ratio (v/v). For example, 0.5 ml of test cells are added to 0.5 ml of 40% PrA-sRBC (thereby yielding a final, working dilution of 20% PrA-sRBC (v/v)). Mix gently, but thoroughly, and apply 100 μl of this cell suspension to the entrance of each Cunningham chamber. This will fill the chamber by capillary action, leaving a small amount at the entrance. Place the slides into humidity chambers and incubate at 37 °C in 5% CO_2/air for 35–45 min. During this period, the PrA-sRBC and human cells settle down on to the slides to create a monolayer. (Do not leave the slides for longer than 45 min at this stage as multilayers will form which impede plaque formation.)

6 Remove excess unattached cells from the chambers at the end of this period by four rapid washes with warm (37 °C) incubation medium (RPMI-1640, supplemented with 0.1% BSA and antibiotics). Do this by placing 50 μl of medium at one entrance to the chamber and draw it through with absorbent paper applied gently to the other side. Using a light microscope, inspect the appearance of the cells remaining in the chamber to check their confluency.

7 Infuse the polyclonal anticytokine at 1/50–1/100 in RPMI-1640 plus 0.1% BSA and antibiotics into the chambers as three 30-μl washes. After the final infusion of antibody, leave a small amount at one entrance to the chamber to avoid excessive drying out of the cells during the subsequent incubation period (i.e. a final volume of 90–100 μl of antibody is needed per slide). Incubate the slides in clean humidity chambers at 37 °C in 5% CO_2/air for up to 12 h.

8 At the end of this period, infuse a solution of 1/50 guinea-pig complement in warm (37 °C) incubation medium into the chambers as three 30-μl washes and incubate in 5% CO_2/air for 20–30 min. Complement-mediated erythrocyte lysis will occur during this period around cytokine-secreting cells (see *Figure 6*).

Protocol 7 continued

9 Check cell viability at this stage using the Trypan Blue exclusion test (NB it is advisable to do this step in the absence of such serum proteins as BSA). Introduce fixative into the chambers (2% glutaraldehyde in PBS) and store at 4 °C until quantitative analysis of individual plaque size and number (this can be done using a simple image-analysis device).

[a] Control experiments to assess the dependency of plaque formation on the secretion of a specific cytokine by cells in the RHPA should include:

• substitution of the polyclonal anticytokine with an equivalent concentration of either an inappropriate antibody, or whole (or if more appropriate, the purified IgG fraction of) non-immune serum from the same species as the donor animal;

• pre-absorption of the polyclonal antibody with the appropriate recombinant or native, purified form of cytokine for 24 h at 4 °C.

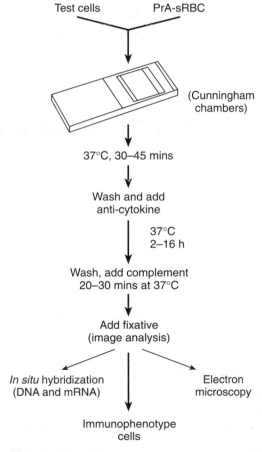

Figure 3 Protocol for the reverse haemolytic plaque assay.

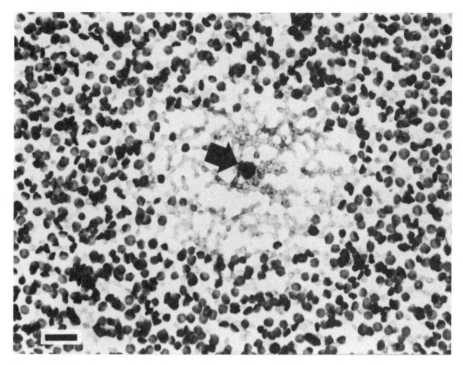

Figure 4 Photomicrograph of a human monocyte (arrowhead) at the centre of an IL-1 plaque area of sRBC lysis in the reverse haemolytic plaque assay. Magnification bar = 20 μm.

Protocol 8

Immunophenotyping cells in the RHPA

Equipment and reagents

- TBS (*Protocol 2*)
- Monoclonal antibody diluted in TBS/0.05% dried milk
- 1/40 rabbit anti-mouse IgG in TBS
- 1/40 rabbit anti-mouse IgG in TBS
- Fast Red substrate
- Haematoxylin
- Aqueous-based mounting medium

Method

1 After infusion of the fixative into the chambers (*Protocol 7*), immerse the slides in TBS and remove the coverslips and the double-sided sticky tape.

2 Rinse the monolayers with TBS for 5 min.

3 Incubate the slides in the appropriate monoclonal antibody for a given human or murine cell-marker (e.g. anti-CD3 for human T cells), diluted 1/10–1/200 in TBS/0.05% dried milk for 2–4 h at room temperature.

4 Wash the slides three times in TBS (do not wash too vigorously as this can dislodge cells).

5 Incubate in a 1/40 dilution of rabbit anti-mouse IgG in TBS for 30 min at room temperature.

6 Repeat step 4.

7 Incubate the slides in a 1/40 dilution of rabbit anti-mouse IgG in TBS for 30 min at room temp.

8 Repeat step 4.

9 Repeat steps 5 and 7, but for only 10 min each.

10 Add Fast Red substrate (see *Protocol 2*, step 11) for 5–60 min at room temperature, after which immunopositively stained cells will appear red in colour. Lightly counterstain the nuclei of stained and unstained cells with haematoxylin and then mount the monolayers in an aqueous-based medium.

3.2 Cell-blot assay

Briefly, this technique visualizes and quantifies subpicogram levels of a given product secreted by cells attached to a protein-binding membrane. The membrane-bound secreted product is then labelled using immunocytochemical methods. Cells surrounded by coloured zones of secreted product are then visualized microscopically and the amount secreted by each cell determined, using computerized image analysis of both the colour intensity and the size of blots (21). Cell blotting was used to demonstrate the release of both the alpha and beta forms of IL-1 by the monocytic leukaemia cell line, THP-1 (22), IL-2 by human lymph node cells and lymphocytes (23), basic FGF by neuroblastoma cells (24), and IFN-γ by human lymphocytes (C. E. Lewis and A. L. Ramshaw, unpublished observations).

Protocol 9

Cell-blot assay (see *Figure 5*)

Equipment and reagents

- Protein-binding membrane (e.g. 'Immobilon-P' supplied by Millipore)
- 25-mm diameter plastic culture wells
- RPMI-1640, 0.025% BSA, plus antibiotics and 2 mM L-glutamine
- TBS (*Protocol 2*)
- 1% BSA in TBS
- Appropriate polyclonal anticytokine (1/1000–1/5000) *or* monoclonal anticytokine (1/100–1/1000) in TBS/1% BSA
- 2% glutaraldehyde (v/v) in phosphate buffer pH 7.2
- 1/1000 mouse anti-rabbit IgG in TBS/1% BSA
- 1/1000 rabbit anti-mouse IgG in TBS/1% BSA
- 1/1000 APAAP in TBS/1% BSA
- Fast Red substrate solution (*Protocol 2*)
- Haematoxylin
- Forceps
- Humidified, 5% CO_2, 37 °C incubator
- *Glass* pipettes

Method

1 Cut the protein-binding membrane into 1.5 cm × 1.5 cm pieces and place the 'structural' side upwards in 25-mm diameter plastic culture wells (inspect the surface appearance of the membrane under a light microscope; the 'structural' side will appear studded along its length). Mark the 'structural' side on each piece of membrane at this stage to aid identification. Use forceps to manipulate the membranes throughout this procedure.

2 Dilute the test cells to a density of 5×10^4/ml in RPMI-1640, 0.025% BSA, plus antibiotics and 2 mM L-glutamine.

3 Aliquot 100 μl of this cell suspension to the centre of each piece of membrane and leave in a humid atmosphere for 4–8h at 37 °C in 5% CO_2.

4 Remove the unattached cells and excess culture fluid carefully with a glass pipette so as not to disturb the cells settled on the membrane. Take care to ensure that the membrane does not flip over during aspiration.

5 Wash the membranes three times with TBS. Do this by lifting out the membrane and placing 1.5 ml of TBS into each well. Position the membrane gently on the surface of the TBS, with the structural surface facing downwards, for 5 min with gentle horizontal shaking. Replace with fresh TBS for each wash. Do not let the membrane dry out between washes or settle face down on the bottom of the culture well.

6 Block unbound protein-binding sites on the membrane with 1% BSA in TBS for 2 h at room temperature.

7 Incubate the membranes in *either* the appropriate polyclonal anticytokine (1/1000–1/5000) *or* monoclonal anticytokine (1/100–1/1000) in TBS/1% BSA for 20–24 h at room temperature (If sodium azide is present remove it by dialysis of the antibody prior to its use in the assay.) Remove protein complexes in the antibody preparations by centrifuging the final working dilution of the antibody at 14 000 g for 10 min at RT. Only apply the supernatants to the membranes.

8 Fix the membranes in 2% glutaraldehyde (v/v) in PBS (pH 7.2) for 15 min at room temperature to help preserve cellular integrity. *Either* do this at this stage *or* after step 16.[a]

9 Aspirate the wells to remove unbound antibody and wash several times in TBS (as in step 5).

10 Incubate membranes in a 1/1000 dilution of mouse anti-rabbit IgG in TBS/1% BSA for 2 h at room temperature

11 Repeat step 5.

12 Incubate the membranes in a 1/1000 dilution of rabbit anti-mouse IgG in TBS/1% BSA for 2 h at room temperature.

13 Repeat step 5.

Protocol 9 continued

14 Incubate the membranes in a 1/1000 dilution of APAAP in TBS/1% BSA for 1 h at room temperature.

15 Incubate the membranes in Fast Red substrate solution (as described in *Protocol 2*, step 11) for 2–4 h to reveal cell blots and/or cellular staining for cytokines.

16 Wash the membranes in TBS and air-dry before inspecting using a light microscope. The cell blots should appear as small, red patches with cells at the centre on the white background.

17 Counterstain the cells at the centre of the cell blots with haematoxylin, dip individual membranes in tap-water and place each one on a glass slide, with the structural surface of the membrane facing upwards. Drop 100 μl of filtered haematoxylin on to each membrane and leave for 2 min. Rinse the membranes in tap-water and air-dry.

[a] Control studies to check for the specificity of the cell-blot assay should include those described for the RHPA in *Protocol 8*.

[b] Application of fixative at the earlier stage of the procedure enhances the preservation and attachment of blot-forming cells, but can also occasionally reduce the antigenicity of the cytokine under study (especially the low levels of secreted cytokine in the blot).

Protocol 10

ELISpot assay (see *Figure 6*)

Equipment and reagents

- Monoclonal anti-human cytokine or hamster anti-mouse cytokine
- PBS
- PBS /1% BSA/0.5% Tween-20
- RPMI-1640 supplemented with 5 mM L-glutamine, 5×10^{-5} M 2-mercaptoethanol, 100 U/ml penicillin, 100 μg/ml streptomycin, and 10% FCS
- PBS/0.5% Tween-20

- Appropriate polyclonal rabbit or monoclonal mouse anticytokine
- 1/1000–1/5000 alkaline phosphatase-conjugated goat anti-rabbit IgG
- Enzyme substrate: 1 mg/ml 5-bromo-4-chloro-3-indolyl phosphate in 2-amino-2-methyl-1-propanol buffer in 0.6% agarose (16)
- 24-well, tissue culture plates
- Humidified, 5% CO_2 in air, 37 °C incubator

Method[a]

NB: Sterile conditions must be employed up to and including step 6.

1 Coat 24-well, tissue culture plates with 500 μl of the optimal dilution (1/200–1/5000) of monoclonal anti-human cytokine or hamster anti-mouse cytokine in PBS at 4 °C for 16–24 h. (96-well tissue culture plates can also be used with the appropriate reduction in coating solution (50–100 μl).)

2 Wash the plates twice with PBS for 5 min each time.

3 Block non-specific protein-binding sites with PBS containing 5% dried milk for 1 h at room temp. Dilute all subsequent antibodies in one of these protein solutions. Wash in PBS.

4 Aliquot the test cells at a density of 10^4 cells/100 μl/well in RPMI-1640 supplemented with 5 mM L-glutamine, 5×10^{-5} M 2-mercaptoethanol, antibiotics, and 10% FCS. Incubate for 2–24 h at 37 °C in a humid atmosphere of 5% CO_2 in air. (The optimal length of this incubation period for good spot formation will vary for different cell types and the level of cytokine-secreting activity.)

5 Remove the cells from the plates by repeated washing with cold PBS/0.5% Tween-20.

6 Add 50 μl of the optimal concentration of the appropriate polyclonal rabbit or monoclonal mouse anticytokine (likely to be in the range of 1/100 to 1/5000) and incubate for 1–2 h at 37 °C.

7 Wash the plates three times with PBS to remove unbound antibody.

8 Add 500 μl of a 1/1000–1/5000 dilution of alkaline phosphatase-conjugated goat anti-rabbit IgG to the wells for 1–2 h at 37 °C.

9 Wash the plates twice with PBS for 5 min each time.

10 Add the enzyme substrate. Note that after 5–10 min this mixture will solidify (do not move the plates during this time) and after 3–5 min at 37 °C, blue spots will appear. Estimate the number of cytokine-secreting cells using a dissecting micro-scope with the plates viewed against a white background.

[a] Controls for the ELISpot assay are essentially those described for the RHPA in *Protocol 8*.

3.3 ELISpot assay

This technique is based on the ELISA-spot assay for the detection of individual antibody-secreting B cells (25). In the reverse form of this assay outlined below, single cells are incubated on a solid surface pre-coated with a specific cytokine antibody, which then binds cytokine secreted during the assay. The cells are washed away and the bound cytokine detected by routine immunocytochemical methods using a second monoclonal antibody which recognizes a different epitope on the cytokine molecule. Numerous studies have described the applica-tion of the ELISpot assay to detect and enumerate cytokine-expressing cells, including, amongst others:

- human lymphocytes secreting IFN-γ (26);
- human T and monocytic cell lines producing IFN-γ and TNF-α (27);
- murine T cells secreting IFN-γ and TNF-α (28);
- murine splenic T cells secreting IL-5 and IFN-γ (29).

Developments in this technique have recently been reviewed in detail (30). Commercial image-analysis equipment and software is now available to analyse the results of ELISpot assays (31).

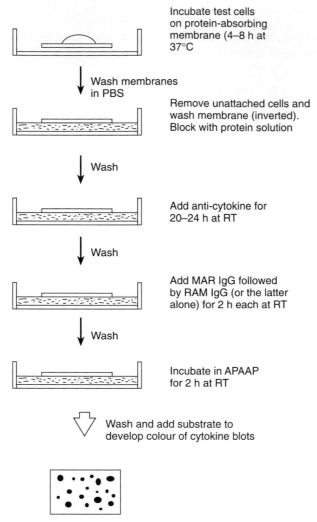

Incubate test cells on protein-absorbing membrane (4–8 h at 37°C

Wash membranes in PBS

Remove unattached cells and wash membrane (inverted). Block with protein solution

Wash

Add anti-cytokine for 20–24 h at RT

Wash

Add MAR IgG followed by RAM IgG (or the latter alone) for 2 h each at RT

Wash

Incubate in APAAP for 2 h at RT

Wash and add substrate to develop colour of cytokine blots

Figure 5 Protocol for the cell-blot assay. MAR IgG, mouse anti-rabbit IgG; RAM, rabbit anti-mouse IgG; APAAP, alkaline phosphatase antialkaline phosphatase; RT, room temperature.

4 Discussion

Although many of the cytokine-release assay protocols outlined in this chapter have been shown to detect cytokines at subpicogram levels, a number of salient points should be noted concerning their general application and interpretation. First, by definition, producer cells in such single-cell techniques are secreting in isolation from their normal intercellular contacts and communication. Thus, the possibility exists that these assays may yield artefactual results. Second, there is considerable debate at present concerning the use of such techniques which detect the antigenic, but not necessarily biologically active, form of cytokines. However, bioassays are equally limited in as much as they are not always

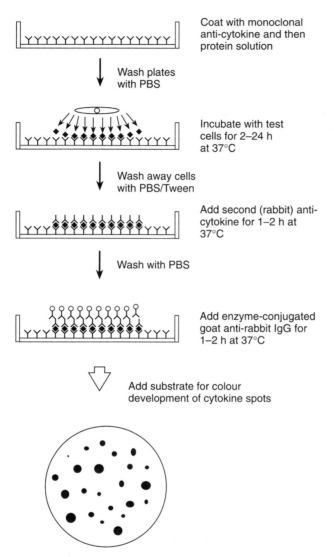

Coat with monoclonal anti-cytokine and then protein solution

Wash plates with PBS

Incubate with test cells for 2–24 h at 37°C

Wash away cells with PBS/Tween

Add second (rabbit) anti-cytokine for 1–2 h at 37°C

Wash with PBS

Add enzyme-conjugated goat anti-rabbit IgG for 1–2 h at 37°C

Add substrate for colour development of cytokine spots

Figure 6 Protocol for the ELISpot assay.

specific for a given cytokine, and when two or more cytokines are present synergistic or antagonistic interactions can also produce confusing data. With this in mind, it may be advisable to use several different forms of cytokine detection in tandem, rather than consider them as alternatives.

Due to space limitations, two methods used recently for quantifying cytokine production by single cells have been omitted here: *in situ* reverse transcription polymerase-chain reaction (*in situ* RT-PCR), a high sensitivity method which visualizes cytokine mRNA; and flow cytometry, which can detect two or more cytokines in single cells (and has been of great utility in the elucidation of T-helper cell subsets). Therefore, the reader is referred to references 30, 32 and 33 for detailed descriptions of how these methods have been adapted for cytokine release. Given the complexity of establishing the *in situ* RT-PCR method in the laboratory, the reader is also referred to specialist works, such as the *In situ PCR* volume in 'The Practical Approach Series', for guidance on how to achieve optimization of this method for a given cytokine mRNA species.

Acknowledgements

CEL's laboratory is funded by the BBSRC, EPSRC, and MRC. BB is funded by Yorkshire Cancer Research. JSL holds a studentship funded by the Special Trustees of the United Sheffield Hospitals Trust.

References

1. Kurt-Jones, E. A., Beller, D. I., Mizel, S. B., and Unanue, E. R. (1988). *Proc. Natl. Acad. Sci. USA*, **82**, 1204.
2. Espevik, T. and Nissen-Meyer, J. (1987). *Immunology*, **61**, 443.
3. Chensue, S. W., Remick, D. G., Shamyr-Forsch, C., Beals, T. F., and Kunkel, S. L. (1988). *Am. J. Pathol.*, **133**, 564.
4. McCall, J. L., Kankatsu, Y., Funamoto, T., and Parry, B. R. (1989). *Am. J. Pathol.*, **135**, 421.
5. Tabibzadeh, S., Poubouridis, D., May, T., and Sehgal, P. B. (1989). *Am. J. Pathol.*, **135**, 427.
6. Cordell, S. L., Falini, B., Erber, W. N., Ghosh, A. K., Abdulaziz, S., Pulford, A. F., Stein, H., and Mason, D. Y. (1984). *J. Histochem. Cytochem.*, **32**, 219.
7. Barkley, D., Feldman, M., and Maini, R. N. (1989). *J. Immunol. Meth.*, **120**, 277.
8. Feldman, M., Brennan, F. M., Chantry, D., Haworth, C., Turner, M., Abney, E., Buchan, G., Barret, K., Barkley, D., Chu, A., Field, M., and Maini, R. N. (1990). *Ann. Rheum. Dis.*, **49**, 480.
9. Andersson, U., Andersson, J., Lindfors, A., Wagner, K., Moller, G., and Heusser, C. H. (1990). *Eur. J. Immunol.*, **20**, 1591.
10. Kazansky, A.,V., Kabotyanski, E. B., Wyszomierski, S. L., Mancini, M. A., and Rosen, J. M. (1999). *J. Biol. Chem.*, **274**, 22484.
11. Jerne, N. K., Henry, A. A., Nordin, H., Fuji, L., Koros, A. M. C., and Leftkovits, S. (1974). *Transplant Rev.*, **18**, 130.
12. Molinaro, G. A. and Dray. S. (1974). *Nature*, **248**, 515.
13. Neill, J. D., Smith, P. F., Luque, E. H., Munoz de Toro, M., Nagy, G., and Mulchahey, J. J. (1987). *Recent Progr. Horm. Res.*, **43**, 175.
14. Allaerts, W., Wouters A., Van der Massen, D., Persons, A., and Denef, C. (1988). *J. Theoret. Biol.*, **131**, 441.
15. Lewis, C. E., McCarthy, S. P. Richards, P. S. M., Lorenzen, J., Horak, E., and McGee, J. O'D. (1990). *J. Immunol. Meth.*, **127**, 51.
16. Palacios, R., Martinez-Mason, O., and De Ley, M. (1983). *Eur. J. Immunol,.* **13**, 221.
17. Lewis, C. E., Leek, R. D., Harris, A. and McGee, J. (1995). *J. Leukoc. Biol.*, **57**, 747.
18. Lewis, C. E., Horak, E., Lorenzen, J., McCarthy, S. P., and McGee, J. O'D. (1989). *Eur. J. Immunol.*, **19**, 2037.
19. Wickenhauser, C., Thiele, J., Lorenzen, J., Schmitz, B., Frimpong, S., Schramm, K., Neumann, I., Zankovich, R., and Fischer, R. (1999). *Leukemia*, **13**, 327.
20. Chauvet, N., Mouihate, A., Verrier, D., and Lestage, J. (1996). *Neuroreport.*, **7**, 2593.
21. Kendall, M. E. and Hymer, W. C. (1987). *Endocrinology*, **21**, 2263.

22. Gaffney., E. V., Stoner, C. R., Lingenfelter, S. E., and Wagner, L. A. (1989). *J. Immunol. Meth.*, **122**, 211.

23. Viselli, S. M. and Mastro, A. M. (1989). *J. Immunol. Meth.*, **125**, 115.

24. Wewetzer, K., Janet, T., Heymann, D., and Unsicker. K. J. (1993). *Neurosci. Res.*, **36**, 209.

25. Sedgwick, J. D. and Holt, P. G. (1983). *J. Exp. Med.*, **157**, 2178.

26. Czerkinsky, C., Abdersson, G., Ekre, H-P., Nilson, L-A., Kloreskog, L., and Ouchterlony, O. (1988). *J. Immunol. Meth.*, **111**, 29.

27. Hutchings, P. R., Cambridge, G., Tite, J. P., Meager, T., and Cooke A. (1989). *J. Immunol. Meth.*, **120**, 1.

28. Skidmore, B. J., Stamnes., S. A., Townsend, K., Glasebrook, A. L., Sheehan, K. C. F., Schreiber R. D., and Chiller, J. M. (1989). *Eur. J. Immunol.*, **19**, 1591.

29. Taguchi, T., McGhee, J. R., Coffman, R. L., Beagley, K. W., Eldridge, J. H., Takatsu, K., and Kiyono, H. (1990). *J. Immunol. Meth.*, **128**, 65.

30. Bienvenu, J. A., Monneret, G., Gutowski, M. C., and Fabien N. (1998). *Toxicology*, **129**, 55.

31. Vaquerano, J. E., Peng, M., Chang, J. W., Zhou, Y. M., and Leong, S. P. (1998). *Biotechniques*, **25**, 830.

32. Gey, A., Hamdi, S., Vielh, P., Mehtali, M., Fridman, W. H., and Tartour, E. (1999). *J. Immunol. Meth.*, **227**, 149.

33. Prussin, C. (1997). *J. Clin. Immunol.*, **17**, 195.

Chapter 10

Flow cytometric detection of intracellular cytokines

Alasdair M. J. Pennycook, Pietro Pala, Steve Matthews
Department of Respiratory Medicine, National Heart and Lung Institute, Imperial College School of Medicine at St Mary's, Norfolk Place, London W2 1PG, UK

Tracy Hussell
Department of Biochemistry, Imperial College, Exhibition Rd, London SW7 2AY, UK

Peter J. M. Openshaw
Department of Respiratory Medicine, National Heart and Lung Institute, Imperial College School of Medicine at St Mary's, Norfolk Place, London W2 1PG, UK

1 Introduction

1.1 Technique background

Recent technological advances in the availability and capability of flow cytometric analysis, coupled with advances in knowledge over the last 10 years, have made intracellular staining for cytokine expression an increasingly ubiquitous technique. It began with the pioneering work of the Anderssons at Stockholm University in the 1980s, who developed a system of cell fixation and permeabilization that left target antigens intact (1). Modifications since then have optimized the technique to allow the detection and further characterization of very few cytokine secreting cells within a heterogeneous population (2, 3).

The basic technique is simple. Any population of cytokine secreting cells can be isolated and stimulated under conditions which prevent protein secretion for a given time. After fixation and permeabilization, cells are incubated with a fluorochrome-conjugated antibody specific for a given cytokine and analysed by flow cytometry. As well as the necessary technical improvements, conceptual advances have made intracellular cytokine staining (ICCS) an especially useful tool. When looking at multiple cytokine responses, for instance in TH1 or TH2 responses, ICCS gives an ease and versatility of analysis that is unrivalled by other methods. This chapter will outline the steps to be taken to stain for any cytokine for which a labelled specific antibody is available, in any secretory cell population.

1.2 Experimental advantages and disadvantages

ICCS has changed the way we view mixed T-cell populations. This is due to several critical advantages over other techniques:

- Single-cell analysis is possible both in terms of frequency and intensity, without the labour required for limiting dilution analysis or ELISpot.
- It is possible to simultaneously detect several cytokines in a single cell.
- Analysis of large cell populations can be achieved quickly and without the need for cloning and prolonged *in vitro* culture.

However, as with any technique, there are also potential hazards and inherent disadvantages:

- Cytokine synthesis is not constitutive, even during vigorous inflammation. *In vitro* re-stimulation is therefore required, increasing the potential for artefacts and bringing associated problems due to activation (see Section 3).
- Even after stimulation, not all cells produce a given cytokine, nor the same cell two different cytokines, with the same kinetics.
- Anatomical information obtainable from *in situ* hybridization or immunohistochemistry is lost (see Chapter 3 in Vol. 1 and Chapter 9 in this volume).
- Cells must be killed for analysis, precluding the possibility of any further functional study.

2 Cell activation

Most studies to date using ICCS have focused on lymphocytes, mainly using density gradient-separated peripheral blood mononuclear cells (PBMC) but whole blood has also been used (4). However, other cell types produce cytokines and the protocols can be readily adapted to such studies (5–7). There are few generally applicable differences between the staining of mouse and human lymphocytes. For clarity, all protocols detailed here are for human PBMC preparations, but are easily adapted for use in mice or other animals.

2.1 Polyclonal activators

There are just a few situations, such as some chronic infections, where unstimulated cells can be studied directly *ex vivo* by ICCS. Some form of activation is usually necessary, the most robust stimulus being a short incubation with phorbol myristate acetate and a calcium ionophore. This is the best method with which to obtain a positive control and the one that should be used first before other activation conditions are considered. However, this is a non-specific activation, and in functional studies it may be more relevant to compare this response with that achieved with more physiologically relevant stimuli (see Section 2.2).

In order to enhance the signal-to-noise (S/N) ratio, it is desirable to add an inhibitor of exocytosis to induce accumulation of intracellular protein. This can be achieved with both monensin and brefeldin A. Users should evaluate both for any advantage in a specific system. Though neither is necessarily preferable, there is some evidence that monensin may be a more robust inhibitor of protein export. Commercial alternatives are also available, based on the same reagents (GolgiPlug (brefeldin A) and GolgiStop (monensin) from Pharmingen). Inhibitors can be added to the cells at the same time as the stimulus, if this provides time for sufficient stimulation, or only for a given period at the end. Reagent toxicity will cause cell death, increasing with prolonged incubation. After 16 hours, brefeldin A at 10 µg/ml will kill around 80% of human PBMC; toxicity is similar with monensin. To minimize this, it is therefore necessary to titrate for the optimal time for both activation and secretion blocking. Dead cells also release DNA that causes cell clumping, which can interfere with cytometric analysis. To prevent this, a DNase treatment step is often desirable.

Different cytokines will be produced with different kinetics, even following PMA stimulation: for instance, IL-4 and -5 detection peaks at 4–6 hours, while IFN-γ peaks at 10 h. Several published studies have therefore used a 4-hour incubation time as a compromise to yield near-optimal results in a workable timeframe (8). In some situations it may be desirable to allow cells to proliferate prior to the addition of PMA and ionomycin. For instance, it has been shown that a given human TH2 T cell does not express IL-4 until it has undergone at least three cycles of division (9). Other cytokines and cell types may require longer or shorter incubation times; cytokine expression in basophils, for example, peaks at around 2 hours.

Protocol 1

Polyclonal activation of T cells for TH1/TH2 phenotyping

Equipment and reagents (All from Sigma unless specified)

- 200 µg/ml Phorbol myristate acetate (PMA) in DMSO
- 10 mM ionomycin Ca^{2+} salt in DMSO (5 mg/0.67 ml)
- 300 mM monensin in methanol (warm to dissolve)
- 3 mg/ml DNase I in PBS
- RPMI-1640 complete medium
- PBS/A: PBS/0.1% NaN_3
- 15 ml conical-bottom tubes, polyethylene or thick-wall polystyrene (Fisher Scientific)

Method

1 Prepare a single-cell suspension of PBMC (10) and resuspend in RPMI-1640 complete culture medium at 10^6/ml in 15 ml tubes (1–2 ml).

2 Add PMA and ionomycin to 10 ng/ml and 100 ng/ml, respectively, and monensin[a] to 10 µM. (Include stimulation controls with monensin alone.)

3 Incubate for 4 h at 37 °C.

4 Add DNase I at a ratio of 1:25 and incubate in a 37 °C waterbath for 5 min.

Protocol 1 continued

5   Add 10 ml of PBS/A to each tube, spin at 500 $\times$ g for 10 min at 4 °C.

6   Resuspend in PBS/A and count the cells.

7   Aliquot to the desired concentration per tube (generally at least 2×10^5 cells are required for sufficient events for each stain; 10^6 is preferable) and spin at 500 g for 10 min at 4 °C.

[a] Use brefeldin A at 10 µg/ml.

2.2 Physiological activators

The general activation stimulus provided by PMA often provokes a more widespread production of cytokines than would be seen in response to antigen. In the case of IFN-γ staining, this may be as much as an order of magnitude or more. This non-specific stimulus represents the potential to produce cytokines at the most basic level, i.e. whether the gene locus is open or closed; however, many more levels of regulation operate *in vivo*. It may therefore be more physiologically relevant to analyse (or at least contrast) the response of T cells to a more 'biological' stimulus. Direct stimulation of the T-cell receptor (TCR) complex can be achieved in a heterogeneous cell population by treatment with solid phase α-CD3 and soluble α-CD28 for 24 hours. The culture may then be expanded with IL-2 and TH1/TH2 skewing cytokines. However, optimization of this process is complex, and is detailed elsewhere (11). If dealing with T-cell clones or lines, it may be preferable to use antigen-presenting cells (APC) loaded with antigen for culture stimulation and expansion. Loaded APCs must have good cell-to-cell contact with responding T cells at an appropriate ratio. This is best achieved by brief centrifugation in round-bottomed tubes. It is possible to use whole antigen-loaded APCs when working with a heterogeneous T-cell population. LPS-primed splenocytes or purified dendritic cells pulsed overnight with whole antigen give limited re-stimulation. APCs are also required if using phytohaemagglutinin (1–10 µg/ml and optionally with α-CD28, 1 µg/ml) or superantigen stimulation (e.g. *Staphylococcus* enterotoxin B, 2 µg/ml).

3 Considerations when surface staining

With the advent of four-colour staining it is now possible to utilize ICCS to extensively phenotype single cytokine-secreting cells by surface antigen expression. Classical surface markers such as CD4 and CD8, as well as novel markers (e.g. T1/ST2 (12)), can distinguish the functional character of cells and allow their correlation with cytokine secretion patterns. In most situations this involves only adding an extra step into the protocol prior to cell fixation. Staining is performed, as it would be in a standard assay; e.g. a 30-min incubation at 4 °C with antibody diluted in PBS/1% BSA, followed by two washes. However, when analysing the results it must be taken into account what has happened to the cells during *in vitro* culture. Even a 4-hour incubation with PMA may result in phenotypic changes.

The most marked example of this is CD4 downregulation following PMA stimulation of human T cells (13, 14). Surface expression of CD4 declines progressively with increasing concentrations of PMA. Therefore, although it is possible to co-localize cytokine production and CD4 expression, the latter marker may no longer delineate the *in vivo* functional CD4 population. The danger is that functional significance is placed on changes that are a result of *in vitro* culture and not *in vivo* differences. There are, however, some possible remedies. Inhibition of phagolysosome degradation can allow the detection of these markers after their endocytosis. Also, CD5+/CD8− or CD3+/CD8− cells may be used as an approximation or in comparison to the CD4 population. In preference, it is possible to stain for surface CD4 prior to the stimulation step. Providing monensin is used throughout stimulation, acidic and proteolytic degradation of the fluorochrome is inhibited and the signal remains detectable (15). Where glycosylphosphatidylinositol anchored markers such as CD14 and CD16 are lost through shedding, the problem is more difficult to overcome. When analysing monocytes, loss of CD14 expression, combined with their tendency to stick to plastic upon activation, makes them a tricky target for analysis. Difficulties of this nature may play a part in determining the optimal titration of PMA concentration and incubation time during activation.

4 Fixation

All published methods for ICCS use an aldehyde-based fixative, generally either formaldehyde or paraformaldehyde. This immobilizes the target antigen within the cell to prevent leakage during the subsequent permeabilization stage. No better fixative has yet been developed, and the two are effectively identical in terms of results, differing only in the preparation of solutions.

Protocol 2

Fixation of activated and surface-stained lymphocytes

Equipment and reagents

For Method A
- 4% fresh paraformaldehyde (PFA); heat to dissolve
- Ice-cold PBS/BSA/A: 1% BSA, 0.05% NaN$_3$ in PBS

For Method B
- 40% formaldehyde
- 1.56 × PBS
- Ice-cold PBS/BSA/A: 1% BSA, 0.05% NaN$_3$ in PBS

A. Paraformaldehyde fixation

1 Pre-warm PFA to 37 °C and pre-cool PBS/BSA/A on ice.
2 Add 500 µl to each tube of stained lymphocytes and leave to stand at room temperature for 5 min.[a] Vortex each tube 3–4 times during this period to avoid clumping.

Protocol 2 continued

3　Add 10 ml of ice-cold PBS/BSA/A and vortex.

4　Centrifuge at 1500 × g for 10 min[b] at room temperature prior to permeabilization.

B. Formaldehyde fixation

1　Add 9 ml of 1.56 × PBS to each stained lymphocyte suspension.

2　Add 1 ml of 40% formaldehyde to each tube and leave to stand at room temperature for 20 min.[a] Vortex each tube at least 3–4 times during the first 5 min to prevent cell clumping.

3　Centrifuge at 1500 × g for 10 min[b] at room temperature. Discard the supernatant and resuspend the pellet in 10 ml of ice-cold PBS/BSA/A.

4　Centrifuge at 1500 × g for 10 min at room temperature prior to permeabilization.

[a] Fixing for an unnecessarily long time increases cellular protein hydrophobicity and can increase the background signal.

[b] The use of BSA in buffers and high-speed centrifugation increases cell recovery since fixed cells pellet poorly.

It may be desirable, especially during large experiments or with unwieldy activation periods, to leave fixed cells at this point. Cells can be stored in the dark at 4 °C in PBS/BSA/A without adverse effects for several days. Alternatively, aliquots can be stored indefinitely at −80 °C in PBS/BSA/A with 10% dimethyl sulfoxide (DMSO). Some commercially available reagents combine the fixation step with permeabilization (e.g. Ortho Permeafix (Ortho), CytoFix/CytoPerm (Pharmingen)) and are acceptable, but they do not provide the required flexibility required in some situations.

Protocol 3

Saponin membrane permeabilization of a fixed lymphocytic cell population

Reagents

- PBS/BSA/A/sap: 1% BSA, 0.05% NaN$_3$, 0.1% saponin[a] in PBS
  Or

- PBS/sap/NFM: 5% (w/v) non-fat milk (NFM), 0.1% saponin[a] in PBS.

Method

1　If using the suspension containing NFM, centrifuge the PBS/sap/NFM at 1500 × g for 30 min and use the clear or slightly opalescent supernatant.

2　Resuspend the fixed and stained PBMC in 100 μl PBS/BSA/A/sap *or* PBS/sap/NFM.

3　Leave to block at room temperature for 10 or 30 min, respectively.

[a] Many protocols use 0.5% saponin in PBS/BSA/A/sap when staining mouse PBMC populations.

5 Intracellular staining

5.1 Permeabilization

Permeabilization of the cell membrane is easily achieved through a short incubation with mild detergent, most often saponin. Saponin is a reversible permeabilization agent and therefore must be included in all reagents in subsequent steps. At this point it is often desirable to add excess blocking protein to decrease the problem of non-specific binding by monoclonal antibodies (mAbs).

The blocking reagent used in this protocol should be used in all subsequent steps (referred to as diluent in *Protocol 4*).

5.2 Cytokine staining

5.2.1 Experimental design

The final stage of the technique, specific staining for intracellular cytokine, is straightforward in itself, but requires the most care during experimental design. The availability of cellular protein for non-specific binding in a permeabilized cell is several orders of magnitude greater than in standard flow cytometric analysis. The blocking step decreases, but does not remove, this problem, thus the importance of proper controls (see Section 5.2.2). Further, the increased availability of target antigen increases the possibility of cross-reaction, as recently illustrated by the demonstration by Singh *et al.* of an IL-6 antibody cross-reacting with histone H2B (16).

Especially for the detection of cytokines such as IL-4, which are fluorescently dim or rarely produced, the optimization of the S/N ratio is paramount. It is technological advances in this area that have allowed ICCS to become so widely applied. Directly fluorochrome-conjugated antibodies with good S/N ratios are increasingly available commercially. Meticulous titration of the antibody concentration (optimum is usually between 0.5 and 5 $\mu g/10^6$ cells) can almost eliminate background staining in some situations. When results are less favourable, it is preferable to use phycoerythrin (PE)-conjugated antibodies, as these usually have the best S/N ratio (in preference to biotinylated antibody then FITC conjugates). Note that biotinylated antibodies cannot be used if the blocking reagent (see *Protocol 3*) contains milk or serum. Use PBS/BSA/A/sap in these situations. Another disadvantage of biotinylated antibodies is that labelled streptavidin is likely to bind to endogenous biotin in cells, increasing the background signal. If working with a weak signal it may be necessary to block the binding capacity of the cellular biotin (incubate cells overnight at 4°C with 10 $\mu g/ml$ of unlabelled streptavidin in PBS/BSA/A/sap) (17).

Protocol 4 is an example of a staining method for IL-4 in human PBMC.

5.2.2 Positive and negative controls

As detailed above, several problems specifically associated with ICCS demand stringent controls in every experiment. Each sample tube should be run with an appropriate control tube. Positive control cells are now commercially available, but certain cell lines stimulated with PMA may make as effective a control.

Protocol 4

ICCS for IL-4 in fixed PBMC preparations

Reagents

- Diluent: PBS/BSA/A/sap *or* PBS/sap/NFM (see *Protocol 3*)
- PE-conjugated mouse IgG1 α-human IL-4, clone 8D4–8 (Pharmingen, 18655A)

Method

1 Dilute 8D4–8-PE to give a final concentration in the staining tube of 0.25 μg/10^6 cells.[a]

2 Add the diluted antibody to fixed and permeabilized PBMC preparation and incubate in the dark at room temperature for 30 min.

3 Add 5 ml of the diluent and centrifuge at 1500 × g for 10 min at room temperature then repeat.

4 Resuspend in 300 μl of PBS for analysis

[a] Antibody can be added directly to the cells after the blocking step (*Protocol 3*), but allowance must be made for the increased volume. To save reagents it may be desirable to centrifuge (1500 × g for 10 min at room temperature) and resuspend the cells.

Protocol 5

Control stain for intracellular IL-4 in human PBMC preparations

Reagents

- Diluent: PBS/BSA/A/sap *or* PBS/sap/NFM (see *Protocol 3*)
- PE-conjugated mouse IgG1 α-human IL-4, clone 8D4–8 (Pharmingen, 18655A)
- Unlabelled clone 8D4–8 (Pharmingen, 18651D)
- PE-conjugated isotype-control IgG1 mouse Ab, clone MOPC21 (Pharmingen, 20605A)

Method

1 Aliquot fixed and permeabilized PBMC preparation (end of *Protocol 3*) into two tubes.

2 Incubate the first tube with 8D4–8 at 5 μg/10^6 cells and the second with the isotype control antibody at the same concentration in diluent, for at least 45 min in the dark at 4 °C.

3 Add labelled antibody[a] (PE-8D4–8) at 0.25 μg/10^6 cells and incubate for a further 30 min in the dark at 4 °C.

4 Wash twice with diluent and resuspend for analysis as in *Protocol 3*.

[a] Note that there is no washing step prior to addition of the labelled antibody.

The process of fixation tends to increase cell autofluorescence, therefore an unstained sample of the cell population should be run to allow for this. As mentioned in Section 3.1, the use of a blocking protein and titration of antibody concentrations can decrease background signal. Fc blocking antibodies (non-specific IgG or α-Fc antibodies) can be used, but seem to be of no advantage when examining T lymphocytes. The use of isotype-matched control antibodies does provide an adequate control, but only when the specificity of both anti-cytokine and isotype mAb is similar. Fixed and permeabilized cells often exaggerate differences in non-specific binding between even closely matched isotype antibodies. Therefore, until a technique is firmly established, it is preferable to use one of the two control protocols detailed below.

Pre-incubating a molar excess of recombinant cytokine with the mAb to block binding provides a rigorous control for specificity. However, this is likely to be highly expensive if large amounts of recombinant protein are required, and should only be performed once as proof of principle, if at all. An alternative is to use an unlabelled version of the mAb to compete-out the binding of the labelled antibody (see *Protocol 5*). Failing this, perhaps the most rigorous test of specificity is showing that two antibodies recognizing different epitopes of the same target antigen consistently give a similar frequency of positive cells. A permeabilization control, i.e. identically treated cells using reagents without saponin, may also be useful to discount surface binding of soluble cytokine.

5.2.3 Flow cytometric analysis

In principle, the analysis of intracellularly stained cells by flow cytometry does not differ from standard surface staining. In both cases, where multiple fluorescence detectors are in use, appropriate compensation using single stained samples is necessary. It is preferable, but sometimes impossible, to use antibodies under conditions that provide clear bimodal distributions on histograms. This may also depend on the cytokine under study; e.g. directly *ex vivo*, IFN-γ will give two distinct peaks, where IL-4 is likely to evidence as a right-shifted 'shoulder' of fluorescence. The use of negative control samples to place statistical gates and collection of sufficient events in this regard is critical. When looking at multiple stains it is usually more informative to use dot or contour plots that allow the visualization of small groupings in the population. Cytokines such as IL-4 and –5 will only be present in a small, but significant, proportion of stimulated fresh PBMC.

The forward- and side-scatter properties of most cell populations remain intact throughout the fixing and permeabilization process. Some evidence of a reduction in forward scatter may be evident, but lymphocyte, macrophage, and granulocyte populations remain easily distinguishable. A surface stain, such as CD4, is useful not only for backgating to identify lymphocyte populations, but may also reduce the S/N ratio by excluding irrelevant events. The results obtained should, in the most part, agree with other assay systems such as ELISpot and ELISA—counterintuitive results are likely to be disproved by rigorous controls.

References

1. Sander, B., Andersson, J., and Andersson, U. (1991). *Immunol. Rev.*, **119**, 65.

2. Jung, T., Schauer, U., Heusser, C., Neumann, C., and Rieger, C. (1993). *J Immunol. Meth.*, **159**, 197.

3. Prussin, C. and Metcalfe, D. D. (1995). *J. Immunol. Meth.*, **188**, 117.

4. Ferry, B., Antrobus, P., Huzicka, I., Farrell, A., Lane, A., and Chapel, H. (1997). *Clin. Exp. Immunol.*, **110**, 410.

5. Kon, O. M., Sihra, B. S., Till, S. J., Corrigan, C. J., Kay, A. B., and Grant, J. A. (1998). *Allergy*, **53**, 891.

6. Rumbley, C. A., Sugaya, H., Zekavat, S. A., El, R. M., Perrin, P. J., and Phillips, S. M. (1999). *J. Immunol.*, **162**, 1003.

7. Kelleher, P. and Knight, S. C. (1998). *Int. Immunol.*, **10**, 749.

8. Hussell, T., Spender, L. C., Georgiou, A., O'Garra, A., and Openshaw, P. J. M. (1996). *J. Gen. Virol.*, **77**, 2447.

9. Bird, J. J., Brown, D. R., Mullen, A. C., Moskowitz, N. H., Mahowald, M. A., Sider, J. R., Gajewski, T. F., Wang, C. R., and Reiner, S. L. (1998). *Immunity*, **9**, 229.

10. Kanot, M. E., Smith, P. D., and Zola, H. (1995). In *Current protocols in immunology* (ed. J. E. Coligan, A. M. Kruisbeck, D. H. Margulies, E. M. Shevach and W. Strober), Chapter 7.1. Wiley, New York.

11. James, S. P. (1995). In *Current protocols in immunology* (ed. J. E. Coligan, A. M. Kruisbeck, D. H. Margulies, E. M. Shevach, and W. Strober), Chapter 7.10. Wiley, New York.

12. Lohning, M., Grogan, J. L., Coyle, A. J., Yazdanbakhsh, M., Meisel, C., Gutierrez-Ramos, J. C., Radbruch, A., and Kamradt, T. (1999). *J. Immunol.*, **162**, 3882.

13. Ruegg, C. L., Rajasekar, S., Stein, B. S., and Engleman, E. G. (1992). *J. Biol. Chem.*, **267**, 18837.

14. Pelchen, M. A., Parsons, I. J., and Marsh, M. (1993). *J. Exp. Med.*, **178**, 1209.

15. Mitra, D. K., De Rosa, S. C., Luke, A., Balamurugan, A., Khaitan, B. K., Tung, J., Mehra, N. K., Terr, A. I., O'Garra, A., Herzenberg, L. A., and Roederer, M. (1999). *Int. Immunol.*, **11**, 1801.

16. Zunino, S. J., Singh, M. K., Bass, J., and Picker, L. J. (1996). *Am. J. Pathol.*, **149**, 653.

17. Elson, L. H., Nutman, T. B., Metcalfe, D. D., and Prussin, C. (1995). *J. Immunol.*, **154**, 4294.

Chapter 11

Development of antibodies to cytokines

S. Poole
Division of Endocrinology, NIBSC, Blanche Lane, South Mimms, Potters Bar, Hertfordshire EN6 3QG, UK

1 Introduction

Antibodies to cytokines can greatly facilitate research on many aspects of these mediators, including: the development of specific and sensitive immunoassays (see Chapter 12); the detection of cytokines in biological fluids, tissues, and cells using immunochemical and immunocytochemical techniques; immmuno-neutralization of biological activities; and delineation of external regions (epitopes) of the cytokines.

2 Choice of immunogen

Recombinant cytokines are generally the immunogens used, although purified native cytokines, conjugates of cytokines to carrier proteins, synthesized peptides with amino-acid sequences corresponding to selected portions of cytokine sequences, and enzymatic digests of cytokines may be used.

2.1 Recombinant cytokines

These offer advantages, in that it is possible to prepare recDNA proteins in large quantities and with low levels of contaminating proteins. Disadvantages for glycosylated cytokines are that non-glycosylated analogues are produced in *Escherichia coli* (*E. coli*) and glycosylation patterns in yeast and in Chinese hamster ovary (CHO) cells are likely to be different from those of the native cytokine. Also, extraction and purification procedures may result in inappropriate folding of these molecules.

2.2 Purified 'natural' cytokines

Purified native cytokines are far more likely to be contaminated with other polypeptides/proteins than recombinant preparations (which are likely to be contaminated with dimers and other oligomers). While it is desirable to immunize with pure preparations of cytokines, this is crucial when the same contaminants are likely to be present in the materials with which the anticytokine antibodies are to be used. When highly purified proteins are initially unavailable for immunization but subsequently do become available, they may then be used for antibody purification by affinity chromatography.

2.3 Conjugates of cytokines

Where there is a high degree of homology between a cytokine and the native cytokine in the species to be immunized, immunogenicity may be enhanced by conjugating the cytokine to a protein carrier. The choice of proteins for conjugation and methods of conjugation are discussed below in relation to small (synthesized) peptide homologues of cytokines. As far as conjugates of the cytokines themselves are concerned, conjugates of recombinant human interleukin-1α (IL-1α), IL-1β, rat IL-1β, and murine IL-1β, when injected into rabbits and guinea-pigs, were less effective than the unconjugated cytokines at generating high-titre, high-affinity antibodies. Cytokines that are poorly immunogenic but which have been produced with a 6×His tag may be bound to Ni–NTA agarose gel to increase immunogenicity (1), as described below for small peptides.

2.4 Small peptide homologues

These are often used when the amino-acid sequence of a cytokine is known but where only limited amounts of pure antigen are available. Also, the use of peptide homologues avoids the circular logic that sometimes arises when characterizing antisera with the same antigens to which they were raised, e.g. a partially purified preparation of a cytokine. A major disadvantage of antipeptide antibodies is that their affinities for the relevant cytokine (i.e. native molecule) are generally much lower than their affinities for the peptides. This renders the antipeptide antibodies generated of little use in developing sensitive immunoassays for the cytokine, although they are sometimes useful for immunochemical/immunohistochemical procedures and for epitope mapping studies. Indeed, the capacity of an antipeptide antibody to immunoprecipitate a cytokine in a liquid-phase assay is the only test that unambiguously defines external sites on the native molecule.

Peptides with molecular weights of less than 2000–3000 are not usually immunogenic, but specific antibodies against these low molecular-weight immunogens can be produced by conjugation to high molecular-weight proteins. A chemical group rendered immunogenic by conjugation is known as a hapten and the process of conjugating it to a larger protein is known as haptenization. Small peptide homologues of cytokines used as immunogens usually comprise 15–20 amino-acid residues and therefore need to be haptenized to generate useful antibodies. An alternative to conjugation is to have peptides synthesized with a 6×His tag, comprising six histidine residues added at either the N-terminus or C-terminus, and to bind them to Ni–NTA agarose gel to increase their immunogenicity (1).

A wide variety of high molecular-weight substances have been used successfully for the haptenization of peptides. These include bovine thyroglobulin (BTG), bovine serum albumin (BSA), ovalbumin (OVA), keyhole limpet haemocyanin (KLH), and purified protein derivative of tuberculin (PPD). It is worth noting that one of the most immunogenic proteins, KLH, is the least soluble and that the methods described below can be used with any of the proteins given above or, indeed, a variety of others. PPD offers several advantages—at least in theory (2). PPD elicits delayed-type hypersensitivity reactions in animals (and in humans) previously exposed to the tubercle bacillus. Thus, animals previously immunized with Bacillus Calmette–Guérin (BCG) are injected subsequently with the peptide–PPD conjugate. PPD provides T-cell help and gives rise to virtually no antibody response in itself: this is particularly useful if it is intended to go on to make monoclonal antibodies, where the presence of significant anticonjugate antibodies are undesirable. The author has found little to choose between the proteins given above, although most workers do have their favourites.

The choice of conjugation reagent is more significant. A number of chemical procedures have been developed for conjugating peptides to proteins. All depend upon the use of cross-linking reagents, which are of two main types: (a) homobifunctional cross-linkers, which have the same functional group at either end and couple via the same amino-acid side chains in peptide and protein, and (b) heterobifunctional cross-linkers, which couple via two different side chains.

2.4.1 Homobifunctional cross-linkers

The most widely used (and easy to use) cross-linker is glutaraldehyde (pentane-1,5 dial). The reaction is complex, involving many different side chains, and produces a heterogeneous, uncharacterized conjugate. With shorter peptides, glutaraldehyde will almost invariably couple via the N-terminal amino group which may be a disadvantage, e.g. if the N-terminal amino acids comprise part of an epitope.

Protocol 1

Conjugation of peptides to KLH with glutaraldehyde

Reagents

- Keyhole limpet haemocyanin (KLH)
- 0.01 M NaOH
- 0.5 M sodium bicarbonate
- DMSO
- 2.5% glutaraldehyde
- PBS
- 1.0 M Tris–HCl pH 8.5
- Magnetic stirrer

Method

1 Dissolve 5 mg of KLH in 1.0 ml of 0.01 M NaOH and then add 1.0 ml of 0.5 M sodium bicarbonate.

2 Dissolve 250 µg of the peptide in 25 µl of DMSO.

Protocol 1 continued

3   Mix 100 μl of the KLH solution with 10 μl of the peptide solution and, while stirring, add 2.5% glutaraldehyde dropwise over 1 h to a final concentration of 0.1%

4   After stirring for further 4 h in the dark, add 0.25 ml of PBS and 25 μl of 1.0 M Tris–HCl, pH 8.5. Store the conjugate below −40 °C.

When a peptide contains a tyrosine group, either as part of the naturally occurring sequence or added during synthesis, a more specific reagent, bis-diazotolidine (BDT), may be used to couple together tyrosine side chains of the peptide and protein.

Protocol 2

Conjugation of peptides to OVA with BDT

Equipment and reagents

- o-Tolidine
- HCl
- Sodium nitrite
- Borate saline pH 9.0
- 0.9% NaCl
- Bis-diazotolidine (which is unstable). Prepare fresh.
- Dialysis membrane system or desalting equipment and reagents
- Magnetic stirrer

Method

1   Dissolve 0.23 g o-tolidine in 45 ml of HCl and place on ice. Dissolve 0.175 g sodium nitrite ($NaNO_2$) in 5 ml of water.

2   Add the $NaNO_2$ solution to the o-tolidine dropwise over 5–10 min with constant stirring, ensure that the mixture remains cold. Note that the colour of the solution changes from clear to yellow, to orangish-red, and back to yellow.

3   Dissolve OVA at 5 mg/ml in borate saline at pH 9.0.

4   Dissolve 5.0 mg peptide in 2.5 ml of the OVA solution.

5   Briskly add dropwise, 1.0 ml freshly prepared bis-diazotolidine (which is unstable).

6   Incubate for 4 h in the dark, and then remove any excess reagents by dialysis or desalting. (Uncoupled peptide is lost through the dialysis membrane 12–14 000 MWCO (Medical International Ltd.). Before immunization dialyse the conjugate into 0.9% NaCl or precipitate with 4 vol. of cold acetone (−70 °C), pellet at 10 000 g, air-dry, and re-disperse in 0.9% NaCl. Store the conjugate below −40 °C.

2.4.2 Heterobifunctional cross-linkers

The water-soluble carbodiimides (e.g. 1-ethyl-3-(3-dimethyl aminopropyl-carbodiimide) couple amino groups to carboxyl groups, and thus form heterogeneous conjugates.

Protocol 3

Conjugation of peptides to bovine thyroglobulin (BTG) with carbodiimide

Equipment and reagents

- 0.1 M sodium bicarbonate
- 0.1 M sodium bicarbonate.
- Carbodiimide
- 0.5 M glycine
- Sephadex G-50 (Pharmacia) column (6 × 100 mm)
- 0.01 M sodium bicarbonate containing 0.9% NaCl as column buffer

Method

1   Dissolve 0.5 mg of the peptide in 0.5 ml of 0.1 M sodium bicarbonate and add to BTG, 1.0 mg in 0.5 ml of 0.1 M sodium bicarbonate.

2   Add 1 mg of carbodiimide and incubate the mixture with stirring for 1 h in the dark at room temperature.

3   Add glycine (0.5 M, 20 μl) to quench unreacted groups and desalt the conjugate on a Sephadex G-50 (Pharmacia) column (6 × 100 mm) using 0.01 M sodium bicarbonate containing 0.9% NaCl as column buffer. Store the conjugate below −40 °C.

When a peptide contains a cysteine residue, either as part of the naturally occurring sequence or added during synthesis, the hetero bifunctional reagent *m*-maleimidobenzoic acid *N*-hydroxy succinimide (MBS) ester may be used to couple sulfydryl to amino groups.

Protocol 4

Conjugation of peptides to keyhole limpet cyanin (KLH) with MBS

Equipment and reagents

- Dialysis system
- 10 mM potassium phosphate buffer pH 7.2
- MBS stock at 3 mg/ml in dimethyl formamide
- 20 ml Sephadex P-30 column
- 50 mM phosphate buffer pH 6.0
- Magnetic stirrer

Method

1   Dialyse KLH against 10 mM potassium phosphate buffer pH 7.2. Adjust the KLH concentration to about 20 mg/ml.

2   Ideally, use freshly weighed out peptide. Note that if using a stock solution of peptide (e.g. in PBS), it may be necessary to reduce the peptide before use. Otherwise, dissolve

the peptide at 5 mg/ml in 10 mM phosphate buffer (4 mg of KLH is required for every 5 mg of peptide).

3 Add 55 μl of 10 mM phosphate buffer to each 4 mg KLH solution.

4 Slowly add 85 μl of the MBS stock at 3 mg/ml in dimethyl formamide to each 4 mg of KLH. Stir for 30 min at room temperature.

5 Desalt the activated KLH on a 10-ml column Biorad 10 DG disposable chromatography Column Cat No 732-2010. Pre-equilibrate and run the column in 50 mM phosphate buffer, pH 6.0. Collect 1-ml fractions (typically about 15). Note that protein elutes as a visible grey peak at the exclusion volume (fractions 6–8), and that about 95% of the KLH is recovered.

6 Add activated KLH to the peptide solution while stirring at room temperature. Adjust the pH to 7.4 and stir at room temperature for 3 h. Store the conjugate below −40 °C.

When a synthesized peptide or recDNA cytokine has been produced with a 6×His tag, the peptide or protein may be bound to Ni–NTA agarose to increase immunogenicity (1).

Protocol 5

Binding of peptides to Ni–NTA agarose gel

Equipment and reagents

- PBS
- Ni–NTA agarose
- Vortex mixer

Method

1 Dissolve the peptide in PBS at about 2 mg/ml.

2 Mix 0.5 ml of this peptide solution with 0.5–1.0 ml of the Ni–NTA agarose that has been washed twice with PBS and resuspended in 4 ml PBS.

3 Allow the peptide to bind to the Ni–NTA agarose at room temperature for 30 min.

4 Vortex and store at −40 °C. After thawing, vortex again before preparing emulsions.

2.5 Enzymatic digests of cytokines

Purified fragments of cytokines offer advantages and disadvantages similar to those of small peptide homologues. Small fragments, i.e. < 3000 kDa, will require haptenization.

3 Choice of animal

Where large quantities of antibodies are required, e.g. for commercial purposes or to provide reference reagents, hybridoma technology has made it possible to produce monoclonal antibodies with predefined binding characteristics, which can be produced in large amounts from immortal cell lines. Another advantage of monoclonal antibodies is that they can be raised against impure immunogens, provided that pure material is available for screening. However, monoclonal antibodies to cytokines often are not neutralizing and (like monoclonal antibodies to most antigens) have lower affinities than polyclonal antibodies to the same antigens. Polyclonal antibodies may also be obtained in quantity from large animals such as sheep, goats, donkeys, and horses.

Rabbits are the first choice when very large volumes of antiserum are not required, provided that sequence homology between the cytokine to be injected and the native rabbit cytokine is not too great. Guinea-pigs will usually be the second choice, although they produce less antiserum and are more difficult to bleed than rabbits.

Whichever of these small species is chosen, it is recommended that several individuals are immunized since individual variation in response can be marked. Groups of at least three, but preferably more, rabbits or guinea-pigs should be used.

4 The adjuvant

A wide variety of substances potentiate the humoral antibody response to injected immunogens. Potentiators include inorganic adsorbents, e.g. aluminium hydroxide, long-chain carbohydrates, resins, mineral oils such as liquid paraffin, and bacterial cell-wall components such as muramyl dipeptide and its analogues. This diversity of materials having adjuvant properties makes it difficult to identify a single mechanism of action. The most important advance in adjuvant technology was the development by Freund and co-workers of adjuvants containing mycobacteria, mineral oil, and emulsifier (3). The simple oil–detergent mixture is termed Freund's 'incomplete' adjuvant (FIA); incorporation of heat-killed *Mycobacterium tuberculosis* or *M. butyricum* (0.5 mg/ml) into the oily mixture yields Freund's 'complete' adjuvant (FCA). The latter is more effective, probably as a result of greater stimulation of the local cellular response. For the immunization schedules described below FCA is used for the primary immunization and FIA for all boosts. For maximum efficiency, it is necessary to prepare a stable, water-in-oil emulsion. This can be achieved in a number of ways, but the simplest is by using the double-hub connector method described in detail by Hurn and Chantler (4)—1 vol. of aqueous immunogen is emulsified in 2–4 vol. of oily adjuvant.

Adjuvants other than Freund's have their advocates, but in the absence of a rigorous comparison of different adjuvants used with the same immunogens it is difficult to make general recommendations. Unfortunately, many reports describing novel adjuvants do not include Freund's as a positive control. In man, only aluminium hydroxide and aluminium phosphate are permitted as adjuvants.

5 Immunization schedules

The protocols described below have proved successful, although scientists in the UK may be required to modify certain of these to comply with current *Home Office guidelines on antibody production: advice on protocols for minimum severity* (5). This will depend upon the procedures permitted under project licences and personal licences held under the *Animals (Scientific Procedures) Act 1986* (6). Consequently, scientists in the UK are advised to discuss immunization protocols with their local Home Office Inspector before commencing immunizations. Similarly, scientists in other countries should ensure that immunization protocols comply with local legislation and ethical considerations before commencing work of this nature.

5.1 Mice

A variety of protocols have proved successful. A protocol which yielded mono-clonal antibodies to IL-1α using BALB/c mice (7) is given below.

Protocol 6

Generation of monoclonal antibodies

Equipment and reagents

- BALB/c mice
- PBS
- FCA
- FIA
- Cytokine or conjugate
- Syringes and needles

Method

1. Emulsify the cytokine or conjugate (25 μg in 0.25 ml of PBS) in FCA (0.75 ml) and inject subcutaneously (SC) into three sites on day 1.

2. On days 30 and 60 after the primary immunization, emulsify 10 μg of the cytokine or conjugate (in 0.1 ml of PBS) in FIA (0.2 ml) and inject intraperitoneally (IP).

3. On day 150 inject the mice intravenously (IV) with 10 μg cytokine or conjugate in PBS (0.3 ml). On day 153 remove the spleens for fusion. A detailed protocol for the production of monoclonal antibodies is given elsewhere (8).

5.2 Rabbits

A series of subcutaneous injections has worked well for a number of rat recDNA cytokines, including IL-1α, recombinant human (rh) IL-1β, IL-6, and a variety of human IL-1β-related peptides.

Protocol 7

Raising rabbit antisera[a]

Equipment and reagents

- Rabbits
- Cytokine or conjugate
- PBS
- FCA

- FIA
- Syringes and needles
- Blood collection pots

Method

1 For three rabbits, emulsify the cytokine or conjugate, about 150–200 μg (in 0.4 ml PBS), in 1.2 ml of FCA for the primary immunization.

2 Make subcutaneous (SC) injections of 0.25 ml of emulsion into each hind limb.

3 Boost the animals by the SC route, 6–8 weeks after the primary immunization and at intervals of 6–8 weeks thereafter. For boosts (for three rabbits), emulsify about 150 μg of the cytokine or conjugate (in 0.4 ml of PBS) in 1.2 ml of FIA and inject 0.25 ml of emulsion SC into each fore limb or into each hind limb, alternately.

4 If desired, take bleeds (20–30 ml) 8–11 days after each boost.

[a] Variations of this protocol have also proved successful (9, 10).

5.3 Guinea-pigs

Although guinea-pigs have responded well to a number of proteins poorly immunogenic in other species, e.g. insulin and parathyroid hormone, the author has not found guinea-pigs to be good responders to human IL-1β-related peptides, nor to rat and mouse IL-1β (possibly because of good sequence homology between rat/mouse IL-1β and guinea-pig IL-1β).

Protocol 8

Raising guinea-pig antisera

Equipment and reagents

- Cytokine or conjugate
- PBS
- FCA

- FIA
- Syringes and needles
- Blood collection pots

Method

1 For three guinea-pigs emulsify about 150 μg of cytokine or conjugate (in 0.4 ml PBS) in 1.4 ml of FCA.

2 Inject 0.15 ml SC (into each of four sites) into the abdominal wall just on either side of the midline.

Protocol 8 continued

3   Boost the animals by the SC route, 4–8 weeks after the primary immunization and at intervals of 4–8 weeks thereafter. For boosts (for three guinea pigs), emulsify about 150 μg of the cytokine or conjugate (in 0.4 ml PBS) in 1.2 ml FIA and inject 0.25 ml of emulsion SC into each hind limb or into each fore limb, alternately.

4   If desired, bleed animals by cardiac puncture, which yields only 3–5 ml of serum, about 8–10 days after each boost.[a]

[a] Because of the low yield of serum and the risk of killing the animals when bleeding by cardiac puncture, it is less practicable to bleed guinea-pigs repeatedly than it is to bleed rabbits. Therefore it is best to immunize a relatively large number of animals for a comparatively long period of time, then bleed them out and select the best antisera.

5.4 Sheep and goats

An intramuscular schedule in sheep and goats has worked well for a number of cytokines (11–14).

Protocol 9

Raising sheep and goat antisera

Equipment and reagents

- Cytokine or conjugate
- PBS
- FCA
- FIA
- Syringes and needles
- Blood collection pots

Method

1   For the primary immunization emulsify about 500 μg of the cytokine or conjugate (in 0.5 ml of PBS) in 1.5 ml of FCA. Inject 0.5 ml of the emulsion intramuscularly (IM) deeply into the haunches and shoulders.

2   Boost with about 250 μg of the cytokine or conjugate (in 0.25 ml of PBS) emulsified in 0. 75 ml FIA, also by the IM route, either into the haunches or shoulders at intervals after the primary immunization of 1–2 months, 4–6 months, 6–8 months, and 10–12 months.

3   Collect bleeds on a regular schedule throughout the immunization.[a] Note that the highest titres occur usually around 10 days after a boost.

[a] Depending on the size of the animal, two or three bleeds of 300–600 ml each may be taken between 1 and 2 weeks after a boost.

6 Screening

Antibodies may be evaluated in a variety of ways depending upon their intended use. Neutralizing activities are usually assessed in specific *in vitro* bioassays (see

Chapter ??). Suitability for use in immunoassays or for delineation of external regions of molecules is usually assessed in solid-phase or liquid-phase binding assays (SPBA and LPBA). SPBAs, which are the basis of the IRMA and ELISA procedures described in Chapter ?? have been described in detail elsewhere (9, 15). Cytokines and related peptides are used at about 10 μg/ml. Incubation steps comprise 1 h at +37°C and ≥1 h at +4°C using ^{125}I-labelled or biotinylated 'second' antibody, i.e. one raised against the immunoglobulin of the species in which the anticytokine antibodies were raised.

LPBAs are the basis of the radioimmunoassays (RIAs) described in Chapter 12, this volume. A procedure used to quantify the antigen-binding activity of poly-clonal antiserum or ascitic fluid is described in *Protocol 10*.

The screening of antibodies to peptides and proteins that incorporate the 6×His tag is described in detail elsewhere (1).

Protocol 10

Liquid-phase binding assay

Equipment and reagents

- LP3 test-tubes
- PBS, pH 7.4, containing 0.5% BSA
- Antiserum at 1/100–1/100 000 final dilution
- ^{125}I-labelled cytokine
- Polyethylene glycol (PEG) 6000
- Bovine gamma-globulin
- Tris–HCl
- Vortex mixer
- Gamma counter equipment and reagents

Method

1 Using LP3 test-tubes, add 100 μl of antiserum at 1/100–1/100 000 (final dilution) to 300 μl PBS pH 7.4 containing 0.5% BSA.

2 Add 100 μl (10 000 c.p.m.) of ^{125}I-labelled cytokine and incubate the mixture at room temperature for 20 h.[a]

3 Separate the bound from the free ^{125}I-labelled cytokine using a polyethylene glycol (PEG)-assisted second antibody procedure. Dissolve 25 g of PEG 6000, 150 mg of bovine gamma-globulin, and 0.788 g of Tris–HCl in 100 ml of deionized distilled water. Add 500 μl of this solution to each tube, vortex the mixture, and incubate for 1 h at room temp.

4 Centrifuge the tubes at 1000 g for 30 min. Aspirate and discard the supernatant. Quantify the radioactivity in the precipitate in a gamma counter.

[a] Labelling methodologies are described in Chapter 12, this volume.

7 Purification of antibodies

Depending upon their intended use, anticytokine sera and monoclonal anti-bodies in ascitic fluid may be used without purification, e.g. for RIA procedures.

However, for many immunochemical procedures, e.g. radiolabelling or enzyme conjugation for use in immunoassays, it is usually necessary to carry out some type of chromatographic technique, e.g. ion-exchange, gel filtration, or affinity chromatography. Mouse and rat immunoglobulins are generally less stable than those of higher mammals and can prove more difficult to purify and successfully fragment. Detailed methods for purifying immunoglobulin and murine monoclonal antibodies are described elsewhere (15–17).

Acknowledgements

The author is grateful to Dr A. F. Bristow (NIBSC) for his help with the preparation of *Protocols 2* and *3*.

References

1. Sheibani, N. and Frazier, W. A. (1998). *Biotechniques*, **25**, 28.
2. Lachman, P. J., Strangeways, L., Vyakarnam, A., and Evans, G. (1986). In *Ciba Foundation Symposium 119*: *Synthetic peptides as antigens*, p. 25. Wiley, Chichester.
3. Freund, J. and McDermott, K. (1942). *Proc. Soc. Exp. Biol. Med.*, **49**, 548.
4. Hurn, B. A. L. and Chantler, S. M. (1980). In *Methods in enzymology*, Vol. 70 (ed. H. Van Vunakis and J. L. Langone), p. 104. Academic Press, New York.
5. Home Office Guidelines.
6. Act of Parliament (1986).
7. Thorpe, R., Wadhwa, M., Gearing, A. J. H., Mahon, B., and Poole, S. (1988). *Lymphokine Res.*, **7**, 119.
8. Bastin, J. M., Kirkley, J., and McMichael, A. M. (1982). In *Monoclonal antibodies in clinical medicine* (ed. A. J. McMichael and J. W. Fabre), p. 503. Academic Press, New York.
9. Limjuco, G., Galuska, S., Chin, J., Cameron, P., Boger, J., and Schmidt, J. (1987). *Proc. Natl. Acad. Sci. USA*, **83**, 3972.
10. Bomford, R., Abdulla, E., Hughes-Jenkins, C., Simkin, D., and Schmidt, J. (1987). *Immunology*, **62**, 543.
11. Poole, S., Bristow, A. F., Selkirk, S., and Rafferty, B. (1989). *J. Immunol. Meth.*, **116**, 259.
12. Taktak, Y. S., Selkirk, S., Bristow, A. F., Carpenter, A., Ball, C., Rafferty, B., and Poole, S. (1991). *J. Pharm. Pharmacol.*, **43**, 578.
13. Rees, G., Ball, C., Ward, H. L., Gee, C. K., Tarrant, G., Mistry, Y., Poole, S., and Bristow, A. F. (1999). *Cytokine*, **11**, 95.
14. Rees, G., Gee, C. K., Ward, H. L., Ball, C., Tarrant, G. M., Poole, S., and Bristow, A. F. (1999). *Eur. Cytokine Netw.*, **10**, 383.
15. Johnstone, A. and Thorpe, R. (1996). In *Immunochemistry in practice*. Blackwell Science, Oxford.
16. Baines, M. G. and Thorpe, R. (1990). In *Methods in molecular biology*, Vol. 10 (ed. M. Manson), p. 79. Humana Press, Clifton, NJ.
17. Baines, M. G., Gearing, A. J. H., and Thorpe, R. (1990). In *Methods in molecular biology*, Vol. 5 (ed. J. W. Pollard and J. W. Walker), p. 647. Humana Press, Clifton, NJ.

Chapter 12

RIA, IRMA, and ELISA for cytokines and their soluble receptors

A. Meager

NIBSC, Blanche Lane, South Mimms, Potters Bar, Hertfordshire EN6 3QG, UK

1 Introduction

The lack of absolute specificity of cultured mammalian cells for the activities of individual cytokines and the often relatively poor reproducibility of cytokine bioassays has created the need for more specific and reproducible, alternative assays. This need has largely been filled by the development of immunoassays for cytokines. Such assays are based on antibodies to each different cytokine and are generally reasonably sensitive and reliable and are quick and easy to perform. Homogeneous cytokines of known protein content can be used to calibrate immunoassays in terms of cytokine concentration (e.g. pg or ng/ml), since the extent of antibody binding is related in a dose-dependent manner to the immunoreactive mass of cytokine present. While the correlation of immunoassay results with biological activity appears possible, such correlations are dependent on a number of variables, including the specificity of antibodies, immunoassay type, and cytokine preparation used for calibration. It is therefore inadvisable to express immunoassay results in units of biological activity (1).

Cell-surface receptors for individual cytokines have been characterized as transmembrane glycoproteins. In addition, it is now known that for the majority of cytokine receptors their glycosylated extracellular domains may be cleaved enzymatically from the cell surface to form 'soluble' receptors. These soluble receptors can enter the circulation and may act as natural physiological 'buffers' of cytokine action since they are still able to bind their respective, cognate cytokine. Alternatively, they may act to transport cytokines to certain cells, tissues, or organs (e.g. to the kidneys for elimination). Levels of particular soluble cytokine receptors, e.g. soluble interleukin-2 receptor (sIL-2R), soluble tumour necrosis factor 75 kDa receptor (sTNF75R), have been found to be raised in various acute and chronic pathological conditions, and hence can be used as disease markers. Their measurement, like cytokines themselves, can be accomplished by the use of appropriate immunoassays.

Broadly speaking, there are three types of immunoassay—radioimmunoassay

(RIA), immunoradiometric assay (IRMA), and enzyme-linked immunoabsorbent assay (ELISA)—that are in regular use for cytokine quantification. All three immunoassays require the availability of monospecific antibodies, i.e. antibodies recognizing only the particular cytokine to be quantified. In addition, RIA requires radiolabelled (e.g. ^{125}I) pure cytokine, whereas IRMA and ELISA require one radiolabelled antibody and one enzyme-linked (or biotinylated) antibody, respectively. Soluble cytokine receptors have mainly been quantified using the ELISA approach, but IRMA may also be used.

It is beyond the scope of the present chapter to describe the production and purification of anticytokine- and soluble receptor-immunoglobulins (Ig); these are adequately dealt with elsewhere (ref. 2 and Chapter 11 in this volume). However, methods for radiolabelling cytokines and anticytokine Ig, and for linking anticytokine Ig to suitable enzymes or biotin are detailed below.

2 Radioimmunoassays (RIA)

These require that the cytokine to be quantified is available as a pure, homogeneous protein (or glycoprotein) and that the latter can be radiolabelled to a high specific activity without untoward structural alterations being induced. There are several ways in which cytokines may be radiolabelled with ^{125}I, but the choice of method largely depends on the robustness of the cytokine to the iodination conditions. For example, chloramine-T (3) will undoubtedly radiolabel cytokines to very high specific activities, but in general it is too denaturing and leads to the loss of biological activity. Other methods therefore are to be preferred, and these include the iodogen (Pierce/Sigma Chemical Co), Enzymobead (Bio-Rad), and Bolton–Hunter (Amersham International) methods. The suitability of these for individual cytokines should, if possible, be determined empirically. As an example, *Protocol 1* details the iodogen method as applied to the radiolabelling of TNF-α.

Protocol 1

The iodogen method for radiolabelling TNF-α

Equipment and reagents

- Eppendorf (or small glass) tube
- 1 mg/ml iodogen (1,3,4,6-tetrachloro-3α, 6α-diphenyl-glycouril) in trichloromethane
- TNF-α
- 0.25 M sodium phosphate buffer pH 6.9
- Carrier-free [^{125}I]Na (100 mCi/ml)
- Disposable 2-ml Sephadex G-25 column
- 2 mg/ml BSA in PBS (BSA–PBS)
- Gamma counter system

Method

1 Coat an Eppendorf (or small glass) tube with 40 μl of iodogen (1,3,4,6-tetrachloro-3α, 6α-diphenyl-glycouril) at 1 mg/ml in trichloromethane, by solvent evaporation.

Protocol 1 continued

2 Add 5 μg of TNF-α in 30 μl of 0.25 M sodium phosphate buffer pH 6.9, together with 10 μl (1 mCi) carrier-free [^{125}I]NaI, to the iodogen-coated tube. Keep on ice for 10 min.

3 Transfer the contents of the tube to a disposable 2 ml Sephadex G-25 column, previously equilibrated with bovine serum albumin (2 mg/ml) in phosphate-buffered saline (PBS). Wash the tube once with 40–50 μl of phosphate buffer and add this to the Sephadex column.

4 Elute the column with BSA–PBS and collect 12 × 200-μl fractions. Count these in a gamma counter and determine the peak of radioactivity (usually in fractions 6–8). Store radiolabelled [^{125}I]TNF-α at 4 °C. (It will be stable for up to 30 days.)

Instructions for ^{125}I-labelling with Enzymobeads (Bio-Rad) and the Bolton–Hunter reagent (Amersham) are supplied by the manufacturers. A further alternative is the N-bromo-succinimide (NBS) method of Reay (4) and this has been successfully applied to the radioiodination of interleukin-1β (5).

Generally speaking, most current radioimmunoassays for cytokines employ a competitive inhibition assay method. In brief, this means that variable amounts of cytokine, as serial dilutions of a standard or in samples, are incubated with a fixed amount of diluted polyclonal anticytokine antiserum, followed by a further incubation period with a fixed quantity of ^{125}I-labelled cytokine. Finally, antibody–cytokine complexes are removed from solution by the addition of a second antibody (to the first species immunoglobulin) or other antibody-binding reagent, e.g. protein A. The amount of the ^{125}I-labelled cytokine bound therefore decreases as the concentration of unlabelled cytokine increases.

An example of this type of radioimmunoassay is given in *Protocol 2*.

Protocol 2

A cytokine radioimmunoassay

Equipment and reagents

- Cytokine standard and samples
- Assay diluent (BSA–PBS, see *Protocol 1*)
- Polystyrene tubes
- Rabbit polyclonal anticytokine
- Benchtop centrifuge
- 1.5% sheep anti-rabbit IgG in 4% polyethylene glycol
- Gamma counter system
- ^{125}I-labelled cytokine tracer (e.g. 10 000 c.p.m.; 100 μCi/mg

Method

1 Add serial dilutions of the cytokine standard or samples in 100 μl of assay diluent (BSA–PBS) to polystyrene tubes containing diluted rabbit polyclonal anticytokine (in 300 μl assay diluent/tube) and incubate for 24–28 h at 4 °C. Pre-determine the dilution of the rabbit polyclonal giving maximum counts per min (c.p.m.) of bound ^{125}I-cytokine (B_o) in the absence of unlabelled cytokine.

2   Add ^{125}I-labelled cytokine tracer (e.g. 10 000 c.p.m.; 100 μCi/mg) in 100 μl of the assay diluent and incubate for a further 20 h at 4 °C.

3   Separate the free and bound cytokine by adding 1.5% sheep anti-rabbit IgG (0.5–1.0 ml) in 4% polyethylene glycol[a] (16–20 kDa). Mix and incubate for 1 h at room temperature, then centrifuge at 1000 g for 30 min.

4   Count the radioactivity (B) pelleted in the assay tubes and express the results as a percentage of B_o ($B/B_o \times 100$; see *Figure 1a*).

[a] The polyethylene glycol separation step can be replaced if the second antibody is immobilized on beads or particles. For example, the Amerlex M system (Amersham International) uses magnetic separation of the second antibody-coated particles.

3 Immunoradiometric assays (IRMA)

In these assays the concentration of cytokine in a sample is determined by the amount of ^{125}I-labelled anticytokine IgG bound to cytokine captured by a first, immobilized, anticytokine antibody (3). Purified antibodies, but not pure cytokines, are therefore required for IRMA. For optimum performance, it is generally necessary to use two cytokine-specific antibodies, each of which recognizes a different epitope or antigenic determinant on the cytokine molecule, particularly when the cytokine is monomeric. Steric separation of the recognized epitopes is essential for the development of highly sensitive assays. Ideally, the use of two complementary anticytokine monoclonal antibodies (mAb) gives the most effective combination for IRMA, although polyclonal anticytokine IgG can also be used in many cases.

For the capture antibody, anticytokine IgG is purified from either (a) ascitic fluid containing anticytokine mAb or (b) polyclonal antiserum.

Protocol 3

Purification of anticytokine IgG

Equipment and reagents

- Saturated ammonium sulfate solution, pH 7.4
- Benchtop centrifuge
- Dialysis membrane Viskingsize 1 MW Cut-off 10 000

- PBS
- Ultragel ACA44 (or Sephacryl 200)
- Elution buffer: 0.1 M sodium phosphate buffer, pH 7.2, containing 0.4M NaCl

Method

1   Add solid ammonium sulfate to 35% saturation and pH 7.4. Centrifuge the precipitate formed at 4 °C at 5000 g for 10 min.

2 Dissolve the protein precipitate in a small volume of PBS and dialyse against PBS overnight at 4 °C.

3 Separate anticytokine IgG by fractionation on Ultragel ACA44 (or Sephacryl 200) using 0.1 M sodium phosphate buffer pH 7.2, containing 0.4 M NaCl, to elute.

4 Test fractions for anticytokine IgG and pool the peak fractions.

This is generally sufficient purification for the capture antibody. However, the antibody to be radiolabelled should be further purified by:

(a) Protein A–Sepharose chromatography (6); *or*

(b) DEAE–Affigel Blue chromatography (7); *or*

(c) HPLC (8).

Protein content may be estimated by the Lowry method (9).

Purified anticytokine IgG may be radiolabelled with ^{125}I using the chloramine-T method (3) (cf radioiodination of cytokines in Section 2) as described below.

Protocol 4

Chloramine-T method for radiolabelling IgG

Equipment and reagents

- mAb IgG
- Eppendorf tubes
- 0.1 M sodium phosphate buffer pH 7.4
- Disposable 2 ml Dowex or Sephadex chromatography column

- 5 mg/ml chloramine T in distilled water
- BSA–PBS (*Protocol 1*)
- 10% sodium azide in PBS
- 0.4 mg/ml L-tyrosine in sodium phosphate buffer

Method

1 Add 10 μg of mAb IgG to an Eppendorf tube containing 10 μl of 0.1 m sodium phosphate buffer pH 7.4 and 10 μl (100 μCi) of [^{125}I]NaI in the same buffer.

2 Add 10 μl of freshly prepared chloramine T (5 mg/ml in distilled water), mix, and stir or agitate the tube contents for 45 sec.

3 Terminate the reaction by adding 50 μl of L-tyrosine (0.4 mg/ml in sodium phosphate buffer).

4 Pass the iodination mixture through a disposable 2 ml Dowex or Sephadex chromatography column, and elute [^{125}I]mAb with BSA–PBS (as previously described). Pool the peak fractions and store with a drop of 10% sodium azide at 4 °C.

A method for carrying out IRMA, essentially that described by Secher (10), is outlined below as applied to the estimation of TNF-α.

Protocol 5

IRMA assay for TNF-α

Equipment and reagents

- Purified capture antibody (an anti-TNF mAb)
- PBS
- Etched polystyrene balls (6.5 mm; Northumbria Biologicals)
- Diluted antibody
- Glass Universal bottles
- 0.1% BSA in PBS
- 0.5% BSA in PBS
- 100, or more, Luckham LP4 tubes Thermoquest Scientific
- TNF-α standard
- Assay diluent: e.g. cell growth medium containing 10% calf serum (see Section 5.2)
- Paper towels
- [^{125}I]anti-TNF-α second mAb
- Gamma counter system

Method

1 Prepare immobilized antibody as follows:

   (a) Dilute the purified capture antibody, an anti-TNF mAb, to approximately 50 μg protein/ml in PBS.

   (b) Add 100, or so, etched polystyrene balls to 14 ml of the diluted antibody in a glass Universal.

   (c) Submerge the beads in the antibody solution overnight at 4 °C, then aspirate the antibody solution and wash four or five times with 0.1% BSA–PBS.

   (d) Store the beads, if desired, under 0.1% BSA–PBS at 4 °C for several weeks.

2 Fill 100, or more, Luckham LP4 tubes with 0.5% BSA–PBS to block any binding to plastic surfaces, and leave overnight at 4 °C. Aspirate the tube contents just prior to setting up the assay.

3 Prepare serial dilutions of the TNF-α standard covering the range 2.5 pg/ml to 25 ng/ml in assay diluent. The latter should be identical, if possible, to the medium of the samples to be tested, e.g. cell growth medium containing 10% calf serum (see Section 5.2 for further discussion). Add 200 μl of TNF-α standard dilutions or samples to the LP4 tubes.

4 Blot the washed antibody-coated beads to dryness on paper towels and add one bead per assay tube. Make sure that the bead is completely submerged and there are no bubbles. Incubate the assay tubes overnight at 4 °C.

5 The following day, aspirate the standard dilutions and samples, and wash the beads extensively with 0.1% BSA–PBS (or simply water) before adding 200 μl of [^{125}I]anti-TNF-α second mAb to all tubes. Dilute the second mAb in 0.1% BSA–PBS so that the resulting solution contains approximately 10^6 c.p.m./ml.

6 Leave the assay tubes for a further 4 h at 4 °C. Aspirate unbound [^{125}I]anti-TNF-α and wash the beads extensively with *either* 0.1% BSA–PBS *or* water.

7 Count the tubes containing the beads in a gamma counter.

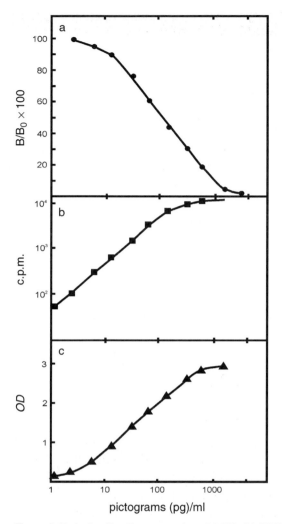

Figure 1 Typical calibration curves from (a) RIA, (b) IRMA, and (c) ELISA, based on in-house data for a human TNF-α standard.

The data so obtained may be plotted as c.p.m. bound (minus negative control, i.e. non-specific binding) versus TNF-α activity/concentration, in pg/ml, either as $\log_{10}$–$\log_{10}$ or semi-$\log_{10}$ plots to generate the calibration curve. Concentrations (pg/ml) of TNF-α in test samples may then be simply interpolated from the calibration curve (*Figure 1b*).

IRMA for soluble cytokine receptors can be carried out in a manner similar to *Protocol 5*, except that:

- the capture anticytokine mAb is replaced by an antisoluble receptor mAb;
- serial dilutions of the cytokine standard are replaced by serial dilutions of purified soluble receptors, preferably a reference preparation of known receptor protein content; and

- the ^{125}I-labelled detector anticytokine mAb is substituted by an appropriate ^{125}I-labelled antisoluble receptor mAb (labelling with ^{125}I is carried out as described in *Protocol* 4).

As an alternative strategy, if capture antisoluble receptor mAbs are available that do not interfere with the binding of cognate cytokine to a soluble receptor, then an ^{125}I-labelled cytokine (^{125}I-labelling is carried out according to *Protocol 1* or similar) may be used instead of a detector ^{125}I-labelled antisoluble receptor mAb, i.e. immobilized mAb–soluble cytokine receptor-[^{125}I]cytokine. The latter guarantees that only functionally active soluble receptors are detected and quantified.

4 Enzyme-linked immunosorbent assays (ELISA)

The principles involved in ELISA are the same as those for IRMA, except that the second anticytokine IgG is:

(a) conjugated to an enzyme;

(b) itself subject to detection with a third antibody–enzyme complex or variable combinations of biotinylated antibodies and streptavidin–enzyme complexes (11).

Purification of anticytokine IgG for ELISA is the same as that described for IRMA (see Section 3). Three enzymes—horseradish peroxidase, alkaline phosphatase, and β-galactosidase—are regularly used for conjugation to a second and third antibody or streptavidin ELISA reagents. Enzyme may be directly coupled to IgG or streptavidin using a variety of methods, the simplest of which involves mixing the reagents with a low percentage solution of glutaraldehyde (12). Alternatively, antibody reagents may be biotinylated using an N-hydroxysuccinimide-biotin ester and detected using streptavidin reagents, which bind with high affinity to biotin molecules (13). Synthetic biotin esters with a 'spacer arm', which ensures that the protein-linked biotin is freely accessible to bind streptavidin, are commercially available (e.g. Amersham International) and it is recommended that the manufacturer's instructions for biotinylation reactions are followed.

When human serum samples are being analysed, it is recommended that Fab fragments of anticytokine IgG are used instead of the second anticytokine IgG, so that problems arising from the presence of heterophilic antibodies (e.g. human anti-mouse IgG) are reduced or eliminated.

Protocol 6 illustrates how various combinations of enzyme-linked and biotinylated reagents may be effectively used in the construction of ELISA.

The use of biotinylated reagents together with multivalent streptavidin–enzyme conjugates may enhance the sensitivity of an ELISA considerably, but may also tend to increase non-specific binding. It is clear that different combinations will have their advantages and disadvantages, and operators should, where possible, use the most suitable combination for a particular need. For example, samples containing large amounts of a cytokine would, in general, require a less sensitive and sophisticated ELISA than for samples containing low cytokine levels.

Protocol 6

ELISA for cytokines

Equipment and reagents

- 96-well micro-ELISA plates
- Anticytokine IgG
- Enzyme-linked (horseradish peroxidase- or alkaline phosphatase-conjugated) second anticytokine IgG
- 0.1 M sodium bicarbonate buffer pH 9.6
- 1% BSA–PBS (*Protocol 1*)
- *Either* 0.05% Tween-20 in PBS (Tween-20–PBS) *or* 0.1% Synperonic F68 (Serva) in PBS
- Cytokine standard
- Test samples
- 0.1 M citrate-phosphate buffer pH 5.0
- ELISA plate reader

For horseradish peroxidase (HRP) conjugates:
- 1 mg/ml orthophenylenediamine (OPD) in citrate-phosphate buffer, 0.006% hydrogen peroxide
- 1 M H_2SO_4

For alkaline phosphatase (AP) conjugates:
- 1 mg/ml *p*-nitrophenylphosphate (*p*NPP) in 1 M diethanolamine buffer, 0.5 mM $MgCl_2$ pH 9.8
- 3 M NaOH

Method

The first two steps are similar in all cases.

1 Coat 96-well micro-ELISA plates with an anticytokine IgG by adding 50–100 μl (depending on the well size) of anticytokine IgG (2.5–10 μg/μl) in 0.1 m sodium bicarbonate buffer, pH 9.6, to each well and incubate the plates for 2 h at 37 °C. Block the remaining sites in the wells by adding 150–200 μl of 1% BSA–PBS per well for at least 20 min. Seal the plates and store at 4 °C until required.

2 Remove unbound anticytokine IgG and blocking buffer by flicking them out. Wash the wells a few times with 0.05% Tween-20–PBS or 0.1% Synperonic F68 (Serva)–PBS (150–200 μl/well). Following the last wash, add serial dilutions of the cytokine standard and undiluted/diluted samples (50–100 μl/well) in duplicate/triplicate and incubate at 37 °C for 1 h. (Note that longer incubation periods may improve the assay sensitivity and reproducibility.)

NB: See Variations 1 and 2 before proceeding with step 3.

3 Wash the wells four times with 0.05% Tween-20–PBS or 0.1% Synperonic–PBS. Add the enzyme-linked second anticytokine IgG, appropriately diluted in 1% BSA–PBS, to all wells (50–100 μl/well) and continue the incubation for a further 1 h at 37 °C.

4 Wash the wells four times with 0.05% Tween-20–PBS or 0.1% Synperonic–PBS. Additional washes with the buffer solution used for making up the enzyme substrate are recommended before adding the substrate solution. For example:

Protocol 6 continued

- *For HRP conjugates*—wash the wells twice with 0.1 M citrate-phosphate buffer, pH 5.0, prior to adding the horseradish peroxidase substrate, orthophenylenediamine (OPD), at 1 mg/ml in the citrate-phosphate buffer containing 0.006% hydrogen peroxide.
- *For alkaline phosphatase conjugates*—wash the wells twice with water prior to adding *p*-nitrophenylphosphate (*p*NPP) at 1 mg/ml in 1 M diethanolamine buffer, 0.5 mM MgCl$_2$ pH 9.8.

5   For most substrates, allow the colour to develop in the dark to avoid the occurrence of non-specific coloration, and thus achieve low background optical densities. Terminate the enzyme reaction, and hence colour development, by adding 1 M H$_2$SO$_4$ in the case of horseradish peroxidase and 3 M NaOH in the case of alkaline phosphatase.

6   Read optical densities (OD) at the wavelengths appropriate to the colour in the wells, e.g. 492 nm for OPD and 405 nm for *p*NPP. Plot data as *OD* versus cytokine activity/concentration in a similar way to that described for IRMA (Section 3, *Figure 1c*).

Variation 1

In step 3, the addition of the enzyme-linked second anticytokine IgG is replaced by the addition of the biotinylated second anticytokine IgG. This generates an extra step 3(a), in which (following the removal of biotinylated IgG and washing the wells with 0.05% Tween-20-PBS) an appropriately diluted streptavidin–enzyme conjugate is added to all wells. Since the binding of the streptavidin reagent is rapid, the incubation time after its addition is 20–30 min at 37 °C. This is followed by step 4 and the protocol continued as previously outlined.

Variation 2

In step 3, the addition of the enzyme-linked second anticytokine IgG is replaced by the addition of the appropriately diluted, unconjugated second anticytokine IgG. Processing this ELISA then entails one or two extra steps: 3(b) the addition of enzyme-linked antispecies IgG (to the second anticytokine IgG); or 3(c) the addition of biotinylated anti-species IgG followed by the further addition of a streptavidin–enzyme conjugate. Each addition is preceded by extensive washing of the wells with 0.05% Tween-20-PBS. Incubation is for 1 h at 37 °C, as in step 3, followed by 30 min at 37 °C for the addition of Streptavidin-enzyme conjugate in the case of 3(c).

ELISA for soluble cytokine receptors may be carried out by following *Protocol 6*; but the anticytokine Ig reagents are replaced by the appropriate antisoluble receptor Ig reagents and the serial dilutions of cytokine standard substituted with those of the relevant purified soluble receptor reference preparation. Alternatively, where anticytokine/antisoluble receptor Ig reagents are available that do not interfere with cytokine binding to a soluble receptor, other ELISA formats are possible, e.g. immobilized antisoluble receptor Ig–(soluble receptor–cytokine complexes)–anticytokine Ig–enzyme. Variations 1 and 2, as outlined above, may also be applied to ELISA for soluble cytokine receptors.

5 Problems

5.1 Calibration

Correct calibration is vital for all types of immunoassays. The standard used for calibration should contain the cytokine or soluble cytokine receptor to be quantified in a molecular form(s) that it is known to be (or predicted to be) representative of the cytokine or receptor molecules present in the samples. For example, a human recombinant IFN-γ standard which contains only non-glycosylated molecules should be used in the immunoassay of samples containing non-glycosylated IFN-γ; such a standard may be unsuitable for calibration when samples containing leucocyte-derived, glycosylated IFN-γ molecules are assayed. Where cytokines exist naturally as mixtures of a number of closely related molecular species, e.g. IFN-α, it may not be possible to exactly duplicate the proportions of these in a standard preparation (2).

Despite this problem of cytokine heterogenicity, there is a clear need for a common *primary standard* with well-characterized and stable antigenic activity for each individual, cytokine-specific immunoassay. Although current WHO international standards (IS) for cytokines are primarily intended for the calibration of bioassays, it has been recommended (1) that they should, if possible, be used as *primary standards* for immunoassays using the nominal mass of cytokine contained in the ampoule for calibration. It should be noted that the mass units assigned to the cytokine standard will not be an 'absolute' mass value, but an experimental value related to a specific method of determination. The primary standard can be used to facilitate comparison when expressing results obtained using different immunoassay procedures or kits. The use of a single primary standard as the immunoassay calibrant has been shown to reduce variability of results (15), a problem associated with the use of multiple, distinct, standards (*Figure 2*). However, the primary standard for each cytokine represents a valuable WHO resource and therefore should not be used on a routine basis. It should be used for the calibration of *secondary* and *working* standards by comparative immunoassay. Large stocks of well-characterized *secondary* and/or *working* standards should be prepared and laid down for future use in the routine calibration of immunoassays.

Where practical, cytokine immunoassays should be appropriately validated using a dilution series rather than single-point determinations for individual samples. Validation studies should also include evaluation of the immunoassay to recognize different molecular forms of a cytokine, immunoassay specificity, reagent stability, interference problems, matrix effects, sensitivity, spiking, and recovery studies, etc. (1). Some of these aspects are dealt with below.

5.2 Mixtures of cytokine and soluble receptors

In some cases, samples can contain a mixture of free cytokine and cytokine–soluble receptor complexes; but immunoassays may only detect the free cytokine because relevant antigenic determinants are hidden by the soluble receptor in

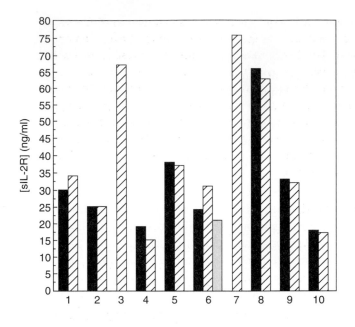

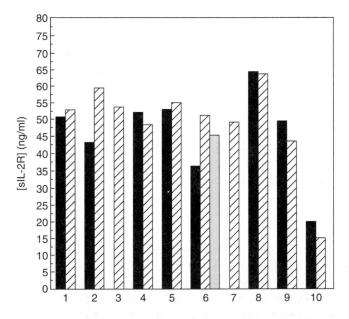

Figure 2 Concentrations of sIL-2Rα measured in 10 different commercial immunoassay kits calibrated with either the sIL-2Rα standard supplied (upper panel) or with a single sIL-2Rα primary standard (lower panel). Where measurements of sIL-2Rα were performed on two or more separate occasions using particular immunoassay kits, results are shown as black- and grey-shaded bars. These data strongly suggest that the use of a single well-characterized soluble cytokine receptor preparation or immunoassay calibrations can reduce variability of results among different immunoassays. (Reprinted with permission of Meager *et al., J. Immunol. Meth.*, **191**, 97–112. © 1996 Elsevier Science Inc.)

the cytokine–soluble receptor complexes. Such samples can lead to difficulties in interpreting the results, even though the correct calibrants have been employed, i.e. it may be concluded that a cytokine is absent or present in much lower levels than actually exist. However, this problem may be overcome by utilizing anticytokine Ig reagents that: (a) recognize epitopes on the cytokine molecule that are not obscured by soluble receptors; or (b) are of high enough affinity to compete with and remove soluble receptors from cytokine molecules. It should be noted that such immunoassays give a measure of the total cytokine content of a sample, but give no indication of the amounts of free (active) and complexed (inactive) cytokine present.

5.3 Assay diluent or matrix

The diluent or matrix for immunoassays should be identical for the cytokine standard or soluble receptor reference preparation and for samples. 'Recognition' of cytokine/soluble receptor is often influenced by the overall concentrations of other molecules, e.g. proteins, mucopolysaccharides (in the matrix) and appropriate precautions should be taken to ensure that these do not unduly influence the results. For example, biological fluids such as sera or synovia may be highly viscous when undiluted and, where possible, it is recommended that these be diluted with an appropriate buffer (or enzyme-treated, e.g. hyaluronidase for synovial fluids) to reduce viscosity before assay. For the estimation of cytokines/soluble receptors in biological fluids, the cytokine standard/soluble receptor reference preparation should be prepared by serial dilution in a comparable fluid, previously shown to give only background or baseline OD in the immunoassay.

5.4 Samples from different sources

Problems are most likely to arise in the assay of differently sourced biological fluids containing very low levels of cytokine together with those where cytokine is actually absent. Here, there will be some variation in the composition of individual samples and it will be virtually impossible to match the matrices of these to that used for standard dilution. This often leads to some scatter about the assay background-OD reading and consequent difficulties in the interpretation of results. Additionally, biological fluids may contain substances other than cytokine which can 'bridge' the first and second anticytokine IgGs and generate false-positives. For example, human sera or plasma occasionally, in varying amount, contain anti-murine IgG and this will bind to the first anticytokine antibody if it is a murine mAb. The second anticytokine IgG can then bind to the Fc portion of human anti-murine IgG to yield a positive result in the immunoassay. This kind of artefact may be reduced or eliminated by either including a low percentage of mouse serum (14) in the assay diluent or by using the Fab fragments of anticytokine IgGs. On the other hand, biological fluids may contain cytokine inhibitors, other than soluble cytokine receptors (see Section 5.2), which can bind to cytokines in such a way that epitopes recognized by anticytokine IgGs are blocked. This will lead to false-negatives. Polyvalent substances such as heparin, which can bind to certain cytokines, e.g. fibroblast growth factors, should therefore not be used in the preparation of plasma, for example.

References

1. Wadhwa, M. and Thorpe, R. (1998). *J. Immunol. Meth.*, **219**, 1.
2. Meager, A. (1987). In *Lymphokines and interferons* (ed. M. J. Clemens, A. G. Morris, and A. J. H. Gearing), p. 105. IRL Press, Oxford.
3. Hunter, W. M. and Greenwood, F. C. (1962). *Nature*, **194**, 495.
4. Reay, P. (1982). *Ann. Clin. Biochem.*, **19**, 129.
5. Poole, S., Bristow, A. F., Selkirk, S., and Rafferty, B. (1989). *J. Immunol. Meth.*, **116**, 259.
6. Ey, P. L., Prowse, S. J., and Jenkin, C. R. (1978). *Immunochemistry*, **15**, 429.
7. Bruck, C., Portelle, D., Glineur, C., and Bolton, A. (1982). *J. Immunol. Meth.*, **53**, 313.
8. Burchiel, S. W., Billman, J. R., and Albert, R. (1984). *J. Immunol. Meth.*, **69**, 33.
9. Lowry, O. H., Rosebrough, N. J., Farr, A. L., and Randall, R. J. (1951). *J. Biol. Chem.*, **193**, 265.
10. Secher, D. S. (1981). *Nature*, **290**, 501.
11. Kemeny, D. M. and Challacombe, S. J. (ed.) (1989). ELISA and other solid phase immunoassays. John Wiley & Sons Ltd, Chichester, UK.
12. Avrameas, S. (1969). *Immunochemistry*, **6**, 43.
13. Guesdon, J-L., Ternynck, T., and Avrameas, S. (1979). *J. Histochem. Cytochem.*, **27**, 1131.
14. Boscato, L. M. and Stuart, M. C. (1986). *Clin. Chem.*, **32**, 1491.
15. Meager, A., Bird, C., and Mire-Sluis, A. (1996). *J. Immunol. Meth.*, **191**, 97.

Chapter 13

Quantitative biological assays for individual cytokines

Meenu Wadhwa, Christopher Bird, Paula Dilger, Tony Mire-Sluis* and Robin Thorpe

Division of Immunobiology, National Institute for Biological Standards and Control, Blanche Lane, South Mimms, Potters Bar, Hertfordshire EN6 3QG, UK

*Genentech Inc. 1 DNA Way, South San Francisco, CA 94080–4990, USA

1 Introduction

Cytokines have often been discovered in complex mixtures by observing their effect on a biological system. This usually becomes the definitive property (or one of several properties) of the cytokine and can become the basis for its bioassay.

Cytokine bioassays are based on various biological effects such as cell proliferation, cytotoxic/cytostatic activity, kinetic effects, antiviral activity, colony formation, or induction of secretion of other cytokine/non cytokine molecules (1).

Bioassays can use primary cultures of cells obtained from animals or, more conveniently, continuous cytokine-dependent or autonomous cell lines (*Table 1*). Biological assays are rarely entirely specific for a particular cytokine and can respond to a number of cytokines and other molecules (e.g. thymocyte assay; assays based on acute myeloid leukaemic cell lines). In these assays, specificity for a particular cytokine can be established using a monospecific neutralizing antibody, and this approach is crucial for confirming the presence of cytokines in many biological (and particularly clinical) samples. In some cases, bioassays may underestimate the cytokine protein content of a biological sample due to the presence of inhibitory molecules, e.g. binding proteins, soluble receptors, receptor antagonists, or inhibitory cytokines such as TGF-β (2–3). It is also possible that bioassays may overestimate the cytokine content of a sample due to synergistic interactions between individual cytokines in the sample (4).

Progress in cytokine science has been very rapid, and there are often a range of useful bioassays available for a particular cytokine. The choice of which assay to adopt can depend on the precise assay information required, the equipment and reagents available, and even on personal choice. This chapter is not intended to present a comprehensive description of all assays available (1, 5), but details

Table 1 Cell lines used in assays for measurement of cytokines

Cytokine	Cell line	Origin	Biological readout	Range (/ml)	Response to cytokines Human	Murine	Refs
IL-1	NOB-1	Murine thymoma	Production of IL-2	0.01–10 IU	TNF	TNF	12
IL-2	CTLL-2	Murine cytotoxic T cell	Proliferation	0.01–10 IU	IL-15, TGF-β_1, TGF-β_2 IL-12,	IL-4, IL-2, IL-15	9
	KIT-225	Human chronic T-lymphocytic leukaemia	Proliferation	0.1–20 IU	IL-7, IL-15, IL-12	IL-12	21
IL-3	MO7e	Human megakaryoblastic leukaemia	Proliferation	0.05–20 IU	GM-CSF, SCF, IL-9, IL-15, TPO, TNF-α, TNF-β, IFN-α, IFN-β, TGF-β_1, TGF-β_2 TGF-β_3	—	29
	TF-1	Human erythroleukaemia	Proliferation	0.02–10 IU	IL-4, IL-5, IL-6, IL-13, IL-15, GM-CSF, NGF, SCF, LIF, Onco M, CNTF, EPO, TNF-α, TNF-β, IFN-α, IFN-β, TGF-β_1, TGF-β_2, TGF-β_3	IL-13, IL-5	31
IL-4	CT.h4S	Murine cytotoxic T cell transfected with HIL-4 receptor	Proliferation	0.1–25 IU	IL-2, TNF-α, TNF-β, IFN-α, IFN-β, TGF-β_1, TGF-β_2	IL-2, IL-4	13
IL-5	TF-1	forementioned	Proliferation	0.1–50 U	forementioned	forementioned	31
IL-6	B9	Murine hybridoma	Proliferation	0.05–5 IU	IL-13, IL-11, Onco M.	IL-4, IL-11, IL-13	14
IL-7	PB1	Murine pre-B cell	Proliferation	20–5000 U	—	—	47
IL-9	MO7e	forementioned	Proliferation	0.5–100 U	forementioned	—	16
IL-10	Ba8.1C1	Murine pro-B cell transfected with hIL-10 receptor	Proliferation	0.5–500 U	—	IL-3	18
IL-11	T10	Murine plasmacytoma	Proliferation	0.5–50 U	IL-6	IL-6, IL-11	15
IL-12	KIT-225	forementioned	Proliferation	0.01–20 U	IL-2, IL-7, IL-15	IL-12	21
IL-13	B9.13	Murine hybridoma	Proliferation	0.3–20 U	IL-6, IL-11	IL-4, IL-11	22
	TF-1	forementioned	Proliferation	0.5–100 U	forementioned		
IL-15	CTLL-2	forementioned	Proliferation	0.2–10 U	forementioned	IL-4, IL-2, IL-15	45
	KIT-225	forementioned	Proliferation	1–1000 U	IL-2, IL-7, IL-12	IL-12	
IL-18	KG-1	Human myelomonocytic leukaemia	Production of IFN-γ	500 ng–1 ng	—	—	26

GM-CSF	MO7e	forementioned	Proliferation	01-10 IU	forementioned	—	29
	TF-1	forementioned	Proliferation	0.01-5 IU	forementioned	forementioned	31
G-CSF	GNFS-60	Murine myeloid leukaemia	Proliferation	0.5-100 IU	IL-6, TGF-β_1, TGF-β_2, M-CSF, Onco M, LIF, IL-13	G-CSF, M-CSF, IL-3, GM-CSF, IL-6, IL-4	32
M-CSF	MNFS-60	Murine Myeloid leukaemia	Proliferation	1.5-150 IU	IL-6, TGF-β_1, TGF-β_2, G-CSF, Onco M, LIF, IL-13	G-CSF, IL-3, IL-6, GM-CSF, M-CSF, IL-4	33
XSCF	O7e	forementioned	Proliferation	1-100 U	forementioned	forementioned	34
	TF-1	forementioned	Proliferation	1-100 U	forementioned	forementioned	1
LIF	TF-1	forementioned	Proliferation	0.05-50 U	forementioned	forementioned	30
TPO	MO7e	forementioned	Proliferation	20 pg-20 ng	forementioned	forementioned	35
	32D/MPL+	Murine myeloid leukaemia transfected with mpl receptor	Proliferation	20 pg-2 ng	forementioned	IL-3, G-CSF	36
Onco M	TF-1	forementioned	Proliferation	0.5-500 U	forementioned	forementioned	
TGF-β	MuLv1	Mink lung fibroblasts	Inhibition of proliferation	10 pg-1 ng	TNF-α, TNF-β	TGF-β, TNF-α	37
	TF-1	forementioned	Inhibition of proliferation	500 fg-1 ng	forementioned	forementioned	38
TNF-α	KYM-1D4	Human rhabdomyosarcoma	Cytotoxicity	0.2-4 IU	TNF-β	TNF-α	40
TNF-β	KYM-1D4	forementioned	Proliferation	1000-1 ng	forementioned	forementioned	
CNTF	TF-1	forementioned	Proliferation	1000-1 ng	forementioned	forementioned	
IFN-α	2D9 + EMCV	Human glioblastoma/encephalomyocarditis virus	Antiviral	0.1 pg-2 pg	IFN-α, IFN-β	—	41
	Daudi	Human B lymphoblastoid leukaemia	Inhibition of proliferation	1 pg-100 pg	forementioned	—	42
IGN-β	2D9 + EMCV	forementioned	Antiviral	0.3 pg-6 ng	IFN-α, IFN-β	—	41
	Daudi	forementioned	Inhibition of proliferation	10 pg-1 ng	forementioned	—	42
IGN-γ	2D9 + EMCV	forementioned	Antiviral	0.005-10 IU	forementioned	—	41
Epo	UT-7/Epo	Megakaryoblastic leukaemia	Proliferation	200 pg-10 ng	TGF-β_1, TGF-β_2	—	46
	TF-1	forementioned	Proliferation	forementioned	forementioned	IL-13	31
BMP-2	W-20-7	Stromal cell line	Induction of alkaline phosphatase	500 ng-0.5 ng	500 ng-0.5 ng	—	39

one or more bioassays that we have found to be reliable, consistent, and suitable for routine use.

1.1 New bioassays

A number of new cytokine bioassays have been devised which use reporter genes and/or cytokine-receptor transfected cell lines to improve assay characterization. Assays based on the KIRA (kinase receptor-activation immunoassays) have also been developed which allow the bioassay of cytokines using a cytokine-sensitive cell line but using an immunoassay (usually ELISA) readout.

In many cases, such assays offer genuine improvements over more conventional methods, e.g. for IL-4. In some cases there is no real alternative to adopting such a method, e.g. for IL-10. However, the methods almost always require reagents, cell lines, etc. which may not be generally available, or are very costly. We have therefore only described these methods where they are indispensable or are particularly advantageous.

1.2 Bioassays compared with immunoassays and receptor binding assays

It seems to be impossible to distinguish between different molecular species of some cytokines using bioassays. The classic example of this is IL-1α and -β, which, although very different structurally, seem to possess apparently identical biological properties, at least on homologous cells. In such instances, immunoassays can be used to specifically quantify the different molecular forms on a protein basis (6). Immunoassays can, in all cases, be used as an alternative to bioassays, although they can detect denatured biologically inactive cytokine molecules and fragments as well as 'inactive' receptor–cytokine complexes (1). Immunoassays need to be very carefully validated to eliminate non-specific artefacts, particularly if they are used for assaying clinical samples (1, 6, 7). WHO/International cytokine society recommendations for the standardization and validation of cytokine immunoassays have been formulated (8). Immunoassays are described in Chapter 12, this volume.

Receptor binding assays are often regarded as a compromise between bioassays and immunoassays as they are based on the ability of cytokine molecules to bind to natural receptors. However, these assays may produce results which do not correlate with bioassay data if some ligand molecules are unable to induce signal transduction following binding to receptor.

2 Biological assays for interleukins

2.1 Bioassay for interleukin-2 (IL-2)

The original bioassays for IL-2 used short-term, lectin-induced, T-cell blasts, but these respond to other cytokines and also to some non-cytokine molecules. IL-2

QUANTITATIVE BIOLOGICAL ASSAYS

can be measured by its proliferative effect on IL-2-dependent cell lines such as HT-2 and CTLL clones (9). The assay based on the CTLL-2 murine T cell line provides a reliable and easy method which responds to IL-2 from most mammalian species.

2.1.1 Maintenance of CTLL cell line

Culture CTLL cells in RPMI-1640 medium containing 10% fetal calf serum (FCS) supplemented with partially purified, rat-splenocyte conditioned medium (or recombinant IL-2) in upright 25 cm^2 flasks. Maintain the cultures using a 2/3-day feeding schedule. Seed the cells at approximately 2×10^4 cells/ml and feed with 1–2% purified conditioned medium (10). This corresponds to a concentration of approximately 15–20 international units (IU/ml) IL-2. After 3 days when the cell density is approximately 2×10^5 cells/ml, split the cultures to 2×10^4 cells/ml and re-feed with IL-2.

Protocol 1

Bioassay for IL-2 using the CTLL cell line

Equipment and reagents

- CTLL cell culture (see Section 2.1.1)
- RPMI-1640 medium
- FCS
- Centrifuge
- 37°C, 5% CO$_2$, humidified incubator
- [^{3}H]thymidine (25 Ci/mmol, 5 mCi/5 ml)
- Cell harvester

- Filter mats
- 96-well microtitre plates
- Trypan Blue
- IL-2 standard (see Section 6 and *Table 2*)
- Test samples
- Scintillation counter, etc.

Method

1 Wash CTLL cells (3 days after feeding) three times with RPMI01640 by centrifuging the cells at 250 × g for 10 min at RT.

2 Determine cell viability, e.g. by Trypan Blue dye exclusion, ^{a}and resuspend the cells to a final concentration of 1×10^5 cells/ml in RPMI-1640 medium containing 10% FCS.

3 Titrate the IL-2 standard (see Section 6 and *Table 2*) in triplicate in 96-well microtitre plates. Start the titration at 20 IU/ml of IL-2 and then make serial twofold dilutions down to 0.019 IU/ml of IL-2. Prepare dilutions of the samples in triplicate. Include a negative control, i.e. culture medium alone. Each well should contain 50 μl.

4 Add 50 μl of the cell suspension to each well and incubate the plates for 18 h at 37°C in a humidified 5% CO$_2$ incubator.

5 Add 0.5 μCi of tritiated thymidine to each well and return the plates to the incubator for approximately 4 h.

Protocol 1 continued

6　Harvest the contents of each well on to filter mats and determine the radioactivity by liquid scintillation counting.

7　Plot a standard curve of c.p.m. versus the concentration of IL-2. To quantitate activity in unknown samples, compare the test results with a standard curve (see Section 6).

[a] Cells should be > 80% viable. The viability test should be routinely conducted for all cell lines (mentioned in this chapter) prior to assay.

2.2 Bioassay for interleukin-1 (IL-1)

Bioassays for IL-1 commonly utilize the ability of this cytokine to induce IL-2 production by T cell lines such as EL4.6.1 and LBRM 33, or in primary cultures of thymocytes (LAF assay). Alternatively, IL-1 can be assayed by measuring its ability to stimulate the proliferation of lines such as the subclone D10S of the murine T-helper cell line D10.64.1 (11). A subclone, NOB-1, of the murine thymoma line EL4.6.1 provides a simple and sensitive bioassay for IL-1. These line produces IL-2 in response to both human and murine IL-1, which is measured using the CTLL-2 cell line-based assay (12).

2.2.1 Maintenance of the EL4/NOB-1 cell line

Culture the cells in RPMI 1640 medium containing 5% FCS in upright 75 cm^2 flasks and feed every 2 to 3 days. Cultures are split 1:5 to 1:10 when the cell density reaches approximately 5×10^5 cells/ml.

Protocol 2

Bioassay for IL-1 using the EL4/NOB-1 cell line[a]

Equipment and reagents

- EL4/NOB-1 cell culture (see Section 2.2.1)
- IL-1 standards (se Section 6 and *Table 2*)
- Equipment and reagents as *Protocol 1*

Method

1　Wash EL4/NOB-1 cells (2–3 days after feeding) twice in RPMI 1640 medium by centrifuging the cells at 250 *g* for 10 min and determine the viability as in step 2 of *Protocol 1*.

2　Resuspend the cells in a final concentration of 2.5×10^5 cells/ml in RPMI 1640 medium containing 5% FCS.

3　Distribute titrations of an IL-1 standard (see Section 6 and *Table 2*) in triplicate in 96-well microtitre plates. Start the titration of the standard at 100 pg/ml of IL-1 (10 IU/ml) and make serial twofold dilutions down to 0.09 pg/ml IL-1 (0.009 IU/ml). Make appropriate dilutions of the samples to be measured for IL-1 activity (either twofold

Protocol 2 continued

or tenfold serial dilutions) in triplicate. Include a culture medium negative control. Each well should contain 100 μl at this stage.

4   Add 100 μl of the washed cell suspension to each well and incubate the plates for approximately 24 h at 37 °C in a humidified 5% CO_2 incubator.

5   Remove 50 μl of the supernatant from each well and determine the IL-2 present using the CTLL-2 bioassay (see *Protocol 1*). Note that the amount of IL-2 in the supernatants will be proportional to the amount of IL-1 in the original samples. Remove supernatants from the EL4/NOB-1 cells and can be stored frozen until the IL-2 can be conveniently assayed.

ᵃ IL-1α and IL-1β can be measured in this assay.

2.3 Bioassay for interleukin-4 (IL-4)

The classical IL-4 assay involves the promotion of cell division of purified B lymphocytes co-stimulated with either anti-immunoglobulin or *Staphylococcus aureus*-Cowan strain 1 or phorbol ester. Alternative assays utilize the ability of IL-4 to augment CD23 expression in the Ramos cell line (B-cell lymphoma) or to induce the proliferation of phytohaemagglutinin (PHA)-activated T lymphocytes, B cell lines such as BALM-4, HFB-1, and L4, or certain haemopoietic progenitor cell lines such as TF-1 or MO-7E (see Section 3.1). However, a human IL-4-responsive cell line, which has been developed by transfecting a murine CTL line with the human IL-4 receptor gene and proliferates in response to human IL-4 (13), provides a highly sensitive and reproducible assay. This assay is described below.

2.3.1 Maintenance of the CT-h4S cell line

Culture the cells in RPMI 1640 medium containing 10% FCS, 2 mM L-glutamine, 1 mM sodium pyruvate, 0.05 mM 2-mercaptoethanol, 10 ng/ml (approximately 100 U/ml) human IL-4 in 25 cm^2 flasks. Cultures are split 1:4 or 1:5 every 2–3 days and refed with fresh medium. (These cells are very sensitive to high pH and diminished 2-ME concentrations, so using fresh medium is important. To split cells, use a sterile cell scraper. Do **not** use trypsin or EDTA.) Cultures are maintained at 37 °C in a humidified 5% CO_2 incubator.

Protocol 3

Bioassay for IL-4 using the CT.h4S cell line

Equipment and reagents

- CT.h4S cell culture (see Section 2.3.1)
- IL-4 standard (see Section 6 and *Table 2*)
- Sterile, cell scraper
- Cell-culture medium: RPMI-1640, 10% FCS
- Equipment and reagents as *Protocol 1*

Protocol 3 continued

Method

1   Distribute titrations of IL-4 in 100 μl volumes in triplicate in 96-well microtitre plates. Start the titration at 10 ng/ml (approximately 100 U/ml) and serially dilute twofold down to 1 pg/ml (0.01 U/ml). Make appropriate dilutions of the samples in 100 μl volumes in triplicate. As a negative control include medium alone.

2   Scrape cells 2–3 days after feeding and count. Wash the cells in RPMI-1640 by centrifuging at 200 g for 10 min at RT.

3   Resuspend the cells to a final concentration of 1×10^5 cells/ml in RPMI-1640 containing 10% FCS.

4   Add 100 μl of the cell suspension to each well and incubate the plates for approximately 44 h at 37°C in a humidified CO_2 incubator.

5   Follow steps 5 and 6 of *Protocol 1*.

6   Plot a standard curve of c.p.m. versus the concentration of IL-4. Compare the test results with the standard curve to estimate the activity in the unknown samples (see Section 6).

2.4 Bioassay for interleukin 5 (IL-5)

Bioassays for IL-5 utilize the ability of this cytokine to stimulate the formation of eosinophil colonies in an agar colony assay or by an estimation of eosinophil peroxidase. Alternatively, IL-5 can be assayed by its proliferative effect on the erythroleukaemic cell line, TF-1 (see Section 3.1).

2.5 Bioassay for interleukin 6 (IL-6)

Most bioassays for IL-6 depend upon the proliferative effect of this cytokine on IL-6-dependent, murine hybridoma cell lines such as MH60, B9, T1165, and 7TD1 (14, 15). Alternatively, IL-6 can be assayed by its ability to enhance differentiation and IgG secretion in Epstein–Barr virus-transformed, human lymphoblastoid cell lines such as CESS. The IL-6-dependent, murine, hybridoma cell line B9 provides a reliable and sensitive assay for measuring mammalian IL-6.

2.5.1 Maintenance of the B9 cell line

Culture B9 cells in RPMI-1640 medium supplemented with 5% FCS and approximately 100 pg/ml (10 IU/ml) of IL-6 (recombinant IL-6 or crude supernant from either IL-1 stimulated fibroblasts or LPS-stimulated monocytes) in 75 cm^2 flasks. Cultures are split 1:5 to 1:10 every 2–3 days and re-fed with IL-6 when the cell density reaches approximately 5×10^5 cells/ml. Cultures are maintained at 37°C in a humidified CO_2 incubator.

Protocol 4

Bioassay for IL-6 using the B9 cell line

Equipment and reagents

- B9 cell culture (see Section 2.5.1)
- IL-6 standard (see Section 6 and *Table 2*)
- Trypan Blue
- XTT dye (Boehringer-Mannheim kit, XTT labelling mixture)
- ELISA reader
- Centrifuge
- 96-well microtitre plates
- Test samples
- 37°C, 5% CO_2 incubator
- FCS
- RPMI-1640 medium without phenol red

Method

1   Wash B9 cells (2 days after feeding) as in *Protocol 1*, step 1 and resuspend to a density of 2.5×10^4 cells/ml in RPMI-1640 medium without phenol red, supplemented with 5% FCS.

2   Distribute an IL-6 standard (see Section 6) as a serial twofold dilution series, in triplicate in 100 μl volumes, in 96-well microtite plates. Start the titration of the standard at 100 pg/ml (10 IU/ml) and dilute down to 0.1 pg/ml (0.01 IU/ml). Make appropriate dilutions of the samples to be measured for IL-6 activity in triplicate in 100 μl volumes. As a negative control include culture medium alone.

3   Add 100 μl of cell suspension to each well and incubate the plates for approximately 96 h[a] at 37°C in a humidified CO_2 incubator.

4   To each well add 50 μl of XTT and return the plates to the incubator for a further 6–7 h. Determine the absorbance at a wavelength of 450 nm using an ELISA reader.

5   Plot a standard curve of absorbance versus the concentration of IL-6. Determine the activity in unknown samples by comparing test results with the standard curve (see Section 6).

[a] Prolonging the incubation to 120 h is sometimes necessary to enhance the signal-to-noise ratio for this assay.

2.6 Bioassay for interleukin 7 (IL-7)

The IL-7 bioassay employs a murine pre-B cell line (PB-1 cells) which is dependent upon exogenous IL-7 for its continuous growth and viability (47). The proliferation induced by human or murine IL-7 is measured by tritiated thymidine incorporation.

2.6.1 Maintenance of the PB-1 cell line

Cells are assayed in incomplete growth medium as follows (all obtained from Sigma): McCoys 5A medium, 15% fetal calf serum, 1 mM sodium pyruvate, 0.4 × MEM non-essential amino-acids (i.e. 1/250 dilution of 100 × stock), 0.4 × MEM essential amino acids (1/125 dilution of 50 × stock), 0.12% sodium bicarbonate, 50 μM beta-mercaptoethanol, 2 mM L-glutamine, 16 μg/ml asparagine, 8.4 μg/ml serine, and 0.4 × MEM vitamins (1/250 dilution of 100 × stock). Cells are maintained in complete growth medium on the addition of 50 ng/ml of recombinant human IL-7. Cultures are passaged when the cells reach a density of 2×10^5 cells/ml and diluted 1/10 with fresh growth medium

Protocol 5

Bioassay for IL-7 using the PB1 cell line

Equipment and reagents

- PB-1 cell line (see Section 2.6.1)
- Cell culture medium (see Section 2.6.1)
- Equipment and reagents as *Protocol 1*
- IL-7 standard (see Section 6 and *Table 2*)

Method

1 Wash the cells as in *Protocol 1*, step 1 and resuspend to a density of 2×10^5 cells/ml in medium containing 5% FCS.

2 Distribute the IL-7 standard in a two-fold dilution series in triplicate in 50 μl volumes in 96-well microtitration plates. Start the titration of the standard at 200 pg/ml (approximately 20 U/ml) and dilute down to 1 pg/ml (0.01 U/ml). Make appropriate dilutions of the samples in duplicate in 50 μl volumes. Include culture medium alone as a negative control.

3 Add 50 μl of the cell suspension to each well and incubate the plates for approximately 3 days at 37 °C in a humidified, 5% CO_2 incubator.

4 Follow *Protocol 1*, steps 5 and 6.

5 Plot a standard curve of c.p.m. versus the concentration of IL-7. Estimate activity in unknown samples by comparison with the standard curve (see Section 6).

2.7 Bioassay for interleukin 8 (IL-8) and other chemokines

Most bioassays for IL-8 rely upon the stimulatory effect of this cytokine on the migration of polymorphonuclear leucocytes. The migration is assessed either by measuring chemokinesis (an enhancement of random movement) or by chemotaxis (a directed locomotion along a concentration gradient). Chemotactic activity can be measured using either a Boyden chamber or a Neuroprobe microchamber, or by using the agarose method. Alternative assays are based on respiratory-burst activity, the elevation of intracellular Ca^{2+} levels, and elastase secretion from activated neutrophils.

2.8 Bioassay for interleukin-9 (IL-9)

This cytokine can be assayed using long-term cultured CD4+ and CD8+ T cell lines and clones, or by its ability to enhance erythroid burst-forming activity in the presence of erythropoietin. Murine IL-9 can stimulate human cells but not vice versa. Alternatively, the MO-7e line proliferates in response to IL-9 (16). This assay is described in *Protocol 12*.

2.9 Bioassay for interleukin-10 (IL-10)

IL-10 is commonly assayed by its ability to inhibit IFN-γ production by activated peripheral blood mononuclear cells (PBMC) or murine TH1 clones, or by its proliferative effect on the murine mast cell line MC/9 (this line also responds to human and murine IL-5 and SCF) (17). Alternatively, B cell lines (e.g. BaF, a murine line which has been transfected with receptors for either human IL-10 or murine IL-10, such as Ba8.1c1, or BaMr respectively) can be used to measure IL-18 (18); assays using these cell lines were found to be highly sensitive and reproducible. Human IL-10 is active on murine cells, but the murine counterpart is inactive on human cells.

2.9.1 Maintenance of the Ba8.1c1 cell line

Culture cells in RPMI-1640 containing 10% FCS (heat-inactivated), 200 mM L-glutamine, 0.05 mM 2-mercaptoethanol, 0.5 mg/ml geneticin (Sigma) and 5% spleen conditioned medium or 1 ng/ml murine IL-3 in upright 75 cm^2 flasks. Cultures are split 1:5 every 2–3 days when the cell density reaches approximately 5×10^5/ml.

Protocol 6

Bioassay for IL-10 using the Ba8.1c1 cell line

Equipment and reagents

- Ba8.1c1 cell culture (see Section 2.9.1)
- Cell-culture medium (see *Protocol* and step 1 below)
- IL-10 standard (see Section 6 and *Table 2*)
- Equipment and reagents as *Protocol 1*

Method

1   Wash cells (2–3 days after feeding) twice as in *Protocol 1*, step 1 and resuspend to a density of 3×10^5 cells/ml in RPMI-1640 containing 2% heat-inactivated FCS and 0.05 mM 2-mercaptoethanol.

2   Titrate the IL-10 standard in triplicate in 96-well microtitre plates. Start the titration at 10 ng/ml (approximately 50 U/ml) and dilute down in a two-fold dilution series to 10 pg/ml (0.05 U/ml) in 50 μl volumes in RMPI-1640 containing 2% heat-inactivated FCS and 0.05 mM 2-mercaptoethanol. Make appropriate dilutions of the samples in triplicate. For a negative control, include culture medium alone.

3   Add 50 μl of the cell suspension to each well and incubate for approximately 44 h at 37°C in a humidified, CO$_2$ incubator.

4   Follow *Protocol 1*, steps 5 and 6.

5   Plot a standard curve of c.p.m. versus the concentration of IL-10. Estimate the activity in unknown samples by comparing test results with a standard curve (see Section 6).

2.10 Bioassay for interleukin-11 (IL-11)

IL-11 can be measured by its stimulatory effect on the proliferation of IL-6-dependent murine plasmacytoma lines such as T1165 (15). A subclone of this cell line, T10, has been developed; the use of this cell line is described in *Protocol 7*. Recently a subclone of the B9 line (see Section 2.5), B9-11, has been derived which shows enhanced sensitivity for IL-11 (19).

2.10.1 Maintenance of the T10 cell line

Culture the cells in RPMI-1640 medium supplemented with 10% FCS, 2 mM L-glutamine, 0.05 mM 2-mercaptoethanol, and 5 ng/ml (approximately 50 U/ml) IL-11 in 75 cm^2 flasks. Cultures are split 1:4 to 1:5 every 2–3 days and re-fed with IL-11. T10 cells are non-adherent, but they do tend to cling to the bottom of the tissue culture flasks. Tap the flask gently to loosen the cells. Maintain the cultures at 37°C in a humidified, 5% CO_2 incubator.

Protocol 7

Bioassay for IL-11 using the T10 cell line

Equipment and reagents

- T10 cells (see Section 2.10.1)
- Cell-culture medium: RPMI-1640, 10% FCS, 2 mM L-glutamine, 0.05 mM 2-mercaptoethanol
- IL-11 standard (see Section 6 and *Table 2*)
- Equipment and reagents as *Protocol 1*

Method

1 Wash T10 cells (2–3 days after feeding) as in *Protocol 1*, step 1 and resuspend the cells to a final concentration of 1×10^5 cells/ml in the culture medium.

2 Distribute titrations of IL-11, in 100 μl volume in triplicate, in 96-well microtitre plates. Start the titration of the standard at 10 ng/ml (approximately 100 U/ml) and make serial dilutions down to 10 pg/ml (0.1 U/ml). Make appropriate dilutions of the unknown samples in triplicate in 100 μl volumes. As a negative control include medium alone.

3 Add 100 μl of the cell suspension to each well and incubate for approximately 44 h at 37°C in a humidified, CO_2 incubator.

4 Follow *Protocol 1*, steps 5 and 6.

5 Plot a standard curve of c.p.m. versus the concentration of IL-11. Estimate the activity in unknown samples by comparing the test results with a standard curve (see Section 6).

2.11 Bioassay for interleukin-12 (IL-12)

IL-12 can be measured by its effect on the proliferation of PHA-activated human lymphoblasts (20). Alternatively, it can be assayed using the IL-2 dependent human T-cell leukaemic line, KIT225/K6-C (21). The murine protein is active on human cells, but not vice versa.

2.11.1 Maintenance of the KIT225/K6-C cell line

Culture the cells in RPMI-1640 medium supplemented with 10% FCS, 2 mM L-glutamine, 0.05 mM 2-mercaptoethanol, and 20 IU/ml of IL-2 in 75 cm^2 upright flasks. Cultures are split 1:5 to 1:10 every 2–3 days and re-fed with IL-2. Cultures are maintained at 37 °C in a humidified, CO_2 incubator.

Protocol 8

Bioassay for IL-12 using the KIT225/K6-C cell line

Equipment and reagents

- Kit 225 cell culture (see Section 2.11.1)
- Cell-culture medium: RPMI-1640, 10% FCS, 2 mM L-glutamine, 0.05 mM 2-mercapto-ethanol, 10 ng/ml (approximately 100 U/ml) recombinant, human (rh) IL-4.
- IL-12 standard (see Section 6 and *Table 2*)
- Equipment and reagents as *Protocol 1*

Method

1 Wash KIT225/K6-C cells (2–3 days after feeding) as in *Protocol 1*, step 1 and re-suspend the cells to a final concentration of 1×10^5 cells/ml in the cell-culture medium.

2 Distribute titrations of IL-12 in 100 μl volumes, in triplicate, in 96-well microtitre plates. Start the titration of the standard at 50 ng/ml and make serial dilutions down to 0.5 pg/ml. Make appropriate dilutions of the unknown samples in 100 μl volumes. As a negative control include medium alone.

3 Add 100 μl of the washed cell suspension to each well and incubate the plates for approximately 72 h at 37 °C in a humidified, CO_2 incubator.

4 Follow *Protocol 1*, steps 5 and 6.

5 Plot a standard curve of c.p.m. versus the concentration of IL-12. Estimate the activity in unknown samples by comparing test results with a standard curve (see Section 5).

2.12 Bioassay for interleukin-13 (IL-13)

This cytokine can be assayed either by its ability to induce the expression of CD23 on B cells of IgE synthesis by purified B cells, or by proliferation of activated human B lymphocytes, as for IL-4 and IL-14 (*Protocol 9*). Alternatively, it can be measured by its proliferative effect on the human erythroleukaemic cell line, TF-1 (described in *Protocol 13*), or the plasmacytoma cell line, B.9.13, a subclone of the B9 cell line (22)

2.13 Bioassay for interleukin-14 (IL-14)

IL-14 can be assayed by its ability to induce proliferation of activated B cells (23). For this, B lymphocytes are purified from peripheral blood or tonsils, using Ficoll–Hypaque separation of mononuclear cells followed by monocyte depletion by adherence and T-cell depletion by E-rosetting. The resulting B cells are then used in the co-stimulatory assay as indicated in *Protocol 9*.

Protocol 9

B-cell co-stimulatory assay for IL-14[a]

Equipment and reagents

- B-cells
- Cell-culture medium: RPMI-1640, 10% FCS
- *Staphylococcus aureus*-Cowan 1 strain (SAC; Calbiochem)
- Ficoll–Hypaque
- PBS
- Equipment and reagents as *Protocol 1*
- IL-14

Method

1 Prepare B cells and resuspend in the cell-culture medium.
2 Incubate the B cells with 1:25 000 dilution of SAC in RPMI-1640 and 10% FCS for 72 h in a 37°C incubator.
3 Remove dead cells by Ficoll–Hypaque separation and cenrifugation at 250 g for 10 min.
4 Wash the cells twice with PBS and resuspend at a concentration of 1×10^6 cells/ml at RT.
5 Distribute titrations of an IL-14 preparation into 96-well microtitre plates in 100 μl volumes. For unknown samples, make appropriate dilutions. For a negative control, include vulture medium alone.
6 Add 100 μl of the cell suspension to each well and incubate the plates for approximately 44 h at 37°C in a humidified, 5% CO_2 incubator.
7 Add 1 μCi of tritiated thymidine to each well and return the culture plates to the incubator for a further 18 h.
8 Follow *Protocol 1*, step 6.
9 Plot a standard curve of c.p.m. versus the concentration of IL-14. Estimate the activity of unknown samples, by comparing the test results with a standard curve (see Section 6).

[a] This assay can be used to measure human IL-4 and human IL-13 by including an appropriate cytokine standard. For measuring activity in samples, neutralizing antibodies should be used to confirm the presence of a particular cytokine.

2.14 Bioassay for interleukin-15 (IL-15)

IL-15 can be measured by its proliferative effect on IL-2-dependent cell lines such as CTLL clones. The assay based on the CTLL-2 murine T cell line provides a reliable and easy method which responds to IL-15 from most mammalian species. Alternatively, the human T cell line, KIT-225 can be used for assaying IL-15 (our unpublished observations).

2.15 Bioassay for interleukin-16 (IL-16)

IL-16 can be measured by its ability to chemoattract CD4 T cells, monocytes, and eosinophils. Alternatively, it can be assayed by its ability to induce the expression of CD25 or MHC class II molecules on T cells.

2.16 Bioassay for interleukin-17 (IL-17)

IL-17 can be measured by its ability to induce the proliferation of T cells in a co-stimulation assay. IL-17 also stimulates the secretation of IL-6 and IL-8 from human foreskin fibroblasts (HFF) and this can be used as an assay for measuring IL-17 as described in *Protocol 10* (24).

2.16.1 Maintenance of HFF

Culture the cells in Dulbecco's Modified Eagle's Medium supplemented with 10% FCS and 2 mM L-glutamine, in 75 cm^2 flasks. Cultures are split 1:5 to 1:10 every 5–7 days using trypsin–EDTA when the cells are confluent. Cultures are maintained at 37 °C in a humidified, CO$_2$ incubator.

Protocol 10

Bioassay for IL-17 using HFF cells

Equipment and reagents

- HFF cells (see Section 2.16.1)
- Cell-culture medium (see Section 1.16.1)
- IL-17
- IL-6 ELISA or bioassay
- 96-well microtitre plates
- Humidified, 37 °C, 5% CO$_2$ incubator
- PBS
- Trypsin–EDTA (Gibco 10 × solution)

Method

1   Harvest cells (5–7 days after feeding) using trypsin–EDTA (diluted 1:10 in PBS) and resuspend to a final concentration of 2×10^5 cells/ml in Dulbecco's Modified Eagle's Medium containing 10% FCS and 2 mM L-glutamine.

2   Add 100 µl of the cell suspension to each well and incubate overnight at 37 °C in a humidified, 5% CO$_2$ incubator.

3   Distribute titrations of IL-17 in 100 µl volumes, in triplicate, in 96-well microtitration plates. Start the titration of the standard at 1000 ng/ml and make serial dilutions.

Make appropriate dilutions of the unknown samples in 100 μl volumes. As a negative control include medium alone. Transfer contents to plates in step 2.

4 Incubate the plates for approximately 24–48 h at 37°C in a humidified, CO_2 incubator.

5 Remove the supernatant from each well and determine the IL-6 produced using a specific ELISA or bioassay for IL-6. Note that the amount of IL-6 in the supernatants will be proportional to the amount of IL-17 in the original samples. Supernatants from the HFF cells can be stored frozen until the IL-6 can be conveniently assayed.

2.17 Bioassay for interleukin-18 (IL-18)

IL-18 or interferon-γ inducing factor (IGIF) can be bioassayed by the ability of this cytokine to induce IFN-γ production from Cona-stimulated PBMC (25). Recently, the human myelomonocytic cell line, KG-1, which produces IFN-γ in response to IL-18, has been used as a simple bioassay for this cytokine (26).

2.17.1 Maintenance of the KG-1 cell line

Culture KG-1 cells in RPMI-1640 medium supplemented with 10% heat-inactivated FCS in 75 cm^2 upright flasks. Cultures are split 1:5 every 3–4 days when the cell density reaches approximately 2×10^6/ml. Cultures are maintained at 37°C in a humidified CO_2 incubator.

Protocol 11

Bioassay of IL-18 using the KG-1 cell line

Equipment and reagents

- KG-1 cells (see Section 2.17.1)
- Cell-culture medium (see Section 2.17.1)
- IL-18
- IFN-γ ELISA
- ELISA plate reader
- 96-well microtitre plates
- Humidified, 37°C, 5% CO_2 incubator

Method

1 Wash KG-1 cells (3–4 days after feeding when the cell density is approximately 2×10^6/ml) once in RPMI-1640 medium by centrifuging the cells at 250 g for 10 min at RT. Determine cell viability as in *Protocol 1*, step 2.

2 Resuspend the cells to a final concentration of 3×10^6 cells/ml in RPMI-1640 medium containing 10% FCS.

3 Distribute titrations of an IL-18 standard (see Section 6 and *Table 2*) in triplicate in 96-well microtitration plates. Start the titration of the standard at 500 ng/ml IL-18 and make serial dilutions down to 0.1 ng/ml of IL-18. Make appropriate dilutions of

Protocol 11 continued

the samples to be measured for IL-18 activity (either twofold or tenfold serial dilutions) in triplicate. Include a negative control of culture medium. Make sure that each well contains 100 μl at this stage.

4   Add 100 μl of the washed cell suspension to each well and incubate the plates for approximately 24 h at 37 °C in a humidified CO_2 incubator.

5   Remove 100 μl of the supernatant from each well and determine the IFN-γ produced using a specific ELISA for IFN-γ. Note that the amount of IFN-γ in the supernatants will be proportional to the amount of IL-18 in the original samples. Supernatants from the KG-1 cells can be stored frozen until the IFN-γ can be conveniently assayed.

3 Bioassays for colony-stimulating factors—interleukin-3 (IL-3), granulocyte colony-stimulating factor (G-CSF), macrophage colony-stimulating factor (M-CSF), granulocyte-macrophage colony-stimulating factor (GM-CSF), stem-cell factor (SCF), thrombopoietin (TPO), and leukaemia inhibitory factor (LIF).

3.1 Introduction

Classically, these factors are assayed by their ability, in soft agar, to stimulate the formation of colonies of differentiated cells from bone-marrow progenitor cells (27). The type of colony produced is obviously dependent upon the factor(s) present in the immediate environment. For example, IL-3 and GM-CSF stimulate the production of mixed colonies of different cell types, whereas G-CSF, M-CSF, and erythropoietin (Epo) are lineage-restricted and produce predominantly granulocyte, monocyte, and erythroid colonies, respectively. In these assays, colonies of more than 50 cells are counted and analysed after 7–14 days using a binocular microscope or by one of the sophisticated image analysers now available. The number of colonies is usually related to the specific activity or concentration of the colony-stimulating factor (CSF) in the agar culture. Morphological analysis, by staining dried and fixed gels, allows proper identification of the colony type. This bioassay is slow, tedious, and not specific and is subject to interference by contaminating factors which may enhance or inhibit colony formation. Alternative assays for CSFs measure the proliferative effect of these factors on cell lines derived from human leukaemias, e.g. AML-193, TALL-101, MO-7e, TF-1 (*Figure 1*), and murine lines such as NFS-60, WEHI 3BD+, and 32DC1 (28–34). Such lines provide rapid, sensitive, and reliable assays. In addition, specificity can be achieved using specific neutralizing antibodies to inhibit the appropriate activity (*Figure 2*). Detailed protocols for some CSFs are described here; these protocols can be applied to measure other cross-reactive cytokines (*Table 1*) by including the appropriate cytokine standard (*Table 2*).

3.1.1 Maintenance of MO-7e/TF-1 cell lines

Culture the cells in RPMI-1640 medium supplemented with 5% FCS and GM-CSF (approximately 4 ng/ml (40 IU/ml) for MO-7e, 2 ng/ml (20 IU/ml) for TF-1) in upright 75 cm^2 flasks. Cultures are split 1:5 every 2–3 days and re-fed with GM-CSF when the cell density reaches approximately 5×10^5 cells/ml. Cultures are maintained at 37 °C in a humidified 5% CO_2 incubator.

Protocol 12

Bioassay using the MO-7e cell line

Equipment and reagents

- MO-7e cells (see Section 3.1.1)
- Cytokine standards (see Section 6 and *Table 2*)
- RPMI-1640 medium 5% FCS
- Equipment and reagents as *Protocol 1*
- FCS

Method

1 Wash MO-7e cells (2–3 days after feeding) as in *Protocol 1*, step 1 and resuspend the cells in RPMI-1640 containing 5% FCS in a final concentration of 5×10^5 cells/ml.

2 Distribute titrations of an appropriate standard (GM-CSF, IL-3, SCF, IL-9, etc., see *Table 2*)[a] in 100 μl volumes in triplicate in 96-well microtitration plates. Start the titration of the standard, e.g. GM-CSF at 1 ng/ml (10 IU/ml) and make serial dilutions (twofold or tenfold) down to 1 pg/ml (0.1 IU/ml). Make appropriate dilutions of the samples in 100 μl volumes in triplicate. As a negative control include culture medium alone.

3 Follow *Protocol 3*, steps 4 and 5.

4 Plot a standard curve of c.p.m. versus the concentration of the particular cytokine standard. Estimate activity in unknown samples by comparison with a standard curve (see Section 6).

[a] This cell line proliferates with different sensitivities to different cytokines, the order being GM-CSF or IL-3 > IL-9 > SCF.

Protocol 13

Bioassay using the TF-1 cell line

Equipment and reagents

- TF-1 cells (Section 3.1.1)
- RPMI-1640, 5% FCS
- Equipment and reagents as *Protocol 12*

Protocol 13 continued

Method

1 Wash TF-1 cells (2–3 days after feeding) as in *Protocol 1*, step 1 and resuspend the cells to a final concentration of 1×10^5 cells/ml in RPMI-1640 containing 5% FCS.

2 Distribute titrations of an appropriate standard (GM-CSF, IL-3, IL-4, etc., see *Table 2*)[a] in 100 μl volumes in triplicate. Start the titration of the standard, e.g. GM-CSF at 1 ng/ml (10 IU/ml) and make serial twofold dilutions down to 0.1 pg/ml (0.001 IU/ml). Make appropriate dilutions of the samples in 100 μl volumes in triplicate. As a negative control include medium alone.

3 Follow *Protocol 3*, steps 4 and 5.

4 Plot a standard curve of c.p.m. versus the concentration of the particular cytokine standard. Estimate activity in unknown samples by comparison with a standard curve (see Section 6).

[a] This cell line exhibits differential sensitivity to different cytokines, the order being GM-CSF or IL-3 > IL-5 > SCF > IL-4.

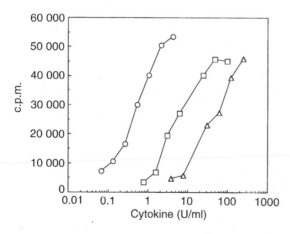

Figure 1 Dose-response curves for human SCF (□, Onco M (△) and Epo (○) using the TF-1 cell line bioassay (as described in *Protocol 13*). [Also refer to *Figure 2* on page 226]

3.1.2 Maintenance of the GNFS-60 and MNFS-60 cell lines

Culture the cells in RPMI-1640 medium supplemented with 5% FCS and 2 ng/ml (200 IU/ml) G-CSF for GNFS-60 and 1000 IU/ml M-CSF for MNFS-60 in upright 75 cm² flasks. Cultures are split 1:5 to 1:10 every 2–3 days and re-fed with G-CSF when the cell density reaches approximately 5×10^5 cells/ml. Cultures should be maintained at 37 °C in a humidified 5% CO_2 incubator.

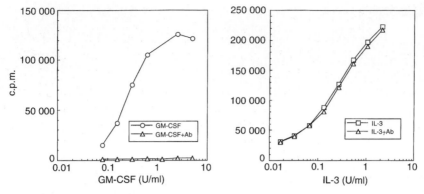

Figure 2 Dose-response curves for (A) human GM-CSF and (B) IL-3 using the TF-1 cell line bioassay. In this experiment, the dose-response experiment was conducted in the presence or absence of a specific neutralizing human antibody for GM-CSF listed in Table 3 (1:250 dilution), illustrating that specificity for a particular cytokine can be achieved using a specific neutralizing antiserum.

Protocol 14

Bioassay of G-CSF using the GNFS-60 cell line

Method and reagents

- GNFS-60 cells (Section 3.1.2)
- Cytokine standards (Section 6 and *Table 2*)
- Equipment and reagents as *Protocol 13*

Method

1 Wash GNFS-60 cells (2–3 days after feeding) as in *Protocol 1*, step 1 and resuspend the cells to a final concentration of 1×10^5 cells/ml in RPMI-1640 containing 5% FCS.

2 Distribute titrations of the G-CSF standard in triplicate in 96-well microtitre plates. Start the titration of the standard at 1 ng/ml (100 IU/ml) and make serial twofold dilutions down to 1 pg/ml (0.1 IU/ml). Make appropriate dilutions of the samples to be measured for G-CSF activity, in triplicate in 100 µl volumes. As a negative control include culture medium alone.

3 Follow *Protocol 3*, steps 4 and 5.

4 Plot a standard curve of c.p.m. versus the concentration of the standard. Estimate activity in unknown samples by comparison with a standard curve (see Section 6).

Protocol 15

Bioassay of M-CSF using the MNFS-60 cell line

Equipment and reagents

- MNFS-60 cells (Section 3.1.2)
- Cytokine standards (Section 6 and *Table 2*)
- Equipment and reagents as *Protocol 12*

Method

1　Wash MNFS-60 cells (2–3 days after feeding) as in *Protocol 1*, step 1 and resuspend the cells to a final concentration of 1×10^5 cells/ml in RPMI-1640 containing 5% FCS.

2　Distribute titrations of the M-CSF standard in 100 μl volumes, in triplicate, in 96-well microtitre plates. Start the titration of the standard at 50 ng/ml (3000 IU/ml) and make serial twofold dilutions down to 10 pg/ml (0.6 IU/ml). Make appropriate dilutions of the samples to be measured for M-CSF activity (either twofold or tenfold serial dilutions) in triplicate in 100 μl volumes. As a negative control include culture medium alone.

3　Follow *Protocol 3*, steps 4 and 5.

4　Plot a standard curve of absorbance versus concentration of standard. Estimate activity in unknown samples by comparison with a standard curve (see Section 6).

3.2 Bioassay for leukaemia inhibitory factor (LIF)

This cytokine can be assayed by its ability to induce differentiation of the monocytic leukaemia cell line, M1. However, a number of other assays have also been developed, e.g. the bone-marrow colony assay (in which LIF synergizes with IL-3 to produce multilineage colonies) or proliferation assays employing either the murine cell line, DA-1a (30) or the human cell line, TF-1 (described in *Protocol 13*).

3.3 Bioassay for thrombopoietin (TPO)

Bioassays for TPO utilize the ability of this cytokine to stimulate the formation of megakaryocytic colonies in a colony assay or to stimulate the proliferation of megakaryocytic cell lines such as HU3 or M-07e (35).

An alternative approach of measuring Tpo is by using a cell line that has been transfected with the human mpl receptor which binds TPO or the c-mpl ligand. An example of this is the 32D/mpl+ cell line (36).

3.3.1 Maintenance of the 2D/mpl+ cell line

Culture the cells in RPMI-1640 medium containing 5% FCS and 1 ng/ml murine IL-3 in upright, 75 cm² flasks. Cultures are split 1:5 every 2–3 days when the cell density reaches approximately 5×10^5 cells/ml. Cultures are maintained at 37°C in a humidified CO_2 incubator.

Protocol 16

Bioassay for TPO using the 32D/mpl+ cell line

Equipment and reagents

- 32D/mpl+ cells (Section 3.3.1)
- TPO

- Equipment and reagents as *Protocol 12*

Method

1   Wash 32D/mpl+ cells (2–3 days after feeding) as in *Protocol 1*, step 1 and resuspend to a concentration of 1×10^5 cells/ml in RPMI-1640 containing 5% FCS.

2   Titrate the TPO standard, in triplicate, in 96-well microtitre plates. Start the titration at 5 ng/ml and serially dilute twofold down to 5 pg/ml in 100 µl volumes of RPMI-1640 containing 5% FCS. Make appropriate dilutions of the samples. As a negative control, include culture medium alone.

3   Follow *Protocol 3*, steps 4 and 5.

4   Plot a standard curve of c.p.m. versus the concentration of TPO. Estimate activity in unknown samples by comparing test results with a standard curve (see Section 6).

4 Bioassays for TGF-β and related proteins

4.1 Bioassay for TGF-β

The classical assay for TGF-β is based on its ability to induce colony growth of fibroblasts in soft agar. For a routine assay, the mink-lung fibroblast line MV-3D9 can be used in a proliferation assay (37). To achieve a greater sensitivity, however, it is better to use the assay based on the ability of TGF-β to inhibit the IL-5-induced proliferation of TF-1 cells (38). Both assays are described here.

4.1.1 Maintenance of MV-3D9 mink-lung fibroblasts

Maintain cells in RPMI-1640 containing 5% FCS in 75 cm² flasks. When confluent (3–4 days), cultures are split 1:7 using 0.01% trypsin.

Protocol 17
Bioassay for TGF-β using the MV-3D9 cell line

Equipment and reagents

- MV-3D9 cells (Section 4.1.1)
- RPMI-1640 without phenol red
- TGF-β standard (Section 6 and *Table 2*)
- FCS
- Equipment and reagents as *Protocol 4*
- Trypsin/EDTA (*Protocol 10*)

Method

1   Trypsinize MV-3D9 cells and resuspend to a density of 5×10^3 cells/ml in RPMI-1640 containing 5% FCS.

2   Distribute titrations of the TGF-β standard, in triplicate, in a separate microtitre plate. Start this at 10 ng/ml and serially dilute twofold down to 10 pg/ml in 100 µl

volumes. Make appropriate dilutions of the samples. For a negative control add culture medium alone.

3 Add 100 μl of the cell suspension to each well and incubate the plates for approximately 120 h at 37 °C in a humidified CO_2 incubator.

4 Follow *Protocol 6*, step 4.

5 Plot a standard curve of absorbance versus the concentration of TGF-β. Estimate activity in unknown samples by comparison with a standard curve (see Section 6).

Protocol 18

Bioassay for TGF-β using the TF-1 cell line

Equipment and reagents
- TF-1 cells (Section 3.1.1)
- Equipment and reagents as *Protocol 12*
- TGF-β standard
- IL-5

Method

1 Prepare cells as described in *Protocol 13*, steps 1 and 2.

2 Distribute titrations of the TGF-β standard, in 100 μl volumes in triplicate, in a 96-well microtitre plate. Start the titration at 1 ng/ml and serially dilute twofold down to 0.1 pg/ml. Make appropriate dilutions of the test samples.[a] As a negative control include medium alone.

3 Add 2 ng/ml (approximately 20 U/ml) of IL-5 to the prepared cell suspension at a density of 1×10^5 cells/ml.

4 Follow *Protocol 3*, steps 4 and 5.

5 Plot a standard curve of c.p.m. versus the concentration of TGF-β. Estimate activity in unknown samples by comparison with a standard curve (see Section 6).

[a] Since TGF-β is initially produced in a latent form, biological samples may require acid-activation by the addition of an equal volume of 2.5 M acetic acid/10 M urea for 10 min at room temperature and neutralization to pH 7.0 with 1 M Hepes/2.7 M NaOH prior to inclusion in the assay.

4.2 Bone morphogenetic proteins

Bone morphogenetic proteins are members of the TGF-β superfamily that are involved in tissue growth and differentiation. They are mainly characterized by their ability to stimulate osteoblast differentiation and bone formation. Bioassays based on these properties are therefore used to measure this particular class of proteins. An assay based on a bone-marrow stromal cell line, W-20-17, is described below (39).

4.2.1 Maintenance of W-20-17 cells

Culture the cells in Dulbecco's Modified Eagle's Medium supplemented with 10% FCS and 2 mM L-glutamine, in 75 cm² flasks. Cultures are split 1:5 to 1:10 every 3–4 days using Trypsin/EDTA when the cells are confluent. Cultures are maintained at 37°C in a humidified CO_2 incubator.

Protocol 19

Bioassay for BMP-2 using the W-20-17 cell line

Equipment and reagents

- W-20-17 cells (Section 4.2.1)
- Cell-culture medium (Section 4.2.1)
- 0.01% trypsin
- 96-well microtitre plates
- PBS
- Glycine buffer: 75 g glycine in approx, 70 ml of distilled water. Adjust to pH 10.3 with 10 M NaOH.

- 12.5% Triton X-100 in 0.9% saline
- $MgCl_2.6H_2O$
- Assay mix: 0.8 ml of 12.5%, Triton X-100, 0.13 g $MgCl_2.6H_2O$, glycine buffer. Make up to 100 ml with dH_2O. Check the pH, filter, and store at room temperature.
- *P*-nitrophenylphosphate (PNPP)
- ELISA plate reader

Method

1 Trypsinize the cells in log-phase growth and dilute to 5×10^4 cells/ml in growth medium.

2 Aliquot 200 μl of cell suspension into each well of a microtitre plate and incubate for 24 h at 37°C, 5% CO_2 humidified atmosphere.

3 Pour out the medium and invert the plate gently on to absorbent paper.

4 Distribute titrations of the BMP standard, in triplicate in 250 μl volumes, in wells of another 96-well plate. Start the titration of the standard at 500 ng/ml and then make serial twofold dilutions down to 0.5 ng/ml. Make appropriate dilutions of the samples in triplicate. For the negative control, add culture medium alone.

5 Transfer 200 μl of medium containing dilutions of standard/samples to plates containing W-20 cells.

6 Incubate the plates for 24 h at 37°C in a 5% CO_2 humidified atmosphere.

7 Pour out the medium and invert the plate gently on to absorbent paper.

8 Wash plates once with 200 μl of PBS/well.

9 Add 50 μl dH_2O/well. Transfer the plates to a –70°C freezer, thaw, refreeze, and then thaw.

10 Prior to use, add PNPP (0.34%) to the assay mix. Add 50 μl of the assay mix to each well.

11 Leave the plates in the dark for 30 min at RT.

12 Carefully agitate the plate until the dye is evenly dispersed throughout the wells and determine the absorbance at 450 nm using an ELISA reader.

13 Plot a standard curve of absorbance versus the concentration of BMP. Estimate activity in unknown samples by comparison with a standard curve (see Section 6).

5 Bioassays for other cytokines

5.1 Bioassay for tumour necrosis factors

The most commonly used bioassay for TNF-α or TNF-β (lymphotoxin) utilizes the cytotoxic action of these cytokines on murine fibroblasts such as L929 or L-M cells; or human cells such as the rhabdomyosarcoma cell line, KYM-1 (40), or its adherent subclone KD4—clone 21 derived from KYM-1. TNF-α and -β can be distinguished from each other by including neutralizing antibodies in the assay.

5.1.1 Maintenance of KD4 cells

Grow cells in DMEM containing 10% fetal calf serum, in 75 cm^2 flasks. Subculture the cells at weekly intervals using 0.01% trypsin and dilute 1:7 in growth medium.

Protocol 20

Bioassay for TNF-α or -β

Equipment and reagents

- KD4 cells (Section 5.1.1)
- Cell-culture medium (Section 5.1.1)
- 0.01% trypsin
- Actinomycin D
- TNF standard (Section 6, *Table 2*)
- 96-well microtitre plate
- FCS
- RPMI-1640 without phenol red

- 3 mM PMS phenazine methylsulphate in 10 ml RPMI-1640 without phenol red + 2% FCS
- MTS (Promega Cell Titre 96 non-radioactive cell proliferation assay
- MTS solution (per plate): 2 ml MTS (2 mg/ml), 100 μl PMSF soln. Prepare immediately before use
- ELISA plate reader

Method

1 Trypsinize the cells in log-phase growth and dilute to 2×10^5 cells/ml in growth medium.

2 Aliquot 100 μl of the cell suspension into each well of a microtitre plate and incubate for 24 h at 37 °C in 5% CO_2 humidified atmosphere.

3 Distribute titrations of TNF standard (see Section 6 and *Table 2*), in triplicate in 100 μl volumes, in wells containing the cells. Start the titration of the standard at 5 IU/ml

Protocol 20 continued

and then make serial twofold dilutions down to 0.001 IU/ml. Make appropriate dilutions of the samples in triplicate. For the negative control, add culture medium alone.

4 Add 100 μl of medium containing 2 μ/ml actinomycin D to the wells.

5 Incubate the plates for 24 h at 37°C in a 5% CO_2 humidified atmosphere.

6 Pour out the medium and invert the plate gently on to absorbent paper.

7 Add 100 μl of the MTS solution per well.

8 Leave the plates for approximately 1 h at 37°C in a 5% CO_2 incubator.

9 Carefully agitate the plate until the dye is evenly dispersed throughout the wells and determine the absorbance at 492 nm using an ELISA reader.

10 Plot a standard curve of absorbance versus the concentration of TNF. Estimate activity in unknown samples by comparison with a standard curve (see Section 6).

5.2 Bioassay for interferons (IFNs)

Interferons are usually assayed by their ability to reduce the viral killing of target cell types by inhibiting the replication of an infecting virus. Generally, cell lines of human origin—2D9, Hep-2/C, WISH, A549—are best for assaying human interferon and cells of mouse origin, e.g. L929 for the assay of mouse interferon. However, certain interferons, e.g. IFN-α, my be measured using heterologous cell lines. The challenge viruses commonly used in these assays are the encephalomycarditis virus (EMCV), vesicular stomatitis virus (VSV) and Semliki forest virus (SFV). These cell–virus combinations have been used in several types of assays for measuring the potency of interferon preparations. The use of the 2D9–EMCV combination, which is sensitive to α, β, and γ forms of interferon is described (41). Also described is the Daudi cell-line assay based on the anti-proliferative effect of IFN-α or -β. IFN-γ does not inhibit the growth of Daudi cells (42). IFN-γ can be assayed by its ability to upregulate MHC class II expression on suitable cells, e.g. Colo 205.

5.2.1 Maintenance of the 2D9 cell line

Culture 2D9 cells in RPMI-1640 medium supplemented with 7% FCS and 1 mM sodium pyruvate in 75 cm^2 flasks. Cultures are split 1:10 every 7 days when the flasks are confluent.

5.2.2 Maintenance of Daudi cell line

Culture Daudi cells in RPMI-1640 supplemented with 7% heat-inactivated FCS, 1 mM sodium pyruvate and 20 μg/ml polymixin B in 75 cm^2 flasks at 37°C in a humidified 5% CO_2 incubator. Cultures are split approximately 1:5 every 3–4 days, reducing the cell concentration to approximately 5×10^4 cells/ml.

Protocol 21

Bioassay for interferons using the 2D9 cell line

Equipment and reagents

- 2D9 cells (Section 5.2.1)
- Cell-culture medium (Section 5.2.1)
- 0.01% trypsin
- IFN standard (Section 6 and *Table 2*)
- 96-well microtitre plates
- EMCV virus
- Trypan Blue

- PBS
- 0.05% amido blue-black stain in 9% acetic acid with 0.1 m sodium acetate filter
- Fixative: 10% formaldahyde in 9% acetic acid with 0.1 M sodium acetate
- 0.1 M NaOH
- ELISA plate reader
- 37°C, humidified, 5% CO_2 incubator

Method

1. Trypsinize 2D9 cells and check the viability. Resuspend the cells to a concentration of 5×10^5 cells/ml in RPMI-1640 containing 7% heat-inactivated FCS and 1 mM sodium pyruvate (Section 5.2.1)

2. Add 100 μl of the cell suspension to each well and incubate overnight at 37°C in a humidified 5% CO^2 incubator.

3. Prepare serial twofold dilutions of the IFN standard, starting at approximately 10 IU/ml (in duplicate in 100 μl volumes) and down to approximately 0.078 IU/ml, add to the wells without disturbing the confluent cells. Make appropriate dilutions of the unknown samples. Incubate overnight, as in step 2.

4. Assign wells for the cell and virus controls, usually lines 1 and 12 are the cell controls. In line 12 are the cell controls and line 11 are the virus controls.

5. Check the plates to ensure that confluent monolayers of cells are present. Remove the growth medium in the wells by flicking and blotting on a paper towel soaked with 70% ethanol.

6. Dilute the EMCV to about 10–30 plaque-forming units/cell in growth medium, or the dilution required to effect a 100% cytopathic effect in unprotected virus controls. Add 100 μl of the viral suspension to all wells except the cell controls. To the latter, add 100 μl of growth medium and return the plates to the CO_2 incubator for another 24 h at 37°C in a humidified CO_2 incubator.

7. Note that the time required for the maximum cytopathic effect (CPE) to develop depends on the specific cell–virus pairings. In the 2D9–EMCV combination, 20–24 h at 37°C are adequate, the A549–EMCV combination requires 30–48 h. Examine monolayers of the virus control wells microscopically to ascertain when maximum CPE is reached. Ideally, the cells should be completely lysed.

8. Remove the medium from all wells by flicking. Blot the plates onto absorbent towels. Wash once with PBS and discard the solution.

9   Add 150 µl of amido blue-black and stain for 30 min at room temperature.

10 Remove the stain solution by flicking out. Fix the cell monolayers with 150 µl of the fixative solution and leave the plates at room temperature for at least 10 min.

11 Flick out the fixative and wash the plates under running tap water for 5 min. Dry the plates at room temperature or at 37 °C.

12 Add 150 µl of 0.1 M NaOH to each well. Make sure that the contents of each well are uniformly distributed by gently tapping the sides of the plates.

13 Measure the absorbance at 620 nm using an ELISA reader.

14 Plot a standard curve of absorbance versus the concentration of interferon. Estimate activity in unknown samples by comparison with a standard curve (see Section 6).

Protocol 22

Bioassay for interferons using the Daudi cell line

Equipment and reagents

- Daudi cells (Section 5.2.2)
- Cell-culture medium (see step 1 below)
- IFN standard (Section 6 and *Table 2*)
- Equipment and reagents as in *Protocol 1*

Method

1   Take Daudi cells 3–4 days after culture, centrifuge at 250 g for 10 min and resuspend the cells to a concentration of 8×10^5 cells/ml in RPMI-1640 with 10% heat-inactivated FCS (no polymixin B).

2   Add the IFN sample standard at approximately 500 IU/ml to the wells, in duplicate in 100 µl volumes, and make serial twofold dilutions down to approximately 0.1 IU/ml in culture medium. Make appropriate dilutions of the unknown samples. Include a negative control, i.e. cells with medium alone.

3   Add 100 µl of the cell suspension to each well and incubate the plates for 72 h at 37 °C in a humidified 5% CO_2 incubator.

4   Follow *Protocol 1*, steps 5 and 6.

5   Plot a standard curve of c.p.m. versus the interferon concentration. Estimate activity in unknown samples by comparison with a standard curve (see Section 6).

5.3 Bioassay for oncostatin-M

This cytokine can be measured by its ability to inhibit the growth *in vitro* of several tumour cell lines, e.g. the A375 melanoma line (43), or by stimulating proliferation of the TF-1 cell line (*Protocol 13*).

5.3.1 Maintenance of the A375 cell line

Culture A375 cells in Dulbecco's Minimal Essential Medium containing 5% FCS, 2 mM L-glutamine, 0.01% non-essential amino-acids, and 1 mM sodium pyruvate. Cells are subcultured twice a week using 0.01% trypsin and seeded at 1×10^4 cells/ml.

Protocol 23

Bioassay for oncostatin-M using A375 cells

Equipment and reagents

- A375 cells (Section 5.3.1)
- Cell-culture medium (Section 5.3.1)
- 0.01% trypsin
- Oncostatin M standard (Section 6 and *Table 2*)

- PBS
- Methanol
- 0.1% crystal violet stain
- 2% Sodium deoxycholate
- ELISA plate reader

Method

1 Trypsinize the cells in log-phase growth and dilute to 2×10^5 cells/ml in growth media.

2 Distribute titrations of the oncostatin-M standard, in 50 µl volumes in triplicate, in 96-well microtitre plates. Start the titration at 5 ng/ml (approximately 250 U/ml) and make serial twofold dilutions down to approximately 5 pg/m (0.25 U/ml). Make appropriate dilutions of the samples to be tested for oncostatin-M activity, in triplicate in 50 µl volumes. As a negative control use culture medium alone.

3 Add 50 µl of the cell suspension to each well and incubate the plates for about 72 h at 37 °C in a humidified 5% CO_2 incubator.

4 Invert and flick the plates over a sink to discard the supernatants.

5 Carefully wash the plates three times with PBS at room temperature.

6 Add 100 µl of methanol to each well and allow to stand at room temperature for 15–20 min. Discard the methanol and blot plates on to absorbent paper.

7 Add 100 µl of 0.1% crystal violet and leave for 5 min at room temperature. Wash the plates gently with tap water until the wash is clear, then blot on to absorbent paper.

8 Add 100 µl of 2% sodium deoxycholate and agitate the plates to disperse stain.

9 Measure the absorbance at 620 nm using an ELISA reader.

10 Plot a standard curve of absorbance versus the concentration of the standard. Estimate activity in unknown samples by comparison with a standard curve (see Section 6).

6 Analysis of results

It is essential that bioassay data is analysed correctly and statistically evaluated. This is particularly important if a valid biological potency is to be assigned to a preparation and if samples are considered to have significantly different cytokine activities. A useful approach for comparing unknown samples with standard

235

preparations is parallel-line analysis. For this, the unknown samples are titrated and then compared to the standard curve of known unitage. The parallel portions of these curves are then used to measure the displacement from the standard, which is proportional to the biologically active cytokine content of the samples. These lines should be parallel if the molecule responsible for the activity in samples/standards is the same. For a detailed account of bioassay analysis, see ref 44. Alternatively, an approximate estimate can be made by taking two or three points from the titration curve and reading the values from the standard curve. 'Single point' determinations are often misleading. Inclusion of reference standards is essential; these can be obtained from the NIBSC or NIAID—see *Tables 2* and *3*. An 'in-house' laboratory standard should be produced for routine use; this should be calibrated directly against the international standard or reference preparation.

Table 2A Availability of Human Cytokine Standards and Reference Reagents

Preparation	Product code	Status[a]	Depository[b]
Interleukin-1 alpha rDNA	86/632	IS	NIBSC
Interleukin-1 beta rDNA	86/680	IS	NIBSC
Interleukin-2 cell line-derived	86/504	IS	NIBSC
Interleukin-2 rDNA	86/564		NIBSC
Interleukin-3 rDNA	91/510	IS	NIBSC
Interleukin-4 rDNA	88/656	IS	NIBSC
Interleukin-5 rDNA	90/586	WRR	NIBSC
Interleukin-6 rDNA	89/548	IS	NIBSC
Interleukin-7 rDNA	90/530	WRR	NIBSC
Interleukin-8 rDNA	89/520	IS	NIBSC
Interleukin-9 rDNA	91/678	WRR	NIBSC
Interleukin-10 rDNA	93/722	WRR	NIBSC
Interleukin-11 rDNA	92/788	WRR	NIBSC
Interleukin-12 rDNA	95/544	WRR	NIBSC
Interleukin-13 rDNA	94/622	WRR	NIBSC
Interleukin-15 rDNA	95/554	WRR	NIBSC
M-CSF rDNA	89/512	IS	NIBSC
G-CSF rDNA	88/502	IS	NIBSC
GM-CSF rDNA	88/646	IS	NIBSC
Leukaemia inhibitory factor rDNA	93/562	WRR	NIBSC
Oncostatin M rDNA	93/564	WRR	NIBSC
Stem-cell factor/MGF rDNA	91/682	WRR	NIBSC
lit 3 ligand rDNA	96/532	WRR	NIBSC
Bone morphogenetic protein-2 rDNA	93/574	WRR	NIBSC
RANTES rDNA	92/520	RR[d]	NIBSC
MCP-1 rDNA	92/794	RR[d]	NIBSC
IFN-alpha leucocyte	94/784	1st IS	NIBSC
IFN-alpha 1 rDNA	83/514	1st IS	NIBSC
IFN-alpha 1/8 rDNA	95/572	1st IS	NIBSC
IFN-alpha 2a rDNA	95/650	2nd IS	NIBSC
IFN-alpha 2b rDNA	95/566	2nd IS	NIBSC

Table 2A Continued

Preparation	Product code	Status[a]	Depository[b]
IFN-alpha 2c rDNA	95/580	1st IS	NIBSC
IFN-alpha n1 lymphoblastoid	95/568	2nd IS	NIBSC
IFN-alpha n3 leucocyte	95/574	1st IS	NIBSC
IFN-alpha consensus rDNA	94/786	1st IS	NIBSC
IFN-omega rDNA	94/754	1st IS	NIBSC
IFN-beta fibroblast	Gb23-902-531	IS	NIAID
IFN-gamma rDNA	Gxg01-902-535	IS	NIAID
TGF-beta 1rDNA	89/514	RR	NIBSC
TGF-beta 2 rDNA	90/696	RR	NIBSC
TGF-beta 3 rDNA	98/608	RR	NIBSC
TNF-alpha rDNA	87/650	IS	NIBSC
TNF-beta rDNA	87/640	RR	NIBSC

[a] IS, International Standard; WRR, WHO Reference Reagent; RR, NIBSC reference reagent.

[b] NIBSC, The National Institute for Biological Standards and Control, Blanche Lane, South Mimms, Potters Bar, Hertfordshire, EN6 3QG, UK. NIAID, The National Institute for Allergy and Infectious Diseases, Solar Building, 6003 Executive Drive, Maryland, USA.

Table 2B Availability of murine cytokine standards and reference reagents

Cytokine	Cytokine standards	
	Status	Source
Interleukin-1 alpha	RR	NIBSC
Interleukin-1 beta	RR	NIBSC
Interleukin-2	RR	NIBSC
Interleukin-3	RR	NIBSC
Interleukin-4	RR	NIBSC
Interleukin-6	RR	NIBSC
Interleukin-7	RR	NIBSC
Interleukin-9	RR	NIBSC
Tumour necrosis factor-alpha	RR	NIBSC
Granulocyte macrophage colony-stimulating factor	RR	NIBSC
Interferon-alpha	IS	NIAID
Interferon-beta	IS	NIAID
Interferon-alpha/beta	2nd IS	NIAID
Interferon-gamma	IS	NIAID

Table 3 Availability of cytokine antibody standards[a]

Cytokine antibody	Status	Source[b]
GM CSF	RR	NIBSC
Interferon-α	RR	NIAID
Interferon-β	RR	NIBSC
Interferon-β	RR	NIAID

[a] These are antibodies (autoantibodies or therapy-induced antibodies) obtained from human sources. RR, NIBSC Reference Reagent.

[b] Refer to *Table 2* for address of sources.

Acknowledgements

We would like to thank the Immunex Corporation, Schering Plough Corporation, Cetus Corporation, Bristol Myer Squibb, Collagen Corporation, R&D Systems, Glaxo Wellcome, Genentech Inc, Sandoz Limited, Genetics Institute, Roche Products Ltd, Chugai Pharmaceutical Company Ltd, Dainippon Pharmaceutical Company Ltd, and Amgen for their generous gift of rDNA cytokines which have been used to develop and characterize some of the assays described in this chapter. We are grateful to L. Pegoraro, T. Kitamura, L. Aarden, P. Lindquist, W. Paul, S. Indelicato, and J. Weaver for providing some of the cell lines described and to Jenni Haynes for preparing the manuscript.

References

1. Thorpe, R., Wadhwa, M., Bird, C. R., and Mire-Sluis, A. R. (1992). *Blood Rev.*, **6**, 133.
2. Hannum, C. H., Wilcox, C. J., Arend, W. P., Joslin, F. G., Dripps, D. J., Heimdal, P. L., Armes, L. G., Sommer, A., Eisenberg, S. P., and Thompson, R. C. (1990). *Nature*, **343**, 336.
3. Ruscetti, F. W. and Palladino, M. A. (1991). *Progr. Growth Factor Res.*, **3**, 159.
4. Wadhwa, M., Dilger, P., Meager, A., Walker, B., Gaines-Das, R., and Thorpe, R. (1996). *Cytokine*, **8**, 900.
5. Wadhwa, M. and Thorpe, R. (1998). *The cytokine handbook* (3rd edn.,), p. 855. Academic Press, London.
6. Thorpe, R., Wadhwa, M., Gearing, A., Mahon, B., and Poole, S. (1988). *Lymphokine Res*, **7**, 119.
7. Wadhwa, M., Thorpe, R., Bird, C. R., and Gearing, A. J. H. (1990). *J. Immunol Meth.*, **128**, 211.
8. Wadhwa, M., Thorpe, R., and participants of the meeting. 91997). *Cytokine*, **9**, 791.
9. Gillis, S., Ferm, M. M., Ou, W. E., and Smith, K. A. (1978). *J. Immunol. Meth.*, **120**, 2027.
10. Schrier, M. H. and Tees, R. (1981). *Immunol. Meth.*, **2**, 263.
11. Orrencole, S. F. and Dinarello, C. A. (1989). *Cytokine*, **1**, 14.
12. Gearing, A. J. H., Bird, C. R., Bristow, A., Poole, S., and Thorpe, R. (1987). *J. Immunol. Meth.*, **99**, 7.
13. Hu-Li, J., Ohara, J., Watson, C., Tsang, W., and Paul, W. E. (1989). *J. Immunol.*, **142**, 800.
14. Aarden, L. A., De Groof, E. R., Schaap, O. L., and Lansdorp, P. M. (1987). *Eur. J. Immunol.*, **17**, 1411.
15. Nordan, R. P. and Potter, M. (1986). *Science*, **233**, 566.
16. Yang, Y. C., Ricciardi, S., Ciarletta, A., Calvetti, J., Kelleher, K., and Clark, S. C. (1989). *Blood,* **74**, 1880.
17. Thompson-Snipes, L., Dhar, V., Bond, M. W., Mosmann, T. R., Moore, K. W., and Rennick, D. M. (1991). *J. Exp. Med.*, **173**, 507.
18. Liu, Y., Wei, S. H., Ho, A. S., de-Waal Malefyt, R., and Moore, K. W. (1994). *J. Immunol.*, **152**, 1821.
19. Lu, Z. Y., Zhang, X. G., Gu, Z. J., Yasukawa, K., Etrillard, M., and Klein, B. (1994). *J. Immunol. Meth.*, **173**, 19.
20. Stern, A. S., Podlaski, F. J., Hulmes, J. D., Pan, Y.-C. E., Quinn, P. M., Wolitzky, A. G., Familletii, P. C., Stremlo, D. L., Truitt, T., Chizzonite, R., and Gately, M. K. (1990). *Proc. Natl. Acad. Sci. USA*, **87**, 6808.
21. Hori, T., Uchiyama, T., Tsudi, M., Umadome, H., Ohno, H., Fukuhara, S., Kita, K., and Uchino, H. (1987). *Blood*, **70**, 1069.

22. Bouteiller, C. L., Astruc, R., Minty, A., Ferrara, P., and Lupker, J. H. (1995). *J. Immunol. Meth.*, **181**, 29.

23. Ambrus, J. L., Jr, Pippin, J., Joseph, A., Xu, C., Blumenthal, D., Tamayo, A., Claypool, K., McCourt, D., Srikiatchatochorn, A., and Ford, R. J. (1993). *Proc. Natl. Acad. Sci. USA*, **90**, 6330.

24. Yao, Z., Painter, S. L., Fanslow, W. C., Ulrich, D., Macduff, B. M., Spriggs, M. K., and Armitage, R. J. (1995). *J. Immunol.*, **155**, 5483.

25. Ushio, S., Namba, M., Okura T., Hattori K., Nukada, Y., Akita, K., Tanabe F., Konishi, K., Micallef M., Fukii, M., Torigoe, K., Tanimoto, T., Fukada, S., Ikeda, M., Okamura, H., and Kurimoto, M. (1996). *J. Immunol.*, **156**, 4274.

26. Konishi, K., Tanabe, F., Taniguchi, M., Yamauchi, H., Tanimoto, T., Ikeda, M., Orita, K., and Kurimoto, M. (1997). *J. Immunol. Meth.*, **209**, 187.

27. Metcalf, D. (1984). *The hemopoietic colony stimulating factors*. Elsevier, Amsterdam.

28. Lange, B., Valtieri, M., Santoli, D., Caracciolo, D., Mavilio, F., Gemperlein, I., Griffin, C., Emanuel, B., Finan, J., Nowell, P., and Rovera, G. (1987). *Blood.*, **70**, 192.

29. Avanzi, G. C., Lista, P., Giovinazzo, B., Miniero, R., Saglio, G., Benetton, G., Coda, R., Cattonetti, G., and Pegoraro, L. (1988). *Br. J. Haematol.*, **69**, 359.

30. Gascan, H., Moreau, J. F., Jacques, Y., and Soulilou, J.P. (1989). *Lymphokine Res.*, **8**, 79.

31. Kitamura, T., Tange, T., Terasawa, T., Chiba, S., Kuwaki, T., Miyagawa, K., Piao, Y., Miyazono, K., Orabe, A., and Takaku, F. (1989). *J. Cell. Physiol.*, **140**, 323.

32. Weinstein, Y., Ihle, J. N., Lavu, S., and Reddy, E. P. (1986). *Proc. Natl. Acad. Sci.*, **83**, 5010.

33. Nakoinz, I., Lee, M., Weaver, J. F., and Ralph, P. (1989). Presented at the *7th International* Congress of Immunology, Abs. 40-23. Gustav Fischer, Stuttgart.

34. Hendrie, P. C., Miyazawa, K., Yang, Y.-C., and Langefeld, C. D. (1991). *Exp. Hematol.*, **19**, 1031.

35. Page, L. A., Thorpe, R., and Mire-Sluis, A. R. (1996). *Cytokine*, **8**, 66.

36. Bartley, T. D., Bogenberger, J., Hunt, P., *et al.* (1994). *Cell*, **77**, 1117.

37. Meager, A. (1991). *J. Immunol. Meth.*, **141**, 1.

38. Randall, L. A., Wadhwa, M., Thorpe, R., and Mire-Sluis, A. R. (1993). *J. Immunol. Meth.*, **164**, 61.

39. Scott-Thies, R., Bauduy, M., Ashton, B. A., Kurtzberg, L., Wozney, J. M., and Rosen, V. (1992). *Endocrinology*, **130**, 1318.

40. Meager, A. (1991). *J. Immunol. Meth.*, **144**, 141.

41. Däubener, W., Wanagat, N., Pilz, K., Seghrouchni, S., Fischer, H. G., and Hadding, U. (1994). *J. Immunol. Meth.*, **168**, 39,

42. Prummer, O., Streichan, U., Heimpel, H., and Porzsolt, F., (1994). *J. Immunol. Meth.*, **171**, 45.

43. Nakai, S., Mizuno, K., Kaneta, M., and Hirai, Y. (1988). A simple, sensitive bioassay for the detection of interleukin-1 using human melanoma A375 cell line. *Biochem. Biophys. Res. Commun.*, **154**, 1189.

44. European Pharmacopoeia (1998). Chapter 5.3, pp. 2–32.

45. Giri, J. G., Ahdieh, M., Eisenman, J., Shanebeck, K., Grabstein, K., Kumaki, S., Namen, A., Park, L. S., Cosman, D., and Anderson, D. (1994). *EMBO J.*, **13**, 2822.

46. Komatsu, N., Yamamoto, M., Fujita, H., Miwa, A., Hatake, K., Endo, T., Okano, H., Katsube, T., Fukumaki, Y., Sassa, S., and Miura, Y. (1993). *Blood*, **82**, 456.

List of suppliers

Accurate Chemical and Scientific Corp., 300 Shames Drive, Westbury, NY 11590, USA

Advanced Biotechnologies Ltd, Units B1-B2, Longmead Business Centre, Blenheim Road, Epsom, Surrey KT19 9QQ
Tel: 01372 723456
Fax: 01372 741414
URL: http//www.abgene.com

Alexis, 3 Moorbridge Court, Moorbridge Road East, Bingham, Nottingham NG13 8QG
Tel: 01949 836111
Fax: 01949 836222
URL: http//www.alexis-corp.com

Amersham Pharmacia Biotech UK Ltd, Amersham Place, Little Chalfont, Buckinghamshire HP7 9NA, UK (see also Nycomed Amersham Imaging UK; Pharmacia)
Tel: 0800 515313   Fax: 0800 616927
URL: http//www.apbiotech.com/
Amersham Pharmacia Biotech, Björkgatan 30, 75184 Uppsala, Sweden

Amersham Corp., 2636 South Clearbrook Drive, Arlington Heights, IL 60005, USA

Anderman and Co. Ltd, 145 London Road, Kingston-upon-Thames, Surrey KT2 6NH, UK
Tel: 0181 5410035
Fax: 0181 5410623

Applied Immune Sciences Inc., 5301 Patrick Henry Drive, Santa Clara, CA 95054-1114, USA

Applied Scientific, San Francisco, CA 944080, USA

Arnold R. Horwell, 73 Maygrove Rd, West Hampstead, London NW6 2BP, UK

Associates of Cape Cod, 704 Main Street, Falmouth, MA 02540, USA

ATCC (American Type Culture Collection), 10801 University Boulevard, Manassas, VA 20110–2209, USA

Autogen Bioclear, Holditch Farm, Mile Elm, Calne, Wiltshire SN11 0PY
Tel: 01249 819008
Fax: 01249 817266
URL: http://www.autogen-bioclear.co.uk

Baxter Healthcare Ltd., Wallingford Road, Compton, Nr Newbury, Berkshire RG20 7QW
Tel: 01635 206 000   Fax: 01635 206 115
URL: http://www.baxter.com

Baxter Healthcare Corporation, Deerfield, IL 60015, USA

BDH Laboratory Supplies, Poole, Dorset BH15 1TD
URL: http://www.bdh.com

Beckman Coulter (UK) Ltd, Oakley Court, Kingsmead Business Park, London Road, High Wycombe, Buckinghamshire HP11 1JU, UK
Tel: 01494 441181   Fax: 01494 447558
URL: http://www.beckman.com/
Beckman Coulter Inc., 4300 N. Harbor Boulevard, PO Box 3100, Fullerton, CA 92834–3100, USA
Tel: 001 714 8714848
Fax: 001 714 7738283
URL: http://www.beckman.com/

Beckman Instruments, Progress Rd, Sands Industrial Estate, High Wycombe, Buckinghamshire HP12 4JL, UK; PO Box 3100, 2500 Harbor Boulevard, Fullerton, CA 92634, USA

Becton Dickinson and Co., 21 Between Towns Road, Cowley, Oxford OX4 3LY, UK
Tel: 01865 748844   Fax: 01865 781627
URL: http://www.bd.com/
Becton Dickinson and Co., 1 Becton Drive, Franklin Lakes, NJ 07417–1883, USA
Tel: 001 201 8476800
URL: http://www.bd.com/

Bellco Glassware (distributed in the UK by Philip Harris Scientific); PO Box 340, Edrudo Rd, Vineland, NJ 08360, USA

Bio 101 Inc., c/o Anachem Ltd, Anachem House, 20 Charles Street, Luton, Bedfordshire LU2 0EB, UK
Tel: 01582 456666
Fax: 01582 391768
URL: http://www.anachem.co.uk/
Bio 101 Inc., PO Box 2284, La Jolla, CA 92038–2284, USA
Tel: 001 760 5987299
Fax: 001 760 5980116
URL: http://www.bio101.com/

Biochrom KG, Leonorenstr. 2-6, D-12247, Berlin, Germany

Biognostik, c/o Chemicon International Ltd, 2 Admiral House, Cardinal Way, Harrow NA3 5UT, UK; 28835 Single Oak Drive, Temecula, CA 92590, USA

Bio-Rad Laboratories Ltd, Bio-Rad House, Maylands Avenue, Hemel Hempstead, Hertfordshire HP2 7TD, UK
Tel: 0181 3282000
Fax: 0181 3282550
URL: http://www.bio-rad.com/
Bio-Rad Laboratories Ltd, Division Headquarters, 1000 Alfred Noble Drive, Hercules, CA 94547, USA
Tel: 001 510 7247000
Fax: 001 510 7415817
URL: http://www.bio-rad.com/

BioWhittaker, BioWhittaker House, 1 Ashville Way, Wokingham RG41 2PL
Tel: 0118 979 5234
Fax: 0800 731 3498
URL: http://www.biowhittaker.com

Boehringer-Mannheim (see Roche Diagnostics)

Brickmann Instruments Inc., 1 Cantiague Rd, Westbury, NY 11590, USA

British Drug Houses (BDH) Ltd, Poole, Dorset, UK

Buck&Holm A/S, Marielundvej 36, DK-2730 Herlev, Denmark

Calbiochem, Boulevard Industrial Park, Padge Road, Beeston, Nottingham NG9 2JR

Campden Instruments, 185 Campden Hill Rd, London W8 1TH, UK

Cappelen Laboratory Technics (CAPP), Kallerupvej 26, PO Box 824, DK-5230 Odense M, Denmark

Carl Zeiss, D-7082, Oberkochen, Germany

CellPro, Inc., Suite 100, 22322-20th Avenue Southeast, Bothell, Washington 982021, USA
Tel: 001 206 485 7644
Fax: 001 206 485 4787

Clontech Laboratories, Unit 2, Intec 2, Wade Rd, Basingstoke, Hampshire RG24 8NE,UK; 1020 East Meadow Circle, Palo Alto, CA 94303, USA

Collaborative Research Inc., Two Oak Park, Bedford, MA 01730, USA

Corning Inc., Corning, NY 14831, USA

Costar/Nuclepore, 1 Alewife Center, Cambridge, MA 02140, USA

Coulter (see Beckman Coulter)

CP Instrument Co. Ltd, PO Box 22, Bishops Stortford, Hertfordshire CM23 3DX, UK
Tel: 01279 757711   Fax: 01279 755785
URL: http//:www.cpinstrument.co.uk/

Dako, Denmark House, Angel Drive, Ely, Cambridgeshire CB7 4ET, UK; 6392 Via Real, Carpinteria, CA 93013, USA

David Kopf, Tujunga, CA, USA

Difco Laboratories Ltd, PO Box 14B, Central Ave, West Moseley, Surrey, KT8 2SE, UK; PO Box 331058, Detroit, MI 48232–7058, USA

Dow Chemicals Company Ltd., Hydrocarbon, 1 Mount Street, London W1

Drummond Scientific Co., 500 Parkway, Broomal, PA 19008, USA

Dupont (**UK**) **Ltd**, Industrial Products Division, Wedgwood Way, Stevenage, Hertfordshire SG1 4QN, UK
Tel. 01438 734000
Fax: 01438 734382
URL: http://www.dupont.com/

Du Pont Co. (Biotechnology Systems Division), PO Box 80024, Wilmington, DE 19880–002, USA
Tel: 001 302 7741000
Fax: 001 302 7747321
URL: http://www.dupont.com/

Dynal (UK) Ltd., 10 Thursby Road, Croft Business Park, Bromborough, Wirral, Merseyside L62 3PW
Tel: 0151 346 1234
Fax: 0151 346 1223
techserve@dynal.u-net.com

Dynal (UK) Ltd., 11 Bassendale Road, Croft Business Park, Bromborough, Wirral CH62 3QL
Tel: 0800 731 9037
Fax: 0151 346 1223
URL: http://www.dynal.net

Dynatech, Daux Road, Billingshurst, West Sussex JRH14 9SJ

Eastman Chemical Co., 100 North Eastman Road, PO Box 511, Kingsport, TN 37662–5075, USA
Tel: 001 423 2292000
URL: http//:www.eastman.com/

Eppendorf, 2000 Hamburg 65–Postfach 650670, Germany

European Collection of Animal Cell Culture, Division of Biologics, PHLS Centre for Applied Microbiology and Research, Porton Down, Salisbury, Wiltshire SP4 0JG, UK

EY Labs, 107-127 N. Amphlett Blvd., San Mateo, California 94401, USA
Tel: 650 342 3296
Fax: 650 342 2648
URL: http//:www.eylabs.com

Falcon (Falcon is a registered trademark of Becton Dickinson and Co.)

Santa Cruz (distributed in UK by Autogen Bioclear)

Savant Instruments, Inc., 100 Colin Drive, Holbrook, NY 11741-4306, USA
Tel: 631 244 2929
Fax: 631 244 0606
URL: http://www.savec.com

Schleicher and Schuell Inc., Keene, NH 03431A, USA
Tel: 001 603 3572398
Schleicher & Schuell GmbH, Hahnestrasse 3, D-37586 Dassel, Germany

Schott Corp., 3 Odell Plaza,Yonkers, NY 10701, USA
Schott Glass, Mainz, Germany

Serva, Novex Experimental Technologies, 11040 Roselle Street, San Diego, CA 92121, USA.
Serva, Novex Electrophoresis GmbH, Brüningstrasse 50, Gebäude C 584, D-65929 Frankfurt am Main, Germany

Shandon Scientific Ltd, 93–96 Chadwick Road, Astmoor, Runcorn, Cheshire WA7 1PR, UK
Tel: 01928 566611
URL: http//www.shandon.com/

Sigma–Aldrich Co. Ltd, The Old Brickyard, New Road, Gillingham, Dorset SP8 4XT, UK
Tel: 0800 717181 (or 01747 822211)
Fax: 0800 378538 (or 01747 823779)
URL: http://www.sigma-aldrich.com/
Sigma Chemical Co., PO Box 14508, St Louis, MO 63178, USA
Tel: 001 314 7715765
Fax: 001 314 7715757
URL: http://www.sigma-aldrich.com/

Sorvall, 31 Pecks Lane, Newtown, CT 06470-2337, USA
URL: http://www.sorvall.com

Sorvall Du Pont Co., Biotechnology Division, PO Box 80022, Wilmington, DE 19880-0022, USA

Spectrum Laboratories (distributed in the UK by Pierce & Warriner Ltd); 23022 La Cadena Drive, Laguna Hills, CA 92653, USA
Spectrum Europe BV, PO Box 3262, 4800 DG Breda, The Netherlands

StemCell Technologies, Metachem Diagnostics Ltd., 29 Forest Road, Piddington, Northampton NN7 2DA
Tel: 01604 870370
Fax: 01604 870194
metachem@skynet.co.uk

Stratagene Ltd., Unit 140, Cambridge Innovation Centre, Milton Rd, Cambridge CB4 44FG, UK
Stratagene Inc., 11011 North Torrey Pines Road, La Jolla, CA 92037, USA
Tel: 001 858 5355400
URL: http://www.stratagene.com/
Stratagene Europe, Gebouw California, Hogehilweg 15, 1101 CB Amsterdam Zuidoost, The Netherlands
Tel: 00800 91009100
URL: http://www.stratagene.com/

Techmate Ltd, 10 Bridgeturn Ave., Old Wolverton, Milton Keynes MK12 5QL, UK.

3M, 3M House, PO Box 1, Bracknell, Berks. RG12 1JU
URL: http://www.3m.com

ThermoQuest Scientific Equipment Group Ltd., Unit 5, The Ringway Centre, Edison Road, Basingstoke, Hampshire. RG21 6YH
Tel: 01256 817282
Fax: 01256 817292

Tissue Culture Services, Boltolph Claydon, Bucks. MK18 2LR

Tommy Nielsen Handels, og Ingeniørfirma, Malervej 6, DK-6710 Esbjerg V, Denmark

UBI (distributed by TCS biologicals)

United States Biochemical (USB), PO Box 22400, Cleveland, OH 44122, USA
Tel: 001 216 4649277

Wallac Finland Oy, Mustionkatu 6, PL 10, 20101 Turku, Finnland

Waters Ltd, The Boulevard, Blackmoor Lane, Watford Hertfordshire, WD1 8YW, UK
Waters Corp., 34 Maple Street, Milford, MA 01757, USA

Wellcome Reagents, Langley Court, Beckenham, Kent BR3 3BS, UK

Wild Leitz UK Ltd, Davy Ave, Knowlhill, Milton Keynes, MK5 8LB, UK

Worthington Biochemical Corporation, Halls Mill Road, Freehold, NJ 07728, USA

Zinsser Analytic, Eschborner Landstr. 135, D-60489 Frankfurt, Germany

Zymed, 458 Carlton Court, S. San Francisco, CA 94080, USA

Index